Public Health and Health Services Research in Traditional, Complementary and Integrative Health Care

International Perspectives

Public Health and Health Services Research in Traditional, Complementary and Integrative Health Care

International Perspectives

Chief Editor

Jon Adams

(University of Technology Sydney, Australia)

Co-Editors

Alex Broom

David Sibbritt

Amie Steel

Gail Hughes

Weizhong Yang

Nelson Filice de Barros

Elizabeth Sommers

Adang Bachtiar

Agustin Kusumayati

W⬤ World Scientific

NEW JERSEY · LONDON · SINGAPORE · BEIJING · SHANGHAI · HONG KONG · TAIPEI · CHENNAI · TOKYO

Published by

World Scientific Publishing Europe Ltd.

57 Shelton Street, Covent Garden, London WC2H 9HE

Head office: 5 Toh Tuck Link, Singapore 596224

USA office: 27 Warren Street, Suite 401-402, Hackensack, NJ 07601

Library of Congress Cataloging-in-Publication Data
Names: Adams, Jon, 1971– editor.
Title: Public health and health services research in traditional,
    complementary and integrative health care : international perspectives /
    Editor-in-chief, Jon Adams (University of Technology Sydney, Australia).
Description: New Jersey : World Scientific, 2019. | Includes bibliographical
    references and index.
Identifiers: LCCN 2018055946 | ISBN 9781786346780 (hc : alk. paper)
Subjects: | MESH: Health Services Research | Delivery of Health Care |
    Public Health | Integrative Medicine | Complementary Therapies
Classification: LCC RA408.5 | NLM W 84.3 | DDC 362.1072/3--dc23
LC record available at https://lccn.loc.gov/2018055946

British Library Cataloguing-in-Publication Data
A catalogue record for this book is available from the British Library.

For any available supplementary material, please visit
https://www.worldscientific.com/worldscibooks/10.1142/Q0202#t=suppl

Desk Editors: Anthony Alexander/Jennifer Brough/Shi Ying Koe

Typeset by Stallion Press
Email: enquiries@stallionpress.com

Foreword

Taking the easy path is rarely the choice that is made by effective academics. The centuries are littered with accusations against those who challenged the status quo. Even the father of modern epidemiology, John Snow, was pilloried in the *Lancet* for arguing cholera was spread by water and not by air. The 'true representatives' accused him of 'treasonable behaviour', for being 'perverse' and 'crochety' and having 'perceptions dimmed in the gloom of the den in which they think and move'.

Research into traditional, complementary and integrative health care sometimes suffers the same sort of accusations from within the contemporary research community. Even so, the popularity of these medicines and approaches to health care has increased significantly in many communities around the world. In response, the use, practice and evaluation of traditional, complementary and integrative health care demands much greater understanding and careful analysis if we are to consider the full spectrum of challenges and opportunities available for improving community health for all.

This book advances our understanding of traditional, complementary and integrative health care within a vast range of contexts and from a wide stable of perspectives. Thanks to careful research and a deep engagement with the topic, the collection offers researchers, health professionals, policymakers and health care users a timely resource to help lead future rigorous investigations, develop appropriate policy, and direct suitable and effective decision-making on what is an increasingly significant area of health care around the globe.

Michael Moore OA
President, World Federation of Public Health Associations (2016–2018)
CEO, Public Health Association of Australia (2008–2018)

About the Editor

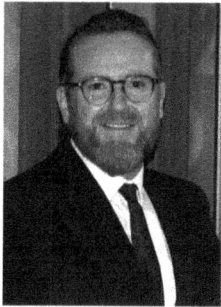

Jon Adams is Distinguished Professor of Public Health, a Fulbright Senior Future Scholar and the Director of the Australian Research Centre in Complementary and Integrative Medicine (ARCCIM) at the University of Technology Sydney, Australia — the only centre in the world dedicated to the public health and health services research of traditional, complementary and integrative medicine and health care. Jon has previously held two NHMRC Fellowships and is currently ARC Professorial Future Fellow. He is also a Senior Fellow and Senior Mentor on the International Oxford Primary Care Research Leadership Program, Nuffield Department of Primary Care Health Sciences, University of Oxford, UK and the National Convenor of the Evidence, Research and Policy in Complementary Medicine Special Interest Group, Public Health Association of Australia (PHAA) (2012–present). He has previously edited/co-edited eight academic research books including Chief Editorship of the first reader collection *Traditional, Complementary and Integrative Medicine: An International Reader* (Palgrave) and has authored over 400 peer-reviewed publications to date. His diverse research interests include examining issues around public health, primary health care, health services research, a range of formal and self-care health-seeking behaviours and practices, and the interface between conventional medical care and traditional, complementary and integrative medicine. More recently, he has been extensively engaged in implementation science, knowledge translation and dissemination research, practice-based research network design and developing strategies and programs in research capacity building and mentorship.

About the Contributors

Gavin J. Andrews is Professor and Graduate Chair of the Department of Health, Aging and Society, McMaster University, Canada. He is a leading health geographer and his wide-ranging research explores the dynamics between space/place and aging, holistic medicine, health care work, phobias, sports and fitness, health histories and popular music. Much of his work is positional and considers the progress, state of the art and future of health geography.

Adang Bachtiar is Professor and Director, Centre for Health Administration and Policy Study, University of Indonesia. He is Chairman of the Advisory Board of the Indonesian Public Health Association (IAKMI) and was President of the Indonesian Public Health Association (IAKMI) from 2008 to 2016.

Adriana Falangola Benjamin Bezerra is Professor at the Social Medicine Department, Universidade Federal de Pernambuco, Cidade Universitária, Recife-PE, Brazil.

Felicity Bishop is Associate Professor in Health Psychology at the University of Southampton, a Fellow of the ARCCIM International Complementary Medicine Research Leadership Program and a Visiting Fellow at the Australian Research Centre in Complementary and Integrative Medicine (ARCCIM), University of Technology Sydney, Australia.

Ryan Bradley is Director of the Helfgott Research Institute at the National University of Natural Medicine, USA. He is also a Fellow of the ARCCIM International Naturopathy Research Leadership Program and a Visiting Fellow at the Australian Research Centre in Complementary and Integrative Medicine (ARCCIM), University of Technology Sydney, Australia.

Alex Breen is Postdoctoral Research Fellow and Technology Lead for Quantitative Fluoroscopy at the AECC University College, Bournemouth, UK. He is also a Fellow of the International Chiropractic Academy for Research Leadership (CARL) Program run by senior academics at the University of Alberta, University of Southern Denmark and University of Technology Sydney.

Alex Broom is Professor of Sociology and Co-Director of the Practical Justice Initiative, Centre for Social Research in Health, University of New South Wales (UNSW), Australia. He is recognized as an international leader in the sociology of health and illness, with a current focus on developing critical analyses of the social dynamics of cancer and palliative care and the global challenge of antimicrobial resistance. Before joining UNSW, he was an ARC Future Fellow at the University of Queensland from 2011–2015.

Caragh Brosnan is Associate Professor at the School of Humanities and Social Sciences, University of Newcastle, Australia. She is also a Fellow of the ARCCIM International Complementary Medicine Research Leadership Program and a Visiting Fellow at the Australian Research Centre in Complementary and Integrative Medicine (ARCCIM), University of Technology Sydney, Australia.

Vincent Chung is Associate Professor at the Jockey Club School of Public Health and Primary Care, Chinese University of Hong Kong. He is an Associate Editor for *BMC Complementary and Integrative Medicine* and *Advances in Integrative Medicine* and serves as an Editorial Board Member of the *European Journal of Integrative Medicine*, *Complementary Therapies in Medicine* and *Scientific Reports*. His research examines health service, public health and policy aspects of integrative medicine, and he advances the evidence-based integration of conventional and complementary health care by promoting rigorous research, policy advocacy and quality education locally, nationally and internationally. Vincent is also a Fellow of the ARCCIM International Complementary Medicine Research Leadership Program and a Visiting Fellow of the Australian Research Centre in Complementary and Integrative Medicine (ARCCIM), University of Technology Sydney, Australia.

Irena Connon is a social anthropologist and transdisciplinary researcher in the fields of political ecology, socio-cultural dimensions of resilience and adaptation to environmental hazard events, environmental sustainability and water security. She specializes in qualitative, ethnographic, transdisciplinary research as well as applied-action and mixed-method research design. Irena is a Research Principal at the Institute for Sustainable Futures, University of Technology Sydney, Australia.

Kieran Cooley is Director of Research at the Canadian College of Naturopathic Medicine, Canada. He is also a Fellow of the ARCCIM International Naturopathy Research Leadership Program and a Visiting Fellow at the Australian Research Centre in Complementary and Integrative Medicine (ARCCIM), University of Technology Sydney, Australia.

Holger Cramer is Research Director at Department of Internal and Integrative Medicine, University of Duisburg-Essen, Germany. He is also a Fellow of the ARCCIM International Complementary Medicine Research Leadership Program and a Visiting Fellow at the Australian Research Centre in Complementary and Integrative Medicine (ARCCIM), University of Technology Sydney, Australia.

Patricia Davidson is Professor and Dean of the Faculty of Nursing at Johns Hopkins University, USA.

Iracema de Almeida Benevides worked as a Technical Advisor, internal and external Consultant of the Brazilian Ministry of Health, Pan American Health Organization and UNICEF from 2001 to 2011. She is also President of the Brazilian Association of Anthroposophic Medicine (ABMA).

Camilla Maria Ferreira de Aquino is Health Administrator at the Pernambuco Health Department and a PhD candidate in Public Health at the Instituto de Pesquisas Aggeu Magalhães (Aggeu Magalhães Research Institute), Fiocruz Pernambuco, Brazil.

Nelson Filice de Barros is Assistant Professor in Sociology, Department of Collective Health, University of Campinas (UNICAMP), Brazil. He is the former Coordinator of the Complementary and Alternative Medicine Work Group, Brazilian Association of Collective Health (ABRASCO), Brazil.

Diana De Carvalho is Assistant Professor of Medicine, Faculty of Medicine, Memorial University of Newfoundland, Canada. She is also a Fellow of the International Chiropractic Academy for Research Leadership (CARL) Program run by senior academics at the University of Alberta, University of Southern Denmark and University of Technology Sydney.

Katie de Luca is a Postdoctoral Research Fellow, Department of Chiropractic, Macquarie University, Australia. She is also a Fellow of the International Chiropractic Academy for Research Leadership (CARL) Program run by senior academics at the University of Alberta, University of Southern Denmark and University of Technology Sydney.

Peter N. DeMaio is reading for the MSc in Evidence-Based Social Intervention and Policy Evaluation at McMaster University, Canada. Peter holds a Combined Honours degree in Health Studies and Gerontology and a Master of Arts in Health Studies and Gerontology from McMaster University. He was awarded the R.C. McIvor Medal as top undergraduate scholar in the Faculty of Social Sciences' graduating class of 2015. Peter has worked for the McMaster Health Forum where his primary responsibilities involved supporting the Health Systems Evidence (HSE) — the world's most comprehensive, free access point for evidence to support policymakers, stakeholders and researchers interested in how to strengthen or reform health systems or in how to get cost-effective programs, services and drugs to those who need them.

Islândia Maria Carvalho de Sousa is a Coordinator of the National Observatory Complementary and Integrative Medicine in the Brazil and member of the Brazilian Association of Collective Health (ABRASCO).

Roger Dunston is Associate Professor in the Faculty of Arts and Social Science and a member of the International Research Centre for Communication in Healthcare (IRCCH), University of Technology Sydney, Australia. Roger's diverse research interests include examination of the nature of professional practice, making change and service redesign, 'patient' participation and co-production, and professional learning. He has led a number of large national development and research projects in these areas.

Andreas Eklund is a Researcher at the Institute for Environmental Medicine, Karolinska Institute, Sweden. He is also a Fellow of the International Chiropractic Academy for Research Leadership (CARL) Program run by senior academics at the University of Alberta, University of Southern Denmark and University of Technology Sydney.

Matthew Fernandez is Lecturer at the Department of Chiropractic, Macquarie University, Australia. He is also a Fellow of the International Chiropractic Academy for Research Leadership (CARL) Program run by senior academics at the University of Alberta, University of Southern Denmark and University of Technology Sydney.

Martha Funabashi is Research Associate and Postdoctoral Fellow, Faculty of Medicine and Dentistry, University of Alberta, Canada. She is also a Fellow of the International Chiropractic Academy for Research Leadership (CARL) Program run by senior academics at the University of Alberta, University of Southern Denmark and University of Technology Sydney.

Daniel Gallego-Perez is a Consultant with the Health Services and Access Unit, Pan American Health Organization (PAHO) and World Health Organization (WHO).

Joshua Goldenberg is a Research Investigator at Bastyr University Research Institute, USA. He is also a Fellow of the ARCCIM International Naturopathy Research Leadership Program and a Visiting Fellow at the Australian Research Centre in Complementary and Integrative Medicine (ARCCIM), University of Technology Sydney, Australia.

Maria Beatriz Guimarães has a degree in Nursing from Uberaba University (2008), Special University of Minas Gerais (2011), a Masters Degree in Health Care from the Federal University of Triângulo Mineiro (2011) and a PhD in Sciences from the Fundamental Nursing Program of the University of Sao Paulo at Ribeirao Preta College of Nursing (2015). She is a Postdoctoral Fellow at the Postgraduate Program in Health Care at the Federal University of Triângulo Mineiro, developing research in evidence-based practice, patient safety and research methods. She is a Professor at the Social Medicine Department, Universidade Federal de Pernambuco, Cidade Universitária, Recife-PE, Brazil.

Helen Hall is a Senior Lecturer and Researcher at the Faculty of Medicine, Nursing and Health Sciences, Monash University, Australia. She is also a Fellow of the ARCCIM International Complementary Medicine Research Leadership Program and a Visiting Fellow at the Australian Research Centre in Complementary and Integrative Medicine (ARCCIM), University of Technology Sydney, Australia.

Joanna Harnett is Associate Lecturer, Faculty of Pharmacy, University of Sydney, Australia, where she teaches and researches the broader area of complementary medicines with a focus upon fostering their appropriate and safe use. She is also a Fellow of the ARCCIM International Naturopathy Research Leadership Program and a Visiting Fellow at the Australian Research Centre in Complementary and Integrative Medicine (ARCCIM), University of Technology Sydney, Australia. Her research projects have focused upon on probiotic use, health literacy and disclosure of complementary medicine use by Australians, pharmacists' role in fostering the safe and appropriate use of complementary medicine, the practice behaviours of complementary medicine health practitioners, and complementary medicine use in specific populations.

Jan Hartvigsen is Professor and Head of the Research Unit for Clinical Biomechanics at the University of Southern Denmark. He is also a Senior Researcher at the Nordic Institute of Chiropractic and Clinical Biomechanics. In addition he is Head of the Graduate Program for Physical Activity and Musculoskeletal Health at the PhD School at the Faculty of Health Sciences, University of Southern Denmark.

Jason Hawrelak is Senior Lecturer in Complementary and Alternative Medicines, Faculty of Health, University of Tasmania, Australia. He is also a Fellow of the ARCCIM International Naturopathy Research Leadership Program and a Visiting Fellow at the Australian Research Centre in Complementary and Integrative Medicine (ARCCIM), University of Technology Sydney, Australia.

Michelle Holmes is a PhD candidate at the University of Southampton and a Lecturer in Research Methods at the AECC University College, Bournemouth, UK. She is also a Fellow of the International Chiropractic Academy for Research Leadership (CARL) Program run by senior academics at the University of Alberta, University of Southern Denmark and University of Technology Sydney.

Gail Hughes is Professor of Public Health and Director, South African Herbal Science and Medicine, University of Western Cape, South Africa. She is also Chair of the Special Interest Group in Integrative, Complementary and Alternative Traditional Health Practice, Public Health Association of South Africa (PHASA) and an active member of the American Public Health Association's Section on Integrative, Complementary and Traditional Health Practices.

Peter Bai James is a trained pharmacy professional and academic researcher with a decade of experience in drug regulation, pharmacovigilance, pharmacy practice and education on drug discovery. Peter is currently a PhD candidate at the Australian Research Centre in Complementary and Integrative Medicine (ARCCIM), University of Technology Sydney, investigating the use of traditional and complementary medicine and conventional medicine in the context of the Ebola epidemic in Sierra Leone.

Melker Johansson is a PhD candidate at the Institute of Sports Science and Clinical Biomechanics, University of Southern Denmark. He is also a Fellow of the International Chiropractic Academy for Research Leadership (CARL) Program run by senior academics at the University of Alberta, University of Southern Denmark and University of Technology Sydney.

Greg Kawchuk is Professor and Canada Research Chair in Spinal Function in the Faculty of Rehabilitation Medicine at the University of Alberta in Edmonton, Alberta, Canada. His field of expertise is biomechanics, and his research interests focus on defining the mechanisms that initiate and sustain spinal disorders so that clinically relevant strategies can be developed toward their prevention or resolution. A major component of his research involves developing new technologies to assess spinal structure and function then using those technologies to evaluate various clinical interventions.

Agustin Kusumayati is the National Chair, Organizational Development at the Indonesian Public Health Association (IAKMI). She is also National Chair of the Special Interest Group in Traditional, Complementary and Alternative Health, Indonesian Public Health Association (IAKMI).

Romy Lauche is a Chancellors Postdoctoral Research Fellow at the Australian Research Centre in Complementary and Integrative Medicine (ARCCIM), University of Technology Sydney, Australia. She is also a Fellow of the ARCCIM International Complementary Medicine Research Leadership Program.

Matthew Leach is Senior Research Fellow at the Department of Rural Health, University of South Australia. He is also a Fellow of the ARCCIM International Complementary Medicine Research Leadership Program and a Visiting Fellow at the Australian Research Centre in Complementary and Integrative Medicine (ARCCIM), University of Technology Sydney, Australia.

Bradley Leech is a PhD Candidate and Research Assistant at the Australian Research Centre in Complementary and Integrative Medicine (ARCCIM), University of Technology Sydney, Australia.

Brenda Leung is the Emmy Droog Chair in Complementary and Alternative Health Care at the School of Medicine, University of Lerthbridge, Canada. She is also a Fellow of the ARCCIM International Complementary Medicine Research Leadership Program and a Visiting Fellow at the Australian Research Centre in Complementary and Integrative Medicine (ARCCIM), University of Technology Sydney, Australia.

Erica McIntyre is a Postdoctoral Research Fellow at the Australian Research Centre in Complementary and Integrative Medicine (ARCCIM), University of Technology Sydney, Australia. Erica has a background in Western herbal medicine and is a Fellow of the ARCCIM International Naturopathy Research Leadership Program. She holds a PhD in psychology, with research interests in the areas of mental health and well-being, health services use, complementary self-care, health communication and decision-making.

Craig Moore is a PhD candidate at the Australian Research Centre in Complementary and Integrative Medicine (ARCCIM), University of Technology Sydney. He is also a Fellow of the International Chiropractic Academy for Research Leadership (CARL) Program run by senior academics at the University of Alberta, University of Southern Denmark and University of Technology Sydney.

Nikki Munk is Assistant Professor of Health Sciences at the School of Health and Rehabilitation Sciences, Indiana University, USA. She is also a Massage and Myotherapy Australia Fellow of the ARCCIM International Complementary Medicine Research Leadership Program and a Visiting Fellow at the Australian Research Centre in Complementary and Integrative Medicine (ARCCIM), University of Technology Sydney, Australia.

Isabelle Page is a PhD candidate at the Département d'Anatomie, Université du Québec à Trois-Rivières, Canada. She is also a Fellow of the International Chiropractic Academy for Research Leadership (CARL) Program run by senior academics at the University of Alberta, University of Southern Denmark and University of Technology Sydney.

Rhiannon Parker is a Postdoctoral Research Fellow at the Practical Justice Initiative, Centre for Social Research in Health, Faculty of Arts and Social Sciences, University of New South Wales, Australia. She specializes in the sociology of health and illness. Her current research explores the social dynamics of cancer, palliative care and antimicrobial resistance. She is currently involved in research investigating what living with cancer means for individuals, communities and families from a migrant background. She is also examining patient and caregiver experiences of palliative care and why antibiotic use continues to elude best-practice guidelines within hospitals. Her further interests include explorations of the role that medical education plays in constructing knowledge about gender and the body.

Wenbo Peng is a Research Fellow in Epidemiology and Public Health at the Australian Research Centre in Complementary and Integrative Medicine (ARCCIM), University of Technology Sydney, Australia and a registered Chinese herbal medicine practitioner, acupuncturist, and Chinese herbal dispenser in Australia. She was awarded the Barbara Gross Award at the 18th Congress of the Australian Menopause Society in 2014. Dr Peng's research focuses upon traditional, complementary and integrative medicine via public health and health services research, practice-based research networks and with a focus upon women's health and chronic illness. She is also currently a member of the Chinese Medical Council of New South Wales, Australia.

Katie Pohlman is a Clinical Research Scientist at Parker University, USA. She is also a Fellow of the International Chiropractic Academy for Research Leadership (CARL) Program run by senior academics at the University of Alberta, University of Southern Denmark and University of Technology Sydney.

Jason Prior is an Associate Professor, Research Director and Associate Director of the Postgraduate Program at the Institute for Sustainable Futures (ISF), University of Technology Sydney, Australia. Jason's program of research focuses on processes of spatial governance through a range of techniques including law, architecture, property rights, planning and environmental management. His more recent collaborations in trans-disciplinary research teams examine the built environment, well-being, chronic illness and ageing.

Rebecca Reid is Associate Director of the Office of Research at the Endeavour College of Natural Health. She is also a PhD candidate and Visiting Fellow at the Australian Research Centre in Complementary and Integrative Medicine (ARCCIM), University of Technology Sydney, Australia and a Fellow of the ARCCIM International Naturopathy Research Leadership Program.

Eric Roseen is a Postdoctoral Research Fellow at the Boston Medical Center's Family Medicine Department, Boston University, USA. He has recently awarded the Ruth Kirchstein National Research Service Award from the National Institutes of Health's National Center for Complementary and Integrative Health.

Janet Schloss is a naturopath and nutritionist who has been in private practice for over 15 years and completed her PhD at the School of Medicine, University of Queensland, Australia, through the Princess Alexandra Hospital. She has also lectured in naturopathy at the Endeavour College of Natural Health, and her main specialty is naturopathy and people who have cancer and chronic diseases, especially those going through conventional medical treatment. Janet is a Fellow of the ARCCIM International Naturopathy Research Leadership Program and a Visiting Fellow of the Australian Research Centre in Complementary and Integrative Medicine (ARCCIM), University of Technology Sydney, Australia.

David Sibbritt is Professor of Epidemiology and Deputy Director, Australian Research Centre in Complementary and Integrative Medicine

(ARCCIM), University of Technology Sydney, Australia. He is a world-leading critical public health researcher focusing upon complementary and integrative health care. David's research focus has been on women's use of complementary medicine to treat chronic illness and for their general well-being. He holds editorial roles for several international peer-reviewed journals.

Elizabeth Sommers is Senior Acupuncturist and Researcher in the Integrative Medicine and Health Disparities Program of Boston Medical Center. She holds degrees from Boston University School of Public Health (1989, 2010) and New England School of Acupuncture (1979). She also coordinates an acupuncture clinic at Tufts Medical Center that provides care for individuals living with HIV/AIDS. Dr. Sommers has been on the research faculty of New England School of Acupuncture (1990–1994) and served as adjunct faculty in Health Policy and Management at Boston University School of Public Health (2015–2018). As an acupuncture researcher, she has published and lectured internationally in the areas of acupuncture detoxification, health economics and treatment of individuals diagnosed with HIV/AIDS. Her book *Acupuncture as an Adjuvant in the Treatment of HIV/AIDS* was published in 2014. Dr Sommers is a member of the editorial board of *The Journal of Alternative and Complementary Medicine* and also serves as the public health editor of the journal *Meridians: Journal of Acupuncture and Oriental Medicine*. She co-edited the special public health issue of the *European Journal of Integrative Medicine* (2013) and also co-edited a 2018 special issue of *Medicines* on acupuncture and cancer care. She is former chair of the American Public Health Association's Section on Integrative, Complementary and Traditional Health Practices (2008–2013), and currently serves on APHA's Governing Council and Intersectional Council Steering Committee. A public health advocate, Dr Sommers is committed to ensuring that healthcare including wellness is a right not a privilege.

Amie Steel is a Senior Research Fellow at the Australian Research Centre in Complementary and Integrative Medicine (ARCCIM), University of Technology Sydney, Australia. She is also a naturopath, educator and researcher with a PhD in the Public Health of Complementary and Integrative Medicine. Amie was the Associate Director of the Office of Research at the Endeavour College of Natural Health from 2015–2018 and also holds an affiliate faculty position at the Helfgott Research Institute, National University of Natural Medicine, Portland, USA.

Tobias Sundberg is an Associated Researcher at the Institute for Environmental Medicine at Karolinska Institute, Sweden. He is also a Fellow of the ARCCIM International Complementary Medicine Research Leadership Program and a Visiting Fellow at the Australian Research Centre in Complementary and Integrative Medicine (ARCCIM), University of Technology Sydney, Australia.

Michael Swain is Lecturer and PhD candidate at the Department of Chiropractic, Macquarie University, Australia. He is also a Fellow of the International Chiropractic Academy for Research Leadership (CARL) Program run by senior academics at the University of Alberta, University of Southern Denmark and University of Technology Sydney.

Charles Dalcanale Tesser is a researcher at the Departamento de Saúde Pública, Centro de Ciências de Saúde, Universidade Federal de Santa Catarina, Brazil.

Claudine Van de Venter is Clinical Data Manager, Desmond Tutu HIV Foundation, University of Cape Town, South Africa. She is also a Fellow of the ARCCIM International Naturopathy Research Leadership Program and a Visiting Fellow at the Australian Research Centre in Complementary and Integrative Medicine (ARCCIM), University of Technology Sydney, Australia.

Naveen Visweswaraiah is Associate Professor at S-VYASA Yoga University, India. He is also a Fellow of the ARCCIM International Naturopathy Research Leadership Program and a Visiting Fellow at the Australian Research Centre in Complementary and Integrative Medicine (ARCCIM), University of Technology Sydney, Australia.

Lesley Ward is Postdoctoral Research Assistant at the Centre for Rehabilitation Research in Oxford, University of Oxford, UK. She is also a Fellow of the ARCCIM International Complementary Medicine Research Leadership Program and a Visiting Fellow at the Australian Research Centre in Complementary and Integrative Medicine (ARCCIM), University of Technology Sydney, Australia.

Jon Wardle is Senior Lecturer in Public Health and a Researcher at the Australian Research Centre in Complementary and Integrative Medicine, University of Technology Sydney, Australia.

Arnold Wong is Assistant Professor in the Department of Rehabilitation Sciences, Hong Kong Polytechnic University, Hong Kong. He is also a Fellow of the International Chiropractic Academy for Research Leadership (CARL) Program run by senior academics at the University of Alberta, University of Southern Denmark and University of Technology Sydney.

Weizhong Yang is Professor and Vice President and Secretary General, Chinese Preventive Medicine Association (CPMA).

Tony Zhang is Associate Professor and Discipline Leader of Chinese Medicine, School of Health and Biomedical Sciences, RMIT University, Australia. He is also a Fellow of the ARCCIM International Complementary Medicine Research Leadership Program and a Visiting Fellow at the Australian Research Centre in Complementary and Integrative Medicine (ARCCIM), University of Technology Sydney, Australia.

Yan Zhang is Associate Professor in Health Services Research and Founding Director of Division of Integrative Medicine at the Department of Family and Community Medicine, Texas Tech University Health Sciences Center, USA. She is also a Fellow of the ARCCIM International Complementary Medicine Research Leadership Program and a Visiting Fellow at the Australian Research Centre in Complementary and Integrative Medicine (ARCCIM), University of Technology Sydney, Australia.

Contents

Introduction

Towards a Public Health and Health Services Research Agenda in Traditional, Complementary and Integrative Health Care

Jon Adams, Alex Broom, David Sibbritt, Amie Steel, Gail Hughes, Weizhong Yang, Nelson Filice de Barros, Elizabeth Sommers, Adang Bachtiar and Agustin Kusumayati

Challenges and Definitions

The task of adequately capturing and reflecting the landscape of any number of emerging and growing health and health care research topics will always face serious challenges. With regard to the public health (PH) and health services research (HSR) of traditional, complementary and integrative medicine/health care (TCIM), these challenges are significantly magnified. On the one hand, both PH and HSR are by their very nature broad-ranging, multi-disciplinary fields of scholarship drawing upon a number of eclectic scientific traditions and perspectives. Also, as previously identified, the interface between PH and HSR is itself not always clear and there is much overlap in focus and approach (Adams, 2008). What is clear is that when considered separately, PH and HSR represent two vast fields of enquiry and when combined, their conceptual and empirical reach is immense.

To add further complexity, TCIM can also be identified as a vast field — to be more accurate, three vast highly related, sometimes overlapping but nonetheless discrete fields (Adams *et al.*, 2012). While not wishing to revisit well-rehearsed debates around definition (Wieland *et al.*, 2011), it is important (especially for those less familiar with the TCIM field) for the purposes of this book that the contours of our interest and focus be clearly outlined. Traditional medicine is defined here as those non-conventional practices, technologies, medicines and approaches to care historically associated with the local indigenous culture (for example, Jamu in Indonesia and Indigenous 'bush' medicine in Australia). Complementary medicine is defined as those non-conventional practices, technologies, products and approaches to care that are imported (not indigenous to the local culture) and are predominantly provided via the private practice of a vast range of complementary medicine practitioners (for example, acupuncture in Europe or North America). Integrative medicine is here defined as the introduction of non-conventional practices, technologies, products and approaches to care alongside conventional medical care and treatments (incorporating varying degrees of integration and building upon interdisciplinary models of practice led by either a medically-qualified practitioner or non-medically qualified practitioner). A final clarification needs to also be introduced; it is important to distinguish between integrative medicine (located in the clinical practices of providers) and integrative health care (which refers to patient-led or community-led integration and/or concurrent use of conventional medical care and non-conventional practices which can often exist beyond the gaze of practitioners).

All three fields — traditional medicine, complementary medicine and integrative medicine — have distinct features and flavours, yet they all embody a common theme: their predominant historical and contemporary location (to varying degrees) beyond the practices, technologies and treatments associated with the dominant medical profession and medical curriculum (Adams *et al.*, 2012). While such a definition could be interpreted or critiqued as one devoid of meaningful content (what features of the many TCIM modalities, practices and technologies positively bind them?), it does nevertheless highlight how crucial the political, cultural, social and economic contexts are to our thinking and orientation towards TCIM and how such titles and locations are themselves open to flux and realignment with respect to time and cultural change. Indeed, it is arguably these wider contexts (the political, cultural, social and economic) which ultimately justify the need for a PH and HSR agenda focused upon TCIM.

Moving Beyond a Limited Research Focus

Unfortunately, while many pockets of multi-disciplinary activity around the PH and HSR of TCIM exist, the bulk of attention, and funding, on TCIM has been far more limited in its focus. The relatively short history — only a few decades — of TCIM research has been dominated by a concern to verify the clinical efficacy of TCIM practices and products (Adams, 2007) and linked to this focus has been a tendency to prioritise clinical trials and other experimental designs. Such an approach is certainly not to be dismissed and can be clearly understood — especially in the face of some within the ranks of the conventional medical field, and related researchers, characterising TCIM as an unscientific clinical field that should either produce hard evidence of efficacy or be ignored/discouraged (Ernst, 2003). Indeed, nobody can claim TCIM is exempt from the wider significant need to ensure health and health care practices be rigorously evaluated and evidence-based. Yet, the heavy focus upon clinical efficacy research and designs has also, intentionally or unintentionally, meant PH and HSR enquiry has been relegated or even neglected as worthy of attention and resource in TCIM research (Adams *et al.*, 2013; Hawk *et al.*, 2015). Such an environment is certainly not healthy for any research field and it is interesting to note the well-established, broad infrastructure that has coalesced around conventional medical and health care concerns that primarily require PH, HSR and other approaches beyond the strictly clinical.

Current Initiatives and Core Elements

Despite the rise of PH and HSR scholarship around TCIM (Adams *et al.*, 2013; Hawk *et al.*, 2015), a co-ordinated, programmatic approach to such work is far less conspicuous. Indeed, a number of the editors and authors of this collection are themselves heading the only dedicated and comprehensive PH/HSR program with TCIM as the exclusive and/or core focus at the Australian Research Centre in Complementary and Integrative Medicine (ARCCIM) at the University of Technology Sydney. ARCCIM houses partnerships across a large pool of both national and international methodologists and researchers — with expertise including epidemiology, biostatistics, health promotion, systematic reviews, meta-analysis and health economics — and a vast range of industry collaborators, professional associations, consumer representative groups and community organizations. The ARCCIM, was founded in 2012 (although the program and collaborations that are core to its success have been active since 2001) and has a mission statement to:

- provide national and international leadership regarding critical public health research and scholarship that contributes to our understanding and evaluation of traditional, complementary and integrative health care use and practice within health care systems;
- help highlight traditional, complementary and integrative health care use and practice as significant public health issues requiring balanced debate and critical academic investigation;
- encourage public health enquiry that subjects traditional, complementary and integrative health care practice and use to rigorous research methods and critical perspectives in order to provide a broad evidence-base for patient care and health policy;
- facilitate research and interventions around traditional, complementary and integrative health and health care that are impactful and which can help inform best world practice and policy;
- help increase the depth and breadth of research capacity in relation to critical public health research in traditional, complementary and integrative health and health care;
- promote partnerships and collaborations with regard to the critical public health of traditional, complementary and integrative health care.

What the ARCCIM program and its core principles reveal is a mature, strong approach to the PH and HSR of TCIM — an approach that moves beyond earlier (and in plenty of cases still current) emotive, partisan appeals from opponents and supporters of TCIM alike (Adams *et al.*, 2012). In contrast, the ARCCIM program rightly subjects knowledge and approaches on both sides of the conventional-unconventional divide to the same exacting consideration, investigation and evaluation. A broad approach that is mirrored in the collection of chapters presented in this book collection.

The Collection and Book Structure

The *Public Health and Health Services Research in Traditional, Complementary and Integrative Health Care* collection has been structured around two interrelated but distinct sections. The opening section of the book (containing Chapters 1–7) introduces and critically reflects upon key disciplinary contributions and methodological advances in contemporary TCIM scholarship within PH/HSR. This section houses chapters exploring TCIM via health geographies, sociology, health economics, policy, regulatory and legal perspectives, in relation to implementation science and with regard to capacity building.

The second section of the collection explores a range of substantive topics and issues important to a PH and HSR of TCIM. These include a number of clinical and practice areas for focus – pregnancy and birthing, cancer care, chronic illness (stroke), low back pain and infectious disease (ebola) — as well as some core themes for enquiry and action — conceptualising TCIM as self-care, exploring TCIM within a broader health system focus, in relation to ecological public health (planetary health) and with attention to health disparities and social justice.

Prospects and Growth

Without doubt, TCIM scholarship is entering a new era — early challenges and concerns around investigating efficacy are being addressed and are also being supplemented and realigned with a much broader, nuanced research gaze that has an ability to cut through overly-simplistic dichotomies and representations of the entire medical and health care landscape.

To draw terminology from Anselm Strauss' highly insightful social worlds analysis (Strauss, 1978; Tovey and Adams, 2001), the boundaries of conventional health care, and provision, TCIM and public health appear to be converging and coalescing, attracting a growing army of stakeholders and supporters — even in the face of lingering but small pockets of opposition. The challenge for scholarship on this topic over coming years is to continue to build a strong program of critical, rigorous and, of equal importance, pertinent investigations and analysis that can appeal to and resonate with those managing, practising and receiving health care from across the entire health system — both formal and informal as well as within and beyond the immediate boundaries of TCIM. Ultimately, PH and HSR focused upon TCIM is an essential component of the ongoing movement towards better health and health care for all across the planet. Our ability as researchers, clinicians, collaborators and supporters to thrive and advance this essential agenda is not going to be without serious challenge but the rewards are far-reaching and well worth the effort.

References

Adams, J. (2004). Exploring the interface between complementary and alternative medicine (CAM) and rural general practice: A call for research. *Health and place*, *10*(3), 285.

Adams, J. (2007). *Researching Complementary and Alternative Medicine*. Routledge, London.

Adams, J. (2008). Utilising and promoting public health and health services research in complementary and alternative medicine: the founding of NORPHCAM. *Complementary Therapies in Medicine*.

Adams, J., Sibbritt, D., Lui, C. W. (2011). The urban–rural divide in complementary and alternative medicine use: a longitudinal study of 10,638 women. *BMC Complementary and Alternative Medicine*, *11*(1), 2.

Adams, J., Andrews, G., Barnes, J., Broom, A., Magin, P. (eds.), (2012). *Traditional, Complementary and Integrative Medicine: An International Reader*. Macmillan International Higher Education.

Adams, J., Sommers E., Robinson, N. (2013). Public health and health services research in integrative medicine: an emerging, essential focus. *European Journal of Integrative Medicine*.

Andrews, G. J. (2003). Placing the consumption of private complementary medicine: everyday geographies of older peoples' use. *Health & Place*, *9*(4), 337–349.

Andrews, G. J., Adams, J., Segrott, J. (2009). Complementary and alternative medicine (CAM): production, consumption, research. *A Companion to Health and Medical Geography*, pp. 587–603.

Ernst, E. (2003). Obstacles to research in complementary and alternative medicine. *Medical Journal of Australia*, *179*(6), 279–279.

Hawk, C., Adams, J., Hartvigsen, J. (2015). The role of CAM in public health, disease prevention, and health promotion. *Evidence-Based Complementary and Alternative Medicine*.

Meyer, S. P. (2010). A geographic assessment of 'total' health care supply in Ontario: complementary and alternative medicine and conventional medicine. *The Canadian Geographer/Le Géographe Canadien*, *54*(1), 104–122.

Strauss, A. (1978). A social world perspective. *Studies in Symbolic Interaction*, *1*(1), 119–128.

Tovey, P., Easthope, G., Adams, J. (2004). *The Mainstreaming of Complementary and Alternative Medicine: Studies in Social Context*. Routledge, London.

Tovey, P., Adams, J. (2001). Primary care as intersecting social worlds. *Social Science & Medicine*, *52*(5), 695–706.

Wardle, J., Lui, C. W., Adams, J. (2012). Complementary and alternative medicine in rural communities: current research and future directions. *The Journal of Rural Health*, *28*(1), 101–112.

Wieland, L. S., Manheimer, E., Berman, B. M. (2011). Development and classification of an operational definition of complementary and alternative medicine for the Cochrane collaboration. *Alternative Therapies in Health and Medicine*, *17*(2), 50.

Section One

Disciplinary Contributions and Methodological Advances

Chapter 1

The Geographies of Traditional, Complementary and Integrative Medicine

Peter N. DeMaio and Gavin J. Andrews

Introduction

Given the popularity of traditional, complementary and integrative medicine (TCIM), there is a growing need for a concentrated research agenda to identify policy priority areas that address the public health and health services dimensions of TCIM production and consumption (Adams *et al.*, 2012; Adams and Robinson, 2013; Andrews *et al.*, 2012; Hawk *et al.*, 2015). Within this broad research agenda, a geography of TCIM can serve to better understand considerations related to place that can influence and inform the coordination of TCIM and conventional health services (Adams and Robinson, 2013; Andrews *et al.*, 2010). To provide an overview of the role of research on place and space in pursuing this goal, the following chapter briefly discusses the development of geographical inquiry as it relates to TCIM. It then further explores the geographies of TCIM at the macro-level, including some of the available research on the epidemiological mapping of TCIM production and consumption. Next, it explores research on micro-level phenomenon related to space and TCIM consumption and production. Finally, it proposes some useful lines of inquiry for future development.

The geographies of TCIM encompasses a range of different topics, contexts and research interests, spanning area-specific traditional/indigenous medicines in low- and middle-income countries to complementary medicines and integrative health care approaches in high-income countries. It also houses a variety of different disciplines, theoretical perspectives and methodological approaches used to study TCIM. With these differences in mind, this chapter aims to provide a broad overview of some of the key issues in geographical research and TCIM.

Emerging Geographical Perspectives

Geographical research in the 1960s largely focused on positivistic approaches aimed at mapping and modelling human behaviour (Andrews, 2002b; Andrews, 2003a; Andrews *et al.*, 2004). A shift occurred during the 1970s and into the early 1980s, with the development of two key bodies of literature placing emphasis on understanding social relations and space (Andrews *et al.*, 2004). A Marxist, radical geography brought attention to the ways spatial relationships reflect and reinforce oppressive class relationships (Harvey, 1973) and humanistic geography emphasized the need to understand the 'sense of place' individuals feel towards social and physical spaces (Tuan, 1976; Relph, 1976). It holds that humans exercise agency within constraints to co-construct their environment through action in relation to constructed meanings and social structures that shape and constrain individuals' intention and action (Gesler, 1992; Williams, 1998). Along with these two important developments came an expansion of sub-disciplines such as medical and health geography, which examine place and its implications for health, health policy and health care delivery (Andrews *et al.*, 2004).

Since the 1980s, post-modern geographies have employed existentialism and phenomenology to better understand the relationships between place, meaning, subjective experience and language (Gregory, 2011). More recently, non-representational theories in geography have attempted to look beyond meaning-making and conscious reflections on external representations (e.g. signs and symbols) towards the pre-cognitive, affective experiences related to place (e.g. Anderson, 2016; Anderson and Harrison, 2010; Cadman, 2009; McCormack, 2008; Thrift, 2008). Throughout this chapter, these approaches in geographical research will be further elaborated to provide a basis for understanding current and future research on the geographies of TCIM.

Geographical Perspectives and TCIM

TCIM research has been an important interest to health (medical) geography since its early development (Andrews *et al.*, 2010). In line with most of medical geography research in the 1970s, Good (1977) emphasized the spatial arrangements of TCIM in relation to accessibility and utilization in urban and rural areas in developing countries. Through these streams of inquiry, Good (1977) sought to inform strategies to improve the availability of conventional medicine through the manpower, resources and access to local populations associated with traditional medicine. Like Good, Anyinam (1990) aimed to direct future medical geography research to address a lack of knowledge about geographic patterns related to TCIM practitioners and consumers. Focusing on Western developed countries, Anyinam proposed that geographers are especially well-situated to study TCIM in relation to its 'spatial organization, change and interrelationships between culture and environmental systems' (Anyinam, 1990, p. 73). Anyinam's proposed research agenda for medical geographers aimed to inform health systems delivery and policy by mapping spatial features of TCIM. These included the geographical distribution of TCIM practitioners, practitioner–population ratios and the locational accessibility to potential users in relation to various conventional medicine practitioners and specialists. To understand the relationships between TCIM and conventional medicine and inform possibilities for future coordination for health service delivery, Anyinam suggested that researchers look to the changing relationships between TCIM and conventional medicine, including analyses of referral networks across TCIM and biomedical practitioners.

At the micro-level, geographical inquiries have examined performances of TCIM, processes of TCIM consumption and the particular kinds of spaces and places in which TCIM takes place (Andrews *et al.*, 2010).

Together, these geographical micro-level considerations shape how TCIM is practiced by providers and how it is experienced by consumers. Informed by humanistic geography and Gesler's (1992) concept of the therapeutic landscape, researchers have sought to understand the meanings associated with the construction of physical spaces in which TCIM is practiced and the ways in which therapies are performed and facilitated through therapeutic relationships (Andrews *et al.*, 2003a, 2010; Williams, 1998). Non-representational theory expands micro-level experiences of place related to TCIM production and consumption. Beyond the physical and cognitive sources of meaningful therapeutic experiences, the relational processes involved with TCIM produce pre-cognitive experiences of place that precede (although may subsequently contribute to) the development of symbolic representations of place (Andrews *et al.*, 2013). These pre-cognitive experiences or 'feeling states' of patients are produced by the 'atmospheres' or 'vibes' (e.g. Massumi, 2002) that are (consciously or unconsciously) engineered by TCIM practitioners to create environments rich in affective possibilities (Conradson and Latham, 2007) and supportive of personal wellbeing (Andrews *et al.*, 2013).

While a nuanced discussion of TCIM delivery and consumption considers both its micro- and macro-level spatial features, such a distinction can nonetheless be helpful for categorizing health geographers' works according to its emphasis (Andrew *et al.*, 2010). At the macro-level, positivistic inquiry aims to quantify distributive features of TCIM production and consumption and to examine the large-scale social relations that shape differences among these features across geographical regions. At the micro-level, geographical research explores subjective meaning, symbolic constructions of place, the phenomenology of place (Andrews *et al.*, 2010; Gregory, 2011) and the pre-cognitive, affective experiences present in places of care and facilitated by therapeutic relationships (Andrews *et al.*, 2003b; Williams, 1998). The remainder of this chapter first explores existing research on the objective, subjective and pre-cognitive features of TCIM production and consumption from a macro-level and micro-level perspective. It then provides an overview of some of the future avenues for geographical contributions to public health and health service research in TCIM.

Macro-level Geographies of TCIM

Consumption patterns across geographical areas

Anyinam (1990) highlighted the importance of understanding spatial differences in attitudes, preferences and the significance attached to TCIM by users. Specifically, how values, belief systems and other socio-cultural characteristics affect these differences. Anyinam proposed mapping patterns of use of various types of TCIM, and trends in increase or decrease of practitioners across areas. Since then, there has been a growing body of literature examining patterns of consumption, attitudes and barriers and drivers to TCIM use.

TCIM consumption is associated with being female, higher income levels, greater educational attainment, higher incidence of chronic illness and lower self-reported health status in both rural and urban areas (Adams *et al.*, 2003, 2018; Conboy *et al.*, 2005; Shreffler-Grant *et al.*, 2007; Wiles and Rosenberg, 2001). Worse health, longer disease duration and increased number of comorbid health problems all predict greater TCIM usage (Wiles and Rosenberg, 2001). Compared to non-users, TCIM users appear to have different attitudes towards health and health seeking behaviours. Even with chronic conditions, TCIM users are more likely to report exercising sufficiently and experiencing greater control over their lives and their health (Wiles and Rosenberg, 2001). Users tend to have a more holistic orientation towards health and are more likely to identify with a cultural group associated with feminism, environmentalism and personal growth psychology and spirituality (Austin, 1998).

Studies examining geographical differences in TCIM consumption suggest larger prevalence rates of TCIM use in rural regions compared to urban areas (Adams *et al.*, 2003, 2011; Barnes *et al.*, 2004; Sibbritt *et al.*, 2005; Nunes and Esteves, 2006). However, there is little evidence that compares the use of specific TCIM modalities between rural and urban areas (Wardle *et al.*, 2012) (see Barnes *et al.*, 2002 for an exception). Self-prescribed TCIM appears to be more common among rural users compared to TCIM use facilitated through consultations with a TCIM practitioner (Wardle *et al.*, 2012). In one study, TCIM users living in remote and very remote areas in Australia were more likely to share information regarding TCIM among their networks and rely more on family, relatives and mass media as sources of TCIM information (Adams *et al.*, 2011). In general, rural residents have been understood to develop resilience, independence and self-reliance in response to limited availability of health and social care services (Leipert and Reutter, 2005; McColl, 2007; Goins *et al.*, 2005). That is, the availability, structure and size of conventional medicine and TCIM practitioners likely shape health-seeking behaviours of rural residents in ways that align them with self-management practices such as self-prescribed TCIM (Wardle *et al.*, 2012).

Production patterns across geographical areas

In his highly influential paper, Good (1977) highlighted several overlapping research streams to be undertaken related to the social and spatial relations of TCIM producers and consumers. He first proposed an initial quantitative mapping of TCIM practitioners (in terms of quantity, types of modalities and practices and their locational attributes). He also proposed that research should aim to analyze and interpret how consumers and providers interact as a geographic and social system (centers of activity, peripheral locations and territorial zones). For example, what are the identifiable patterns of illness-related behaviour in territorial zones, and how might these be shaped by distance to conventional medical practitioners versus TCIM practitioners? Anyinam (1990) highlighted the need for quantitative data on the local, regional and national distributions of TCIM practitioners, their referral networks, their catchment areas and their relationships to biomedical services. Due to the vast range of TCIMs and the areas in which they are provided, very few studies have addressed these issues directly (Andrews *et al.*, 2010) (For exceptions see Verheij *et al.*, 1999; Williams, 2000). Researchers have studied some of the patterns of TCIM production across geographical location and the structures that shape these patterns. For example, a number of studies have examined regulatory practices within clearly-defined areas of political jurisdiction (Boon, 2002; Gilmour *et al.*, 2002). In one such study, Gilmour *et al.* (2002) explored the ways naturopaths, traditional Chinese medical practitioners and homeopaths navigated regulatory frameworks and socio-political environments to achieve statutory self-regulation in Ontario, Canada.

Studies have also examined TCIM provision and consumption within and across places at the regional and national level (Sherwood, 2000; Wilkinson and Simpson, 2001), municipal and township level (Chacko, 2003) and even within and between individual institutions and clinics (Chen and Chang, 2003; Sternberg *et al.*, 2003; Johnston *et al.*, 2003). However, the spatial features of these studies are not central to their research focus and analysis (Andrews *et al.*, 2010).

The size and structure of TCIM practices encompasses the pathways to TCIM care, organization of private practices, the location of the practices and types of therapies offered. In their study on older adults who use TCIM, Andrews (2003b) found that the size/structure of TCIM practices was related to the mean number of TCIM modalities used per week, with older adults attending larger group practices using a larger number of modalities per week than those who attended individual practices. Older adults were found to have a fairly high level of market knowledge and appeared to seek out greater treatment availability from the larger group practices (Andrews, 2003b). As a result, the mean distance travelled to the larger group practices was substantially longer than those travelling to individual therapists. Larger group practices attracted the majority of their older clients from outside the towns in which the practice was based, while individual therapists attracted only 5% of their clients from outside their home towns. In general, the scope of practice among rural TCIM providers may be broader compared to urban providers (Wardle *et al.*, 2012). For example, chiropractic patients from rural areas were found to be close to twice as likely to present with non-musculoskeletal problems when compared with urban patients (Hawk *et al.*, 2001).

From a systems perspective, scholars have examined the ways in which TCIM is geographically regulated, formalized and systematized (e.g. Del Casino, 2004). Both the geographical characteristics on a macro-level, such as the distribution of TCIM and the spaces in which it is provided, as well as the geographical features of space and place at a micro-level are important to understanding how TCIM operates from a health services and systems perspective (Andrews *et al.*, 2010). Often, both macro- and micro-level geographical features of TCIM production and consumption change as its relationship with biomedicine changes. Del Casino (2004) describes Thailand's partial integration of traditional medicine within the public health care system. Traditional medicine became offered in hospitals, changing not only the location of its delivery, but at the same time changing the organization, packaging and protocols for the preparation and provision of its medicinal materials to better suit the 'sterility and scientific precision' (pp. 68–69) of the hospital.

Barriers and drivers of TCIM consumption and practice

To date, some of the key barriers and drivers of TCIM consumption and practice studied relate to referral networks and knowledge of and attitudes about TCIM or conventional medicine. One common barrier to TCIM use includes a lack of referrals from conventional health care practitioners (Wardle *et al.*, 2012). This barrier may be more common in urban areas, as a study in New Zealand suggests that conventional practitioners in rural areas may be more likely to refer their patients to TCIM services than their urban counterparts (Hider *et al.*, 2007). Another commonly cited barrier is patients' skepticism regarding TCIM treatment effects or a lack of knowledge about TCIM (Wardle *et al.*, 2012). Conversely, research has indicated that TCIM users are motivated by their dissatisfaction with conventional medicine because they find it does not meet their needs or desire greater control over the healing process and a more holistic/individualized approach (Wiles and Rosenberg, 2001). However, other research has indicated that most users seem to report that they use TCIM in conjunction with conventional medicine (Barnes *et al.*, 2004; Wiles and Rosenberg, 2001).

Geographical differences, such as differences in distance towards TCIM practices and differences in features of urban and rural life may also change the way consumers approach TCIM. Travel difficulties and time constraints have been highlighted as barriers for a number of TCIM modalities (Wardle *et al.*, 2012). In one study, women from major cities were found to enjoy greater access to TCIM practitioners and information about TCIM compared to those in other regions (Adams *et al.*, 2011). However, some studies suggest that a lack of availability of local TCIM in rural localities is not always a decisive barrier, and that rural patients are often willing to travel to receive TCIM services (Nichols *et al.*, 2012; Wiles and Rosenberg, 2001). The availability of conventional medicine has also been explored as a potential driver of TCIM consumption. Research suggests that reduced availability of conventional health care services is an important driver of TCIM consumption in rural settings (Barish and Snyder, 2008; Leipart *et al.*, 2006; Trangmar and Diaz, 2008). Differences in characteristics of TCIM practices among rural and urban areas may also change the way TCIM is consumed. Compared to rural and remote areas, major cities in Australia have been found to have higher costs for TCIM consultations and a lower sense of community (Adams *et al.*, 2011). This may align with findings that rural residents are more likely to use their community networks as a source of knowledge of TCIM (Adams *et al.*, 2011).

Micro-level Geographies of TCIM

While there has been an emphasis on macro-scale production and consumption of therapeutic places in relation to social, cultural and economic interests, a growing body of literature has shifted to encompass micro-level interactions of the way in which therapeutic landscapes are experienced (e.g. Andrews, 2003b, 2004, Andrews *et al.*, 2013; Doel and Sergrott, 2004; Williams, 1998, 2002). As qualitative research has grown within geographical research, concepts such as Gesler's (1992) 'therapeutic landscape' have been employed to understand the healing qualities of place and how space is managed or constructed as a source of healing. The overlap between TCIM and humanistic geography is present in the ways in which research has explored symbolic landscapes and the symbolic meanings embedded in medical systems and the way health and illness is structured, named, interpreted and treated (Kleinman, 1973; Williams, 1998). Non-representational theories can inform geographers' understandings of the relational environment, affect and the pre-cognitive features of therapeutic landscape as well as how bodies both acquire affective capacities (Duff, 2010) and simultaneously transmit affect, such that they continuously produce the relational environment (Andrews *et al.*, 2013). With these perspectives in mind, this section touches briefly on the healing qualities of place, the management and construction of space in relation to performances of TCIM, and TCIM's extension of health and wellbeing into the realm of everyday spaces.

Healing qualities of place

For many TCIM users, place is imbued with healing qualities. Researchers such as Williams (1998, 2000) and Andrews (2002b, 2003, 2004) have explored how the spaces in which TCIM is practiced may themselves promote healing or wellbeing. Williams (1998) discusses the physical and psychological aspects of therapeutic landscapes created by practitioners to not only heal but to maintain health and wellbeing. The 'authentic' or 'caring' environments that promote the healing process consist of the physical attributes of the spaces in which care is delivered as well as the meaningful interpersonal relationships built and maintained within them. Similarly, Andrews (2002b) notes that healing is often experienced through physical, emotional and/or spiritual connection to place (hot springs, remote wilderness or holiday destinations). A 'sense of place' often provides psychological rootedness to TCIM users in ways that support their belief systems and everyday lifestyles related to health and wellbeing (Williams, 1998; Andrews, 2003b).

Management and construction of space in TCIM

Complementing studies on place in relation to the construction of meaning in TCIM practice, geographical research has explored the spaces in which TCIM is practiced, particularly the ways they are produced, arranged and challenged. Notably, Doel and Segrott (2004) examine the importance of materials in relation to therapeutic practice and the encounters between practitioners and clients. The authors draw from post-structuralist approaches to understand TCIM as unique events that are 'always unexpected', materialized in unique socio-spatial settings through the interactions between patients, practitioners and medicines and specific to each encounter. For example, materials such as essential oils and herbal remedies play a signature role within, and even shape, the therapeutic encounter. As such, Andrews *et al.,* (2013) hold that networks of relations between spaces should be thought of as an ongoing process, rather than complete. They are constantly 'coming into being' as material, symbolic and emotional influences continuously shape their development (Darling, 2010). Place is also constructed as a performance of relationships that depend on the specific relational configurations that support them (Anderson and Harrison, 2010). That is, networks of place are not fixed but continuously changing in their development as a result of the relational influences that shape them.

TCIM therapists employ many materials within their practices to support various modalities. Doel and Segrott (2004) distinguish three kinds of materials used in TCIM practice: the 'signature materials' that make each therapy unique (e.g. aromatherapy's essential oils), 'supplementary materials' that facilitate the practice of TCIM itself (e.g. treatment equipment) and the 'marginalia' that facilitate the unique use of such materials for the individual client. Beyond physical materials, Andrews *et al.*, (2010) describe the 'tools' of TCIM as including imagination and visualization, as well as materials, to extend the concept of the therapeutic landscape beyond physical spaces to places and spaces within one's imagination. Andrews (2004) and Williams (1998) examine the ways in which TCIM therapists actively rely on imagination and visualization, including imagining places, as part of the healing process.

Finally, the therapeutic experience, including affective and symbolic experiences, are embedded in and facilitated by structural features and the relationships developed between the user and their therapist (Andrews, 2003b). Andrews (2003b) found that older TCIM users perceived larger TCIM practices more as centres of therapeutic activity, while individual therapists were perceived more as a convenient, local resource. For both larger TCIM practices and individual therapists, users felt a sense of loyalty to their therapist and practice setting. According to Williams (1998), therapeutic relationships create a strong sense of place in relation to the meeting places for therapeutic activity such as offices and waiting rooms, which can augment the healing process. Additionally, clinics are embedded within locations imbued with tradition, lifestyles, spiritualism (organic food shops, health food shops, new age and alternative shops and social spaces) that support life styles associated with (and even part of) TCIM treatment (Andrews, 2003b).

TCIM in everyday spaces

With TCIM consumption associated with various alternative lifestyles or philosophical commitments (Andrews, 2003b; Austin, 1998; Wiles and Rosenberg, 2001), it is no surprise that TCIM consumption often extends outside designated therapeutic spaces and into the realm of everyday life. Andrews *et al.* (2010) describe the spatial diffusion of TCIM as concerned with the delivery of therapies across a range of new spaces, and largely attributable to the increase in self-treatment materials (e.g. homeopathic preparations, acupuncture pens, manuals and self-help book and so forth). Similarly, Doel and Segrott (2003a) the way in which TCIM users transform everyday activities into therapeutic practices. In their study of TCIM in British mass media, they found that the editors of magazines largely focus on the medical efficacy of TCIM, its ability to address a much broader range of activities and everyday spaces in relation to health and wellbeing, and its association with a more natural or alternative lifestyle. As integrative efforts between conventional medicine and TCIM grow, TCIM has also expanded into spaces of conventional medicine (e.g. Del Casino, 2004; Joos *et al.*, 2011). However, little is known about the experiences of users and TCIM practitioners who operate in these spaces.

Future Investigation

Future research objectives related to TCIM relate to several geography sub-disciplines (Andrews *et al.*, 2010). Together, these lines of inquiry can help provide insight into the contexts under which TCIM and conventional health services are provided, considerations related to TCIM users and providers, and the coordination of TCIM and conventional health services. For example, medical and health geographies of TCIM can further explore health-related work, workplaces and concepts and practices related to TCIM and conventional care. Social geographies of TCIM, in addressing TCIM as a broader social phenomenon, can continue to examine how space and place shape the consumption of TCIM within and across social groups and help better understand the social context in which providers, businesses and overlapping sectors support the production of TCIM. Such insights may prove valuable for coordinating public health and other health services delivery initiatives for both TCIM and conventional health services. Similarly, the cultural geographies of TCIM can help understand the consumer and production cultures that should be considered when coordinating health services.

Complementing the social and cultural perspectives described above, political geographies of TCIM can understand spatial considerations related to policy, legal and regulatory issues. For example, at the macrolevel, such research may examine the regulation and training of TCIM practitioners, the legal status of TCIM modalities and national policies related to TCIM. At the micro-level, political geographies can help understand political factors and various levels of state influence that can influence the role of place in shaping practitioners' decisions about the production of TCIM. It can better understand the nuanced interactions between different scales of political places, and the ongoing processes of their production and interpretation. Geographical research in TCIM can help understand four fields of economic research related to TCIM (Andrews *et al.*, 2010). First, it can describe the flow of capital to TCIM, both from public and private sources. Second, it can help understand the international, regional and local labour markets that shape the distribution of TCIM practitioners. Third, it examines the social power relationships that occur in work spaces, including the cultures and counter cultures in everyday interactions and labour relations. Finally, it can offer insight into the experiences of consumption of TCIM and the experiences of place during the negotiation of care. Together, a better understanding of the political and economic geographies of TCIM can help tailor health services to places in relation to their local, regional and national political, economic and policy contexts.

Three other sub-disciplines that can lend help to inform health service delivery related to TCIM are urban and rural geographies, feminist geographies and historical geographies. Urban and rural geographical perspectives can help understand issues related to service access, such as the different modalities available and the extent to which they are provided in rural and urban locations. It can also contribute insight into the various cultures associated with the production and consumption of TCIM and their location in rural and urban spaces (Andrews, 2003b). To date, feminist geographies have noted that certain TCIM modalities are largely produced by women, and that different consumption patterns exist across modalities for men and women (Adams *et al.*, 2018; Andrews, 2002a). What is still missing is research exploring the ways in which space and gender shape TCIM consumption and production. That is, to not only understand the distributive features of TCIM production and consumption between genders, but also why these different patterns occur (Andrews *et al.*, 2010). Feminist geographies should also aim to understand how gender shapes experiences of conventional and TCIM in spaces where they are integrated (Doel and Segrott, 2003a). Finally, historical geographies of TCIM can further explore how TCIM is embedded in histories of place and historical identities of communities, regions and nations. Such lines of inquiry may also uncover how TCIM helps shape the development of places where TCIM is accepted, disputed, or otherwise used in the formation of local, group-based, or national identity.

References

Adams, J., Andrews, G., Barnes, J., Broom, A., Magin, P. (eds.), (2012). *Traditional, Complementary and Integrative Medicine: An International Reader*. Palgrave Macmillan, Basingstoke, Hampshire, UK.

Adams, J., Robinson, N. (2013). Public health and health services research in integrative medicine: An emerging, essential focus. *European Journal of Integrative Medicine*, 5(1), 1–3.

Adams, J., Sibbritt, D., Broom, A., Loxton, D., Pirotta, M., Humphreys, J., Lui, C. W. (2011). A comparison of complementary and alternative medicine users and use across geographical areas: A national survey of 1,427 women. *BMC Complementary and Alternative Medicine*, *11*(1), 85.

Adams, J., Sibbritt, D., Easthope, G., Young, A. F. (2003). The profile of women who consult alternative health practitioners in Australia. *Medical Journal of Australia*, *179*, 29–300.

Adams, J., Sibbritt, D., Lui, C. (2011). The urban–rural divide in complementary and alternative medicine use: A longitudinal study of 10,638 women. *BMC Complementary and Alternative Medicine, 11*(1), 2.

Adams J., Steel, A., Broom, A., Frawley, J. (eds.), (2018). *Women's Health and Complementary and Integrative Medicine*. London, Routledge.

Anderson, B., Harrison, P. (2010). *The Promise of Non-representational Theories*. Ashgate, Farnham, Surrey, UK.

Anderson, B. (2016). *Taking-place: Non-representational Theories and Geography.* Routledge, London, UK.

Andrews, G. J. (2002a). Private complementary medicine and older people: service use and user empowerment. *Ageing and Society*, *22*(3), 343–368.

Andrews, G. J. (2002b). Towards a more place-sensitive nursing research: an invitation to medical and health geography. *Nursing Inquiry*, *9*(4), 221–238.

Andrews, G. J. (2003a). Locating a geography of nursing: Space, place and the progress of geographical thought. *Nursing Philosophy*, *4*(3), 231–248.

Andrews, G. J. (2003b). Placing the consumption of private complementary medicine: Everyday geographies of older peoples' use. *Health and Place*, *9*(4), 337–349.

Andrews, G. J. (2004). (Re) thinking the dynamics between healthcare and place: Therapeutic geographies in treatment and care practices. *Area*, *36*(3), 307–318.

Andrews, G. J. (2009). Complementary and Alternative Medicine. In Kitchin, R. and Thrift, N. (eds.), *The International Encyclopaedia of Human Geography*, Elsevier, Oxford.

Andrews, G. J., Boon, H. (2005). CAM in Canada: Places, practices, research. *Complementary Therapies in Clinical Practice*, *11*(1), 21–27.

Andrews, G. J., Adams, J., Segrott, J. (2010). Complementary and alternative medicine (CAM): production and consumption. In Brown, T., McLafferty, S. and Moon, G. A., (eds.), *Companion to Health and Medical Geography.* Blackwell, Chichester, UK.

Andrews, G. J., Evans, J., McAlister, S. (2013). 'Creating the right therapy vibe': Relational performances in holistic medicine. *Social Science and Medicine*, *83*, 99–109.

Andrews, G. J., Segrott, J. Lui, C. W., Adams, J. (2012). The geography of complementary and alternative medicine. In Adams, J., Andrews, G. J., Barnes, J., Broom, A. and Magin, P. (eds.), *Traditional, Complementary and Integrative Medicine: An International Reader.* Palgrave MacMillan, London.

Andrews, G. J., Wiles, J., Miller, K. L. (2004). The geography of complementary medicine: Perspectives and prospects. *Complementary Therapies in Nursing and Midwifery*, *10*(3), 175–185.

Anyinam, C. (1990). Alternative medicine in western industrialized countries: An agenda for medical geography. *The Canadian Geographer/Le Géographe Canadien*, *34*(1), 69–76.

Austin, J. (1998). Why patients use alternative medicine. *Jama*, *279*(19), 1548–1553.

Barish, R., Snyder, A. E. (2008). Use of complementary and alternative health-care practices among persons served by a remote area medical clinic. *Family and Community Health*, *31*(3), 221–227.

Barnes, P.M., Powell-Griner, E., McFann, K., Nahin, R. L. (2004). Complementary and alternative medicine use among adults: United States, 2002. *Seminars in Integrative Medicine*, *2*(2), 54–71. WB Saunders.

Boon, H. (2002). Regulation of complementary/alternative medicine: A Canadian perspective. *Complementary Therapies in Medicine*, *10*(1), 14–19.

Cadman, L. (2009). Nonrepresentational theory/nonrepresentational geographies. *International Encyclopedia of Human Geography*, *7*, 456–463.

Chacko, E. (2003). Culture and therapy: Complementary strategies for the treatment of type-2 diabetes in an urban setting in Kerala, India. *Social Science and Medicine*, *56*(5), 1087–1098.

Chen, Y. F., Chang, J. S. (2003). Complementary and alternative medicine use among patients attending a hospital dermatology clinic in Taiwan. *International Journal of Dermatology*, *42*(8), 616–621.

Conboy, L., Patel, S., Kaptchuk, T.J., Gottlieb, B., Eisenberg, D., Acevedo-Garcia, D. (2005). Sociodemographic determinants of the utilization of specific types of complementary and alternative medicine: An analysis based on a nationally representative survey sample. *The Journal of Alternative and Complementary Medicine: Research on Paradigm, Practice, and Policy*, *11*(6), 977–994.

Conradson, D., Latham, A. (2007). The affective possibilities of London: Antipodean transnationals and the overseas experience. *Mobilities*, *2*(2), 231–254.

Darling, J. (2010). "Just being there": Ethics, experimentation and the cultivation of care. In Anderson, B. and Harrison, P. (eds.), *Taking Place: Nonrepresentational Theories and Geography*. Farnham, Ashgate.

Del Casino, V. J. (2004). (Re) placing health and health care: Mapping the competing discourses and practices of 'traditional' and 'modern' Thai medicine. *Health and Place*, *10*(1), 59–73.

Doel, M. A., Segrott, J. (2003a). Beyond belief? Consumer culture, complementary medicine, and the disease of everyday life. *Environment and Planning D: Society and Space*, *21*(6), 739–759.

Doel, M. A., Segrott, J. (2003b). Self, health, and gender: Complementary and alternative medicine in the British mass media. *Gender, Place and Culture: A Journal of Feminist Geography*, *10*(2), 131–144.

Doel, M. A., Segrott, J. (2004). Materializing complementary and alternative medicine: Aromatherapy, chiropractic, and Chinese herbal medicine in the UK. *Geoforum*, *35*(6), 727–738.

Duff, C. (2010). Towards a developmental ethology: Exploring Deleuze's contribution to the study of health and human development. *Health*, *14*(6), 619–634.

Gesler W. (1992). Therapeutic landscapes: Medical issues in the light of the new cultural geography. *Social Science and Medicine*, *34*(7), 735–746.

Gilmour, J., Kelner, M., Wellman, B. (2002). Opening the door to complementary and alternative medicine: Self-regulation in Ontario. *Law and Policy*, *24*(2), 149–174.

Goins, R. T., Williams, K. A., Carter, M. W., Spencer, S. M., Solovieva, T. (2005). Perceived barriers to health care access among rural older adults: A qualitative study. *The Journal of Rural Health*, *21*(3), 206–213.

Good, C. M. (1977). Traditional medicine: An agenda for medical geography. *Social Science and Medicine*, *11*(14–16), 705–713.

Gregory, D. (2011). Human geography. In: Gregory, D., Johnston, R., Pratt, G., Watts, M. and Whatmore, S. (eds.), *The Dictionary of Human Geography*, 5th Edition, John Wiley & Sons.

Harvey, D. (1973). *Social Justice and the City*, Edward Arnold, London.

Hawk, C., Adams, J., Hartvigsen, J. (2015). The role of CAM in public health, disease prevention, and health promotion. *Evidence-Based Complementary and Alternative Medicine*, *2015*, 1–2.

Hawk, C., Long, C. R., Boulanger, K. T. (2001). Prevalence of nonmusculoskeletal complaints in chiropractic practice: Report from a practice based research program. *Journal of Manipulative and Physiological Therapeutics*, *24*(3), 157–169.

Hider, P., Lay-Yee, R., Davis, P. (2007). Doctors, practices, patients, and their problems during usual hours: A description of rural and non-rural primary care in New Zealand in 2001–2002. *The New Zealand Medical Journal* (Online), *120*(1253).

Johnston, G. A., Bilbao, R. M., GrahamBrown, R. A. C. (2003). The use of complementary medicine in children with atopic dermatitis in secondary care in Leicester. *British Journal of Dermatology*, *149*(3), 566–571.

Joos, S., Musclmann, B., Szecsenyi, J. (2011). Integration of complementary and alternative medicine into family practices in Germany: Results of a national survey. *Evidence-Based Complementary and Alternative Medicine*, *2011*, 1–8.

Kleinman, A.M. (1973). Medicine's symbolic reality: On a central problem in the philosophy of medicine. *Inquiry*, *16*(1–4), 206–213.

Leipert, B. D., Matsui, D., Rieder, M. J. (2006). Women and pharmacologic therapy in rural and remote Canada. *Canadian Journal of Rural Medicine*, *11*(4), 296–301.

Leipert, B. D., Reutter, L. (2005). Developing resilience: How women maintain their health in northern geographically isolated settings. *Qualitative Health Research*, *15*(1), 49–65.

Massumi, B. (2002). *Parables for the Virtual: Movement, Affect, Sensation*. Duke University Press, Durham, UK.

McColl, L. (2007). The influence of bush identity on attitudes to mental health in a Queensland community. *Rural Society*, *17*(2), 107–124.

McCormack, D. P. (2008). Geographies for moving bodies: Thinking, dancing, spaces. *Geography Compass*, *2*(6), 1822–1836.

Nichols, E., Weinert, C., Shreffler Grant, J., Ide, B. (2012). Complementary and alternative medicine providers in rural locations. *Online Journal of Rural Nursing and Health Care*. *6*(2), 40–46.

Nunes, B., Esteves, M. S. (2006). Therapeutic itineraries in rural and urban areas: A Portuguese study. *Rural and Remote Health*, *6*(1), 394.

Relph, E. (1976). *Place and Placelessness*, Vol. 1, Pion, London: Pion.

Sherwood, P. (2000). Patterns of use of complementary health services in the South-West of Western Australia. *Australian Journal of Rural Health*, *8*(4), 194–200.

Shreffler-Grant, J., Hill, W., Weinert, C., Nichols, E., Ide, B. (2007). Complementary therapy and older rural women: Who uses it and who does not? *Nursing Research*, *56*(1), 28–33.

Sibbritt, D. W., Adams, J., Young, A. F. (2005). A longitudinal analysis of mid-age women's use of complementary and alternative medicine (CAM) in Australia, 1996–1998. *Women and Health*, *40*(4), 41–56.

Sternberg, S. A., Chandran, A., Sikka, M. (2003). Alternative therapy use by elderly African Americans attending a community clinic. *Journal of the American Geriatrics Society*, *51*(12), 1768–1772.

Thrift, N. (2008). *Non-representational Theory: Space, Politics, Affect*. Routledge, London, UK.

Trangmar, P., Diaz, V. A. (2008). Investigating complementary and alternative medicine use in a Spanish-speaking Hispanic community in South Carolina. *The Annals of Family Medicine*, *6*(Suppl 1), S12–S15.

Tuan, Y. F. (1976). Humanistic geography. *Annals of the Association of American Geographers*, *66*(2), 266–276.

Verheij, R. A., de Bakker, D. H., Groenewegen, P. P. (1999). Is there a geography of alternative medical treatment in The Netherlands? *Health and Place*, *5*(1), 83–97.

Wardle, J., Lui, C. W., Adams, J. (2012). Complementary and alternative medicine in rural communities: Current research and future directions. *The Journal of Rural Health*, *28*(1), 101–112.

Wiles, J., Rosenberg, M. W. (2001). 'Gentle caring experience': Seeking alternative health care in Canada. *Health and Place*, *7*(3), 209–224.

Wilkinson, J. M., Simpson, M. D. (2001). High use of complementary therapies in a New South Wales rural community. *Australian Journal of Rural Health*, *9*(4), 166–171.

Williams, A. (2002). Changing geographies of care: Employing the concept of therapeutic landscapes as a framework in examining home space. *Social Science and Medicine*, *55*(1), 141–154.

Williams, A. (1998). Therapeutic landscapes in holistic medicine. *Social Science and Medicine*, *46*(9), 1193–1203.

Williams, A. M. (2000). The diffusion of alternative health care: A Canadian case study of chiropractic and naturopathic practices. *The Canadian Geographer/ Le Géographe Canadien*, *44*(2), 152–166.

Chapter 2

The Social Science of Traditional, Complementary and Integrative Medicine

Alex Broom, Rhiannon Parker and Jon Adams

Why Do We Need a Sociology of TCIM?

Sociologists have traditionally taken a different approach to the study of traditional, complementary and integrative medicine (TCIM) than other academic disciplines (Broom and Tovey, 2008a), and in this chapter we will outline several key areas of emphasis. The broad approach taken within sociological work in TCIM is constructivist in character. That is, seeking an understanding of *why* people use what they do rather than *what* is used and by whom. In this way, the sociology of TCIM focuses on making sense of the life-worlds of people who are using various therapeutic options and of the clinicians involved in their care. Sociology thus utilises certain forms of 'evidence' in seeking an understanding of the life-worlds of persons using TCIM and/or biomedicine, and is often qualitative in character, utilising interviews, ethnography, surveys and focus groups (Broom, 2005). Survey research is a common means for examining the question of why people engage with TCIM and their perceptions around these practices across time and locale (Frawley *et al.*, 2014). What binds the broad umbrella of TCIM social science to date is an emphasis on systematically *exploring the subjective experiences* of patients, consumers and communities of therapeutic practices rather than *assessing the bio-physical outcomes* of care (however intertwined these may be). In this sense, the sociology of TCIM emphasizes understanding and incorporating *subjective experience* and mapping societal-level *structural dimensions* that shape who uses what practices, when and where (e.g. class, ethnicity, gender, locale, etc.). The sociology of TCIM seeks higher-level explanations — *or theoretical models* — for interpreting why TCIM and/or biomedicine are consumed and delivered in particular ways across time, place and communities (e.g. Meurk *et al.*, 2013). In this way, a sociology of TCIM is *critical* (in that it unravels the taken-for-granted that can impede deeper analysis), *multi-stakeholder* and *theory-generating* (e.g. Hirschkorn and Bourgeault, 2005; Broom and Tovey, 2007a, 2007b, 2008a, 2008b). It engages, for example, how such things as identity, culture, economy, politics and emotions can shape medicines (and their reception in societies) (e.g. Sointu, 2005, 2006a, 2006b, 2011). A critical sociology of TCIM thus plays an important role in the field, bridging the forms of skepticism that can plague medical analysis of TCIM while also avoiding the valorization of TCIM — a common feature of the complementary medicine field more broadly. Below, we outline examples of how sociological explanations have been deployed to understand the rise and ongoing engagement with TCIM across place, locale and time, and forms of resistance to this rise.

Sociologies of TCIM in 'Western' Contexts

In some respects, TCIM was a natural concern for social scientists given the embeddedness of concerns of therapeutic development with relations of power, ideology, modernity and broader social transformations (Cant and Sharma, 2004). Beyond what continued to occur in non-OECD countries (more on that below), what was evident in the 'West' was a resurgence of — or perhaps a curious persistence in — interest in non-biomedical care, despite the major advances seen in biomedicine over the 19th and 20th Centuries. Yet, biomedicine in all its forms and functions was an entrenched mechanism of the modern state, and fully institutionalized

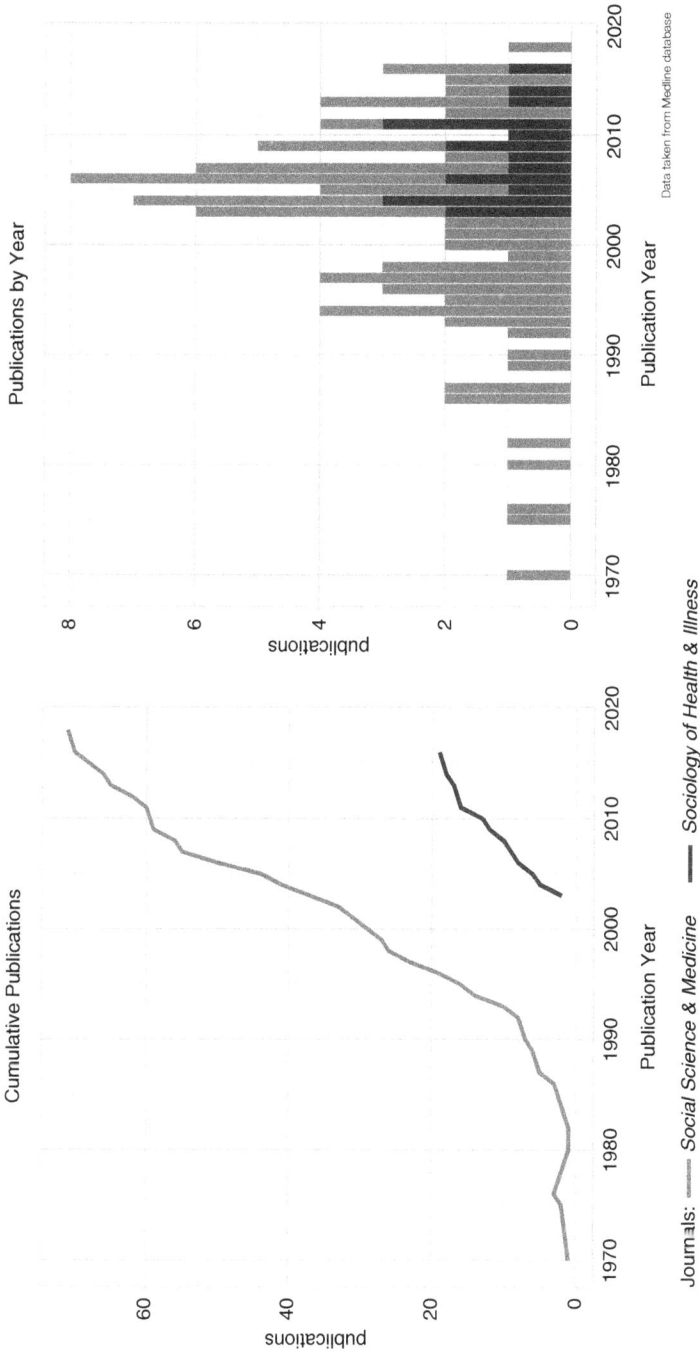

Figure 1.   TCIM-related publications in *Social Science and Medicine* and *Sociology of Health and Illness* from 1970 till today.

as the dominant form of care. Science, as determined by particular structures of knowledge production, dominated what filtered into the institutionalized 'biomedicine' creating an increasingly rigid system of structures which essentially placed TCIM (at least many modalities therein) precariously in relation to structures of authority. From a sociological perspective, this was intriguing in that lay practice (Williams and Calnan, 2013) was not reflecting expert perspectives (and in enduring ways) and that this was becoming a political, economic and ideological struggle. As shown in Figure 1, where we merely select articles published in two prominent health sociology journals, what results is a steady increase in social science interest in TCIM (in western contexts) from the 1980s onwards.

Sociology of Professions

The 'original' sociology of TCIM tended to focus on inter-professional dynamics (e.g. Kelner *et al.*, 2004; Coulter and Willis, 2004; Adams, 2000). The field has moved beyond constructing TCIM in contrast to professional or medical dominance (Willis, 1989), which was a popular approach in the 1980s and 1990s given that TCIM was not mainstreamed in Western societies (as perhaps we could say it is today) (Adams *et al.*, 2017). This was a period of considerable inter-professional tussle, at least within countries such as Australia, the UK and the US, between 'conventional' systems of knowledge and their professional groups and TCIM. This resulted in a long period of what many social scientists called *boundary work* — the attempt to prevent the penetration of TCIM into conventional medical systems and forms of (State and non-State) funding (Broom, 2002; Winnick, 2005). In this context, much of the sociological analysis centred on attempts by various conventional medical groups and organizations to exclude TCIM (Allsop and Saks, 2003; Cant and Sharma, 1996).

Sociology of Knowledge

The sociology of knowledge offered subtlety to the debates around TCIM and biomedicine as it was articulated in western industrialized contexts (e.g. Hollenberg and Muzzin, 2010). This sphere of social science introduced debate around the distinctions between TCIM and biomedicine with regard to such topics as how we collect knowledge of what works and what does not work (*vis-à-vis* whether it works) (Prior, 2003). This shifted the debate from issues of protection of professional territory to questions about the nature of knowledge (Hess, 2004; Keshet, 2009). Rather than TCIM popularity being temporary and public engagement waning over time, social scientists observed its rising popularity and a disjunction between formalized medical knowledge (of what works) and individual beliefs about what works. As a result, work on what can broadly be termed epistemology — the study of knowledge or knowledge production — emerged with a focus on what counts as data in studies of TCIM (Brosnan, 2016; Mizrachi *et al.*, 2005). While many other spheres of TCIM research wanted to reproduce a biomedical epistemology (knowledge produced through trials), social scientists wanted to explore whether the assumptions about knowledge creation in health and medicine were a 'good fit' with what TCIM was 'doing' for people in the community (Keshet, 2010). Much of this work intersected with an emerging interest in persons (rather than patients) and holism (rather the biophysical reductionism) that was gaining traction both in the public sphere and across forms of medicine in the late 20th Century. Somewhat erroneously for many TCIM modalities, but still interestingly, for social scientists, the debate around TCIM and biomedicine was infused with these broader political debates and shifts around holism and person-centeredness. In turn, the shift to market capitalism in many nation States made way for (often) private TCIM funding within a deregulated private health insurance environment (at least in Australia), illustrating how the way the health care system is funded and the level of state intervention shapes what counts as effective (Kelner and Wellman, 1997). That is, what counted as legitimate knowledge (of effectiveness) in the mid-20th Century started to shift subtly from a biomedical evidence base to a set of intermingling ideas about what is of value in the (now) 21st Century (driven by many dynamics around consumerism, individualism, autonomy, holism, vitalism, neoliberalism and so on). As noted, social scientists have been agnostic about this process, observing these trends rather than celebrating or denigrating the rise or mainstreaming of TCIM therein. What is clear within this body of work is that TCIM practices are embedded in social, cultural, political and historical conditions which shape their highly variable levels of acceptability, traction and consumption in our communities.

Sociology of the Body

Sociologists also explore in considerable detail the micro-relations of TCIM, not merely the structural conditions within which they are delivered (Baarts and Pedersen, 2009). For example, and broadly under the umbrella of the 'sociology of the body', social scientists have sought to augment professions/knowledge-directed analysis with a focus on what actually happens in various TCIM encounters (e.g. Sointu, 2006a). While TCIM is a highly varied plethora of practices and logics, and one must be very careful in making broad claims as to the benefits or features of such encounters, there are some shared dispositions or approaches that have been commonly observed in social science studies of the 'pull' of TCIM encounters (Gale, 2011). Broadly, arguments have been offered around the value and importance of different features of the therapeutic encounter in the search for healing or wellness. Gale articulates, for example, body work and body-talk as key components of the TCIM emphasis on narrative, touch, intuition and the embodied patient, not as a passive recipient of health care, but as communicative, thus raising the acute importance of the therapeutic encounter in healing and care. Interwoven with work in the sociology of knowledge (i.e. how does a practitioner 'know' what a person needs within an encounter) is engagement with the forms of therapeutic exchange, healing, care and sites of 'success' (often beyond a biomedical lens, or even from the perspectives of many in the TCIM community) that are unexplainable within the current paradigm of assessment of how things work. In sum, this 'body' of sociological work challenges splits between mind–body–society (adding society in from the traditional Cartesian split) that imbue assessments of value and effectiveness, asking whether we know what is really occurring within healing practices. Patient and community perspectives are viewed as powerful in understanding this facet of TCIM engagement.

Sociologies of TCIM in the 'Developing World'

An interesting feature of the sociology of TCIM has been its western centricity despite the reality that many of the TCIM practices routinely utilized in western contexts have non-western histories and even origins. While this is not exclusively the case, it represents an interesting paradox in the sociology of TCIM and its tendency to emphasize the locales where there is a clash between biomedical sensibilities and TCIM. Or perhaps in turn, the bias of the academy toward the concerns of western modernity, rather than the global South. Regardless, the majority of the world's population utilise TCIM as routine health care. While the level of knowledge of the reach of TCIM use across economically poorer nations is fairly poor, what is clear is widespread ongoing use of TCIM across populations (albeit varied across communities — more on this below). As shown in Figure 2, in author A's (Broom) work in South Asia focussing on cancer patients use of TCIM, use ranged between 34 and 84%, illustrating high use of TCIM even in contexts of (more privileged) populations who have access to conventional cancer care. While the data on TCIM use has been varied, even across WHO reports (e.g. WHO, 2005), a recent study (see Figure 3) showed relatively low levels of consultations in middle-income countries, suggesting much of TCIM is self-prescribed

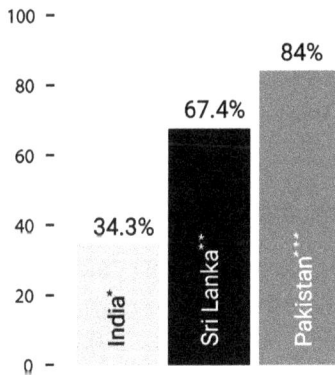

Figure 2.   Use of TCIM by cancer patients.

Sources: *Broom *et al.* (2009). **Broom *et al.* (2010). ***Tovey *et al.* (2005).

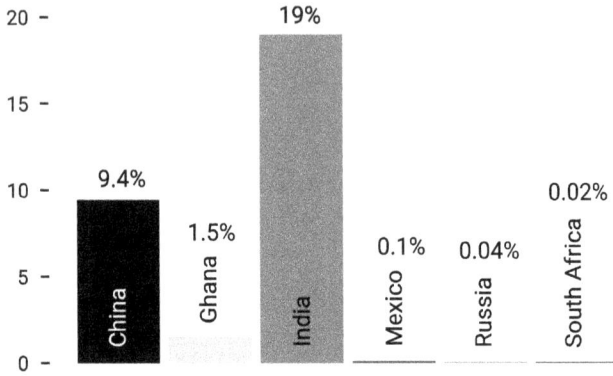

Figure 3.   Reports of low traditional medicine use according to consultations with traditional medicine providers and health care providers within middle-income countries (Oyebode *et al.*, 2016).

(Oyebode *et al.*, 2016). Regardless, in the context of many developing countries — of which South Asia becomes the focus here — there exist a multiplicity of therapeutic practices and a close intersection of culture, identity and health care choices and practices (Broom *et al.*, 2018; Broom and Doron, 2013). This requires a different, albeit complementary, series of conceptual considerations for making sense of the inter-relationships between different spheres of medicine across contexts and locales. Below, we outline just some considerations in the sociology of TCIM, as pertinent to economically poorer countries, using specific examples from South Asia.

Tradition, Identity and Medicine as Social Practice

Work in sociology tends to conceptualise 'medicine' as a discrete facet of everyday life — a mechanism for staying healthy or ameliorating illness and/or suffering. This, in some respects, articulates the western tendency to compartmentalise health and illness from everyday life (another split that has emerged from the institutionalization of illness). This ensures the 'treatment' of medicine, as a social category, as distinct from other facets of the social, including issues of taste, identity, culture and shared histories. Yet, as is shown in scholarship focused on traditional medicines in developing countries (e.g. Broom *et al.*, 2009a, 2016; Broom and Doron, 2013), these distinctions do not hold up in practice and in fact shape some of the many reasons why people make choices about using particular practices, practitioners and modalities. This theme centres on the embeddedness of *TCIM use in intersecting spheres of self, identity and community*, rather than on (biomedical) evidence of its effectiveness (as emergent in clinical studies). From a sociological perspective, this does not mean that TCIM decision-making is non-evidence based, but rather, that in thinking about use, benefit and support for particular practices, we need to consider the breadth of dimensions that shape the ongoing support for a wide range of therapeutic practices. Whether in relation to HIV in Africa (Batisai, 2016; O'Brien and Broom, 2014) or cancer in India (Broom *et al.*, 2009a, 2009b), what we can see is how *solidarity is articulated in care* and preferences. In the India context, Ayurveda, for example, has a deep pre-colonial and post-colonial history that is deeply embedded in the national psyche. Similarly, a recent world yoga tour by the Prime Minister of India, Modi, illustrated the embeddedness of 'medicine' (in this case, self-care) in national identity, cultural narratives and post-colonial identity work. Thus, from a sociological perspective, *TCIM use represents a form of biopolitics* (see also Fries, 2008; Wahlberg, 2006) — a reassertion of Indian sociality and solidarity and, in the context of Ayurveda, a locally scientific/credentialized medical system (however contested this might be in other realms). *Biopolitics* in this context refers to dynamics of authority, resistance and epistemological challenge (what counts as credible knowledge and 'know-how'). What we can see is the sociology of knowledge coming into play again, but with different dimensions in developing countries. This illustrates that TCIM should not be viewed as merely 'medicine' but as part of the social fabric and that people's investment in therapies is a complex and evolving combination of benefit, identity, commitment, community and historical associations. This is clearly shown in the excerpts shown in Table 1 from our study of pluralism in cancer in India, whereby we asked oncologists for their views on why patients engage with TCIM. We note that the medicine-as-culture argument also holds for biomedicine in western contexts although this point has been under-emphasized in relation to TCIM in developing

Table 1.   Medicine-as-culture.

Clinician 5: (Consultant, Medical Oncologist)	Because you are born [in India] with so many things in place, even the spices that you use for, in food for example. Steadily I learned that each of them also has some kind of medicinal use. I mean, turmeric and cumin, yeah, that's what we've been hearing about (in the literature). The traditional medicines are our way of life without our even knowing it
Clinician 8: (Consultant, Head and Neck Surgeon)	Alternative medicines are ingrained in our social and cultural system. Even, you see, at home, if you have some abdominal discomfort or headache, you don't go to a doctor, they'll say 'try some home remedies'. Even your elders within the family will give you some medicines, or they'll go, take you to the Homeopath or Ayurvedic, or some practitioner
Clinician 10: (Specialist Oncology Nurse)	Ayurvedic, I personally use it for jaundice. We take out the leaves of that plant, and we make it a paste, and you take it with milk, every morning for 1 week. After that I checked my bilirubin count. With jaundice, it is effective

countries. This, we note, does not diminish the significant of TCIM nor reify its importance, but rather inserts a social angle on the multiple reasons underpinning the prominence and continued popularity of TCIM in, for example, India, despite the now widespread availability of biomedicine.

Inequalities, Structural Violence and the Socioeconomic (Mediations) Medical Pluralism

An important mediating factor in the aforementioned dynamics is the reality that medical pluralism is a highly unequal process, both across and within nations (Broom *et al.*, 2009a; Cant and Sharma, 1999). Access to health care remains poor across much if not all the developing world and it is thus important to embed any understanding of TCIM within and beyond developing countries in an understanding of inequitable access and social justice considerations. In western contexts, as mentioned above, purchasing TCIM is largely out-of-pocket and based on choices made by the consumer (albeit also mediated by capacity to pay). Yet there is broad access to a baseline form of public health care across most of the

OECD context. In many developing countries, with India being a prime example once again, the capacity to pay strongly influences what exactly will be used. In this context, families may, for example, choose not to seek biomedical care if necessary finances are not available. Compared to biomedical resources, TCIM may offer a more cost-effective, accessible or acceptable alternative and may even be the only available option. While this is rarely the case — TCIM and biomedical options are usually used equally or together — it is vital to ensure that the *polarization in access to forms of medicine* informs all sociological work on TCIM. In this way, we need to add to the dimensions of identity, community and taste, the *day-to-day realities of structural violence* as a mediating factor in the 'choices' people make in relation to medicine.

Such statements shown in Table 2 clearly raised serious issues for social justice, but they also point to the importance of embedding

Table 2. Structural determinants within TCIM use.

Clinician 13: (Consultant, Haematologist)	… in India, generally, I would say the females would be using a lot more alternative medicine because they don't even come to the hospital, actually. I mean, we have a huge disparity in sexes for all the patients that we treat, for every disease. In Hodgkin's, it's something like twenty to one, in leukaemia, it's easily ten to one because, for a female, they would not even be bringing the patient to a tertiary care hospital. I mean, they would be lost somewhere along the way *Interviewer*: Tell me why? Basically because, why would you spend so much money on a female child, or a female relative? I mean, see in India, you have a breadwinner. That breadwinner is the most important person, and everything is spent on maintaining the breadwinner's health because without him (sic), the whole family is going to suffer, but if a female dies, you can always have a second wife or you can have another daughter
Clinician 1: (Consultant, Medical Oncologist)	There's son wise difference and delay in (presentation) and all those things. They (women) do not have that freedom to go and express themselves, they do not have access to the lady doctors in the community, in which they can go and talk to them

understandings of TCIM in a social determinants approach. That is, without dismissing TCIM use as a practice of the poor or uneducated, understanding that opportunity for different forms of care and access to practitioners is highly varied in economically poorer contexts. What this means is that in seeking to promote development, we need to accommodate an understanding of both preference and belief, but in turn, access and opportunity.

Research Agenda in the Sociology of TCIM

The sociology of TCIM has evolved considerably over the course of the last 30–40 years, and this has included a wide range of approaches that have provided insight into importance dimensions of this (health) social movement. With the rise of China and India, among other middle-income countries, globally mobile populations, and cosmopolitan environments in many countries, medical pluralism is only likely to increase into the 21st Century, thus requiring sustained attention (and new frameworks) from social scientists. With biomedical health systems struggling to live up to public expectations in many OECD countries, the profile of TCIM practices as health care 'beyond-the-state' and 'out-of-pocket' care seems unlikely to wane (and likely to accelerate). A contracting welfare state, aging population, and focus on patient preference in the current milieu will foster this movement.

While it may appear somewhat obvious to those within social science that the topic of TCIM should be a core focus for health enquiry and scholarship, especially considering the fact that TCIM has historically occupied a 'fringe' and 'outsider' status in terms of the public health care system, such a proposition is not necessarily a given. Fortunately, alongside (and in many ways, in support of) the broadened focus resulting from public health and health services research around TCIM, latter-day scholarship is beginning to accommodate, advance and appreciate the unique contributions the social sciences offer our understanding of contemporary issues relating to TCIM.

References

Adams, J., Tovey, P., Easthope, G. (2017). *Mainstreaming Complementary and Alternative Medicine: Studies in Social Context*. Routledge, London.

Adams, J. (2000). General practitioners, complementary therapies and evidence-based medicine: The defence of clinical autonomy. *Complementary Therapies in Medicine, 8*(4), 248–252.

Allsop, J., Saks, M. (2003). *Regulating the Health Professions.* Sage, London.

Baarts, C., Pedersen, I. K. (2009). Derivative benefits: Exploring the body through complementary and alternative medicine. *Sociology of Health and Illness, 31*(5), 719–733.

Batisai, K. (2016). Towards an integrated approach to health and medicine in Africa. *SAHARA-J: Journal of Social Aspects of HIV/AIDS, 13*(1), 113–122.

Broom, A. (2002). Contested territories: The construction of boundaries between "alternative" and "conventional" cancer treatments. *New Zealand Journal of Sociology, 17*(2), 215–34.

Broom, A. (2005). Using qualitative interviews in CAM research: A guide to study design, data collection and data analysis. *Complementary Therapies in Medicine, 13*(1), 65–73.

Broom, A., Tovey, P. (2007a). Therapeutic pluralism? Evidence, power and legitimacy in UK cancer services. *Sociology of Health and Illness, 29*(3), 551–569.

Broom, A., Tovey, P. (2007b). The dialectical tension between individuation and depersonalisation in cancer patients' mediation of complementary, alternative and biomedical cancer treatments. *Sociology, 41*(6), 1021–1039.

Broom, A., Tovey, P. (2008a). *Therapeutic Pluralism: Exploring the Experiences of Cancer Patients and Professionals.* Routledge, London.

Broom, A., Tovey, P. (2008b). Exploring the temporal dimension in cancer patients' experiences of non-biomedical therapeutics. *Qualitative Health Research, 18*(12), 1650–1661.

Broom, A., Doron, A., Tovey, P. (2009a). The inequalities of medical pluralism: Hierarchies of health, the politics of tradition and the economies of care in Indian oncology. *Social Science and Medicine, 69*(5), 698–706.

Broom, A., Nayar, K., Tovey, P., Shirali, R., Thakur, R., Seth, T., Chhetri, P. (2009b). Indian cancer patients' use of Traditional, Complementary and Alternative Medicine (TCAM) and delays in presentation to Hospital. *Oman Medical Journal, 24*(2), 99–102.

Broom, A., Wijewardena, K., Sibbritt, D., Adams, J., Nayar, K. (2010). The use of traditional, complementary and alternative medicine in Sri Lankan cancer care: Results from a survey of 500 cancer patients. *Public Health, 124*(4), 232–237.

Broom, A., Doron, A. (2013). Traditional medicines, collective negotiation, and representations of risk in Indian cancer care. *Qualitative Health Research*, *23*(1), 54–65.

Broom, A., Chittem, M., Bowden, V., Muppavaram, N., Rajappa, S. (2016). Illness experiences, collective decisions, and the therapeutic encounter in Indian oncology. *Qualitative Health Research, 27*(7), 951–963.

Broom, A., Kenny, K., Bowden, V., Muppavaram, N., Chittem, M. (2018). Cultural ontologies of cancer in India. *Critical Public Health*, *28*(1), 48–58.

Brosnan, C. (2016). Epistemic cultures in complementary medicine: Knowledge-making in university departments of osteopathy and Chinese medicine. *Health Sociology Review*, *25*(2), 171–186.

Cant, S., Sharma, U. (1996). Demarcation and transformation within homoeopathic knowledge. A strategy of professionalization. *Social Science and Medicine*, *42*(4), 579–588.

Cant, S., Sharma, U. (2004). *A New Medical Pluralism: Complementary Medicine, Doctors, Patients and the State*. Routledge, London.

Coulter, I. D., Willis, E. M. (2004). The rise and rise of complementary and alternative medicine: A sociological perspective. *Medical Journal of Australia, 180*(11), 587–589.

Frawley, J., Adams, J., Broom, A., Steel, A., Gallois, C., Sibbritt, D. (2014). Majority of women are influenced by nonprofessional information sources when deciding to consult a complementary and alternative medicine practitioner during pregnancy. *The Journal of Alternative and Complementary Medicine, 20*(7), 571–577.

Fries, C. J. (2008). Governing the health of the hybrid self: Integrative medicine, neoliberalism, and the shifting biopolitics of subjectivity. *Health Sociology Review*, *17*(4), 353–367.

Gale, N. K. (2011). From body-talk to body-stories: Body work in complementary and alternative medicine. *Sociology of Health and Illness*, *33*(2), 237–251.

Hess, D. J. (2004). Medical modernisation, scientific research fields and the epistemic politics of health social movements. *Sociology of Health and Illness*, *26*(6), 695–709.

Hirschkorn, K., Bourgeault, I. (2005). Conceptualising mainstream health care providers' behaviours in relation to complementary and alternative medicine. *Social Science and Medicine*, *61*(1), 157–70.

Hollenberg, D., Muzzin, L. (2010). Epistemological challenges to integrative medicine: An anti-colonial perspective on the combination of complementary/alternative medicine with biomedicine. *Health Sociology Review*, *19*(1), 34–56.

Kelner, M., Wellman, B. (1997). Health care and consumer choice: medical and alternative therapies. *Social Science and Medicine*, *45*(2), 203–212.

Kelner, M., Wellman, B., Boon, H., Welsh, S. (2004). Responses of established healthcare to the professionalization of complementary and alternative medicine in Ontario. *Social Science and Medicine*, *59*(5), 915–930.

Keshet, Y. (2009). The untenable boundaries of biomedical knowledge: Epistemologies and rhetoric strategies in the debate over evaluating complementary and alternative medicine. *Health*, *13*(2), 131–155.

Keshet, Y. (2010). Hybrid knowledge and research on the efficacy of alternative and complementary medicine treatments. *Social Epistemology*, *24*(4), 331–347.

Meurk, C., Broom, A., Adams, J., Sibbritt, D. (2013). Rurality, mobility, identity: Women's use of complementary and alternative medicine in rural Australia. *Health and Place*, *20*, 75–80.

Mizrachi, N., Shuval, J. T., Gross, S. (2005). Boundary at work: Alternative medicine in biomedical settings. *Sociology of Health and Illness*, *27*(1), 20–43.

O'Brien, S., Broom, A. (2014). HIV in (and out of) the clinic: Biomedicine, traditional and spiritual healing in Harare. *SAHARA-J: Journal of the Social Aspects of HIV*, *11*(1), 94–104.

Oyebode, O., Kandala, N., Chilton, P., Lilford, R. (2016). Use of traditional medicine in middle-income countries: A WHO-SAGE study. *Health Policy and Planning*, *31*(8), 984–991.

Prior, L. (2003). Belief, knowledge and expertise: The emergence of the lay expert in medical sociology. *Sociology of Health and Illness*, *25*(3), 41–57.

Sointu, E. (2005). The rise of an ideal: Tracing changing discourses of wellbeing. *The Sociological Review*, *53*(2), 255–274.

Sointu, E. (2006a). Recognition and the creation of well-being. *Sociology*, *40*(3), 493–510.

Sointu, E. (2006b). The search for wellbeing in alternative and complementary health practices. *Sociology of Health and Illness*, *28*(3), 330–349.

Sointu, E. (2011). Detraditionalisation, gender and alternative and complementary medicines. *Sociology of Health and Illness*, *33*(3), 356–371.

Tovey, P., Broom, A., Chatwin, J., Ahmad, S., Hafeez, M. (2005). Use of traditional, complementary and allopathic medicines in Pakistan by cancer patients. *Rural and Remote Health*, *5*(4), 447.

Wahlberg, A. (2006). Bio-politics and the promotion of traditional herbal medicine in Vietnam. *Health*, *10*(2), 123–147.

Williams, S. J., Calnan, M. (eds.), (2013). *Modern Medicine: Lay Perspectives and Experiences*. Routledge, London.

Willis, E. (1989). *Medical Dominance: The Division of Labour in Australian Health Care*. Allen & Unwin, Sydney.

Winnick, T. A. (2005). From quackery to "complementary" medicine: The American medical profession confronts alternative therapies. *Social Problems*, *52*(1), 38–61.

World Health Organization. (2005). National policy on traditional medicine and regulation of herbal medicines: Report of a WHO global survey.

Chapter 3

Health Economic Evaluation of Traditional, Complementary and Integrative Medicine

Islândia Maria Carvalho de Sousa,
Adriana Falangola Benjamin Bezerra and
Camilla Maria Ferreira de Aquino

Introduction

Throughout the world, the advancement of health technologies has increased the cost of health care systems and compromised their sustainability (Birch *et al.*, 2015). There is therefore a demand for studies that examine the effectiveness and cost of treatments in health care systems. However, most of the methods employed in economic evaluation are built upon closed mathematical models and their use for evaluating more complex health practices such as TCIM is challenging. This chapter explores the importance of using economic evaluation in traditional, complementary and integrative medicine (TCIM) research as well as the limitations and potential regarding the application of economic evaluation models in this area.

Why is it Important to Undertake Economic Evaluation Research in TCIM?

Growing health sector spending is a concern in many countries, especially in those cases where health services are public. However, as the needs and demands of patients grow exponentially, resources become proportionately scarcer (Gurgel Jr *et al.*, 2017). In view of this, techniques for rationalization of expenditure, such as health economic evaluation, may be employed in an attempt to meet health needs, without disregarding the financial viability of public health care systems. Health care systems are thus forced to re-examine the costs and benefits of their actions in order to ensure effective implementation of interventions and efficient allocation of resources (Brasil, 2009; Thomas and Chalkidou, 2016).

Recently, there has been a tendency for health professionals and managers to use economic evaluation such as cost-effectiveness (CEA) and cost-utility (CUA) (Ford *et al.*, 2010; Clement *et al.*, 2009). Economic evaluations (CEA and CUA) do not assign a monetary value to outcomes of health interventions. The outcomes are measured in terms of the most appropriate outcome units. These measurement units may include the number of diseases and complications prevented, the number of hospitalizations prevented, the number of cases of a disease detected, and/or the number of lives or life years saved (Brasil, 2009).

Across the various types of economic evaluation available, the main differences concern: (1) the types of outcome considered, (2) the implications of the various evaluation techniques employed and (3) the scope of the analysis. The resources used are always measured in monetary units, but the ways of measuring outcomes differ, according to four types of analysis: cost–benefit, cost-minimization, cost-effectiveness and cost-utility. A fifth form of measurement is currently also gaining attention: cost and consequences analysis (Brouselle *et al.*, 2011) (Table 1). The decision as to which form of analysis to employ will depend on the purpose and the availability of data and other resources.

In short, economic evaluations compare interventions or technologies in terms of both costs and outcomes. They are thus based on opportunity cost — an application of resources in certain programs and technologies may entail not providing resources for other programs and technologies

Table 1. Classification of economic evaluations.

Type of Analysis	Type of Outcome	Evaluation Technique
Cost-Effectiveness Analysis (CEA)	Life-years saved, patient-years free of symptoms, complications prevented	Final measurement unit is the Incremental cost-effectiveness ratio (ICER) The ICER assesses the cost per unit of achieving the outcome by different means
Cost-Utility Analysis (CUA)	Utility or general well-being; can be converted into quality adjusted life years (QALYs) or disability adjusted life-years (DALYs)	This is a sophisticated form of CEA (which also has an ICER), in which outcomes are measured in terms of impact on both the quantity and the quality of life
Cost-Minimization Analysis (CMA)	None. The outcome is assumed to be the same for each intervention and not separately assessed	Explores the cost of achieving the same outcome by different means
Cost-Benefit Analysis (CBA)	Infer monetary values for CEA or CUA outcomes	Employs the same evaluation method as CEA or CUA
Cost-Consequence Analysis (CCA)	Uses CEA and/or CUA outcomes	Examination of the cost of each intervention and comparison of the differences between each of the relevant outcome measures

Sources: Adapted from Hulme and Long (2005), Brasil (2009), Brouselle *et al.* (2011).

(Thomas and Chalkidou, 2016). The actual cost of an activity does not therefore correspond to resources spent alone but also to the value of all other activities no longer provided (Howard-Wilsher *et al.*, 2016).

In the case of TCIM, assimilation into a public health system is justified by its specific characteristics. TCIM practices are based on a concept of the whole person, are less invasive, promote self-care and harness the body's natural ability to heal itself (Sousa and Vieira, 2005) and, furthermore, expend fewer resources (Yu Su *et al.*, 2015). They also require a lower level of technological resources (i.e. low use of equipment by professionals during care) (Sousa and Vieira, 2005). In the case of Brazil, TCIM services are less likely to require referral of patients for specialized services, diagnosis or tertiary treatment. When offered by a public health system, TCIM thus combines the possibility of more extensive care (conventional biomedical practices and TCIM) with sustainable cost (Neto *et al.*, 2016).

Reflections on the cost-effectiveness of health systems is of fundamental importance for achieving a full commitment to optimization of the quality of life of all citizens. Disputes regarding how best to allocate scarce resources — both with regard to conventional medical care and TCIM services and treatments — necessitate investigation of cost-effectiveness (Solomon *et al.*, 2013), in a manner that takes into consideration all health-seeking behaviour and practices, including both conventional medical care and TCIM services and treatments.

What are the Possibilities of Applying Economic Evaluation Models in TCIM?

The field of TCIM is extremely varied and contains a wide range of modalities, practices and healing rationalities (Adams *et al.*, 2012). It thus generates a diversity of possible outcome measurements. Nevertheless, one feature common to many TCIM is the promotion of vitalism (Coulter, 2003) and the espousal of an approach involving personalized care adapted to the individual and his or her needs (Ford *et al.*, 2010). Consequently, many TCIM treatment approaches rarely follow pre-established clinical protocols — a situation that constitutes a challenge to the application of economic evaluation (Hulme and Long, 2005).

In fact, the prevailing paradigm within health economics (and cost calculation) is a positivist one appropriate for a clinical evaluation, as performed in conventional medicine (Ford *et al.*, 2010). Randomized, observational studies and even some case and control studies investigate the effectiveness of an intervention in a controlled environment (Cohen *et al.*, 2015). The aim is to identify the true and single effect of the object of study on the health of individuals and thereafter employ this technology in different environments and at different times. Patterns and associations are thus sought out as a way of enabling a generalization of the results. When establishing health care protocols with a fixed order of actions and resources — exams, medications and procedures — that should be followed, there is therefore a generalization of individuals' needs with regard to a given health problem.

However, generalization is a major challenge in TCIM, where every patient is viewed as unique. Furthermore, TCIM often comprises a combination of modes of care derived from different health models (Ayurveda, Traditional Chinese Medicine, homeopathy) and consequently, involves different possible interventions and therapeutic effects which may be difficult to quantify and can occur over a long time period (Ford *et al.*, 2010). The plurality of TCIM in terms of the manner of care poses a challenge, not only for cost calculations but also for subsequent CEA/CUA outcome analysis.

When conducting economic evaluations in TCIM, researchers insist on using methods that have been shown to be limited in evaluating the effects of a holistic approach. But when TCIM is subject to the same standard assessments developed for biomedical practices, which search for outcomes not intended by the TCIM practice under evaluation, the method cannot be considered appropriate (Ostermann *et al.*, 2011; Kim *et al.*, 2016). This explains the limited or inconclusive effectiveness found by studies that have employed biomedicine-based designs, such as randomized trials and case-control designs (Herman *et al.*, 2014).

A recent systematic review of international studies of health economic assessment has shown TCIM to be potentially cost-effective or cost saving (Yu Su *et al.*, 2015, Howard-Wilsher *et al.*, 2015). However, such findings are somewhat controversial. Some comparisons undertaken have shown cost-effective health improvements for TCIM in relation to usual treatment, but a previous systematic review indicated that some TCIM interventions may increase costs without providing further health benefits (Howard-Wilsher *et al.*, 2015).

Another design feature of commonly performed economic evaluation of TCIM in the international literature is the evaluation of a specific TCIM, for example, acupuncture, homeopathy or tai chi, since it is often relatively convenient and straightforward to follow the users of such discrete practices in some health services (Ford *et al.*, 2012). This approach assumes that a patient receives only one TCIM in isolation at a given time (when we know this is in many circumstances not the case, especially in the case of integrative TCIM care (Adams *et al.*, 2013)). It is often a challenge to clearly establish which outcomes may be associated with which TCIM or conventional medical practice/intervention when TCIM is in nearly all cases practiced and used alongside or concurrent to other TCIM or conventional medical practices (Reid *et al.*, 2016; Sibbritt and Adams, 2010). This is a situation that is common across specialist care services and primary health care services, the latter being the predominant setting for TCIM integration in Brazil.

Towards a CAE of TCIM in Brazil: A Contemporary Case Study

With a view to developing research designs and methodology that are able to adjust TCIM cost-effective studies to planning and health management processes and thereby contribute to the evidence-base, a group of multi-disciplinary researchers — constituting the Health Policy Economics Research Group (GPEPS) at the Federal University of Pernambuco (UFPE) and the Health Knowledge and Practices Research Group (GPS) at the Oswaldo Cruz Foundation (Fiocruz) — carried out a number of studies of health services specializing in TCIM. These studies enabled the researchers to begin to design and refine a number of early steps needed for the application and use of economic evaluation with regard to TCIM.

A multicenter study (Bezerra *et al.*, 2016) was conducted in two public health services specializing in TCIM in two State capitals in the Northeast of Brazil (Assunção, 2016; Neto *et al.*, 2016). One was chosen on account of it being a pioneer of Brazilian TCIM Policy and the second due to its considerable reach and breadth of service as well as physical infrastructure. Both of these public health services are funded by local government and specialized in TCIM, but do not offer conventional medical services. The study aimed to access the cost-effectiveness of TCIM services in general and their cost-effectiveness in the care of common psychosomatic disorders, referred to as "diffuse suffering" by Valla (2002).

Information regarding the resources needed and their cost were collected by way of face-to-face interviews with the administrators and practitioners who work with providing TCIM health services. Information about the effectiveness of the care was collected through interviews with the professionals and investigation of the patients' records. The study was approved by the Brazilian Ethics Committee (CAAE: 07270212.4.0000.5208). The professionals at the service either had training in conventional medicine (as nurses, doctors, physiotherapists, psychologists, pharmacists) and specialized in TCIM or were trained primarily as TCIM therapists.

Two hundred and one patients with diffuse suffering were identified at the two health services, most of them female and young adults. The most common complaints were anxiety, insomnia and pain. In only one of the services did the professionals register the patients' follow-up in the charts, thereby enabling analysis of the results. The reports indicate improved health outcomes. The most frequent forms of TCIM used for individuals with diffuse suffering were acupuncture, Bach florals and homeopathy.

A mathematical model specific to prospective analysis of TCIM was first developed. As the target population were patients identified with diffuse suffering (a chronic disease) a cyclical model was selected as being the most appropriate and a Markov model was employed (Kryscio, 2013). However, it soon became clear that to create a hypothetical model would necessitate constructing an average patient profile (a step in the Markov model) and designing a single model progression. From the position of a modality based on both integral care and the uniqueness of the patient, like TCIM, such an approach is highly challenging, even inconceivable. Each patient is unique even if he or she has the same disease and a standard progression of care cannot therefore exist.

Furthermore, in a Markov model, the described disease states are mutually exclusive, with an individual unable to be in more than one state of illness at any one time. This constitutes a limitation when illness is considered a complex and multifactorial problem, as it is by much of TCIM (Sato, 2010). This outcome analysis method was therefore discarded, although the objective remained the same. Cost analysis was conducted (absorption costing) and the effectiveness analysis considered data from the medical registry, containing the description of symptoms and treatment evolution.

Brouselle *et al.* (2011) do not propose an aggregate indicator (cost-effectiveness ratio) for the cost and measurement of effectiveness/consequence of the intervention analyzed. Instead, the relationship between costs and consequences, are to be interpreted by the decision-maker based on the information presented.

Two effectiveness analyses were employed to interpret the results of specialized TCIM services in our study. A number of selected outcomes related to the patient, such as: the number of TCIMs employed by patients; the number of TCIM consults undertaken until a sensation of well-being or healing had been achieved; and the total number of TCIM consults prior to the patient being discharged from care. Other outcomes were possible measures of the effectiveness of TCIM in treating diffuse suffering (the number of times the individual left home, decreased medication use, reported improvements in self-perceived health, adherence and follow-up over time). The TCIM therapies available, the types of TCIM offered, the total number of patients who attended and the total number of activities (group practices or individual consults) were also considered. It was, however, necessary to change the scope of the study from TCIM care to TCIM service, owing to difficulties regarding the records of patients being accompanied by the study. The information registry did not make it possible to measure all the possible effectiveness results that had been planned (Assunção, 2016; Neto *et al.*, 2016).

Towards a Cost-Effectiveness Analysis (CEA) of TCIM: Outlining Steps and Safeguards

Drawing upon our recent empirical studies (Bezerra, 2016; Assunção, 2016; Neto *et al.*, 2016) we here outline a number of steps and safeguards that should be considered by those seeking to undertake and advance CEA in TCIM. Economic assessment compares competing technologies or

Table 2.   Health economic analysis perspectives and related costs input.

Adopted Perspective	Related Costs Input	Costs Examples
Individual, Patient or Client	Costs incurred by patients and/or their families	Travel expenses; drugs; professional caretakers; lost days of work and lost income
Institutional or Service Provider or Third-Party Payer	Costs related to patient care and service maintenance sustained by health institutions, employer, government or insurance	Health professionals' fees; drugs; hospitalizations (health materials and equipment, building and equipment maintenance, electricity and water bills)
Society	Costs considered from both an individual and institutional viewpoint, but also from that of other parties not directly related to the health condition	Costs for other government sectors; losses related to unproductive time away from work

Sources: Adapted from Hulme (2005); Ford *et al.* (2010); Drummond *et al.* (2015).

interventions as a way of providing support for decision-making. The decision as to which costs will be considered and measured is directly related to the viewpoint — or perspective — to which the economic evaluation is related or focused (Table 2). The choice of a particular perspective depends on the purpose of the study and the individual performing the evaluation. Societal and third-party payer perspectives are commonly employed, while the least used perspective is that of the patient, as an individual (Drummond *et al.*, 2015).

The result of CEA comparisons is calculated as an Incremental Cost-Effectiveness Ratio (ICER), which aims to determine the quantity of financial resources required to attain one unit-measure of the selected outcome, considering the new/competing case (B) and the baseline/control option (A) (Figure 1).

$$ICER = \frac{Cost\ B - Cost\ A}{Outcome\ B - Outcome\ A}$$

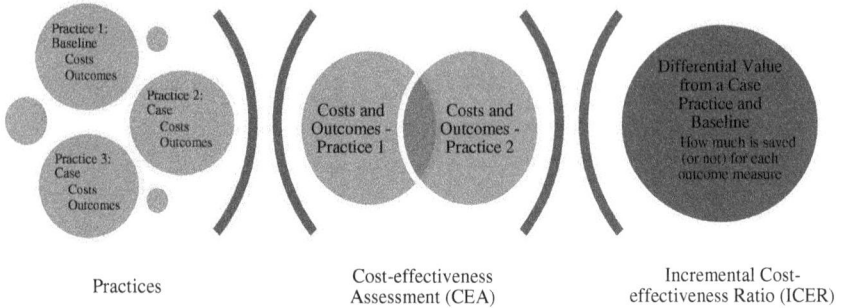

Figure 1.   Cost-effectiveness assessment steps, for various practices/activities selected for analysis, with variables (costs and outcomes) and the ratio resulting from a comparison of practices.

Table 3.   Examples of cost categories identified in economic evaluations.

Human Resources	Materials	Equipment	Infrastructure
Administrative staff; medical staff; other health professionals (nurses, psychologists, nutritionists and so forth); TCIM therapists, etc.	Needles; drugs; surgical gloves, etc.	Stethoscopes; X-ray machines; tables, etc.	Rent of premises; electricity; water and so forth

Although the costing analysis and effectiveness measurements/analysis occur concurrently, for the sake of simplicity, let us assume that the evaluative process starts with the costing process. Regardless of the object of study — albeit a technology, program, intervention, health care service or health policy — the resources used (human resources, equipment or infrastructure) are quantified and monetarily valued and then assigned to the following categories: costs related to human resources; costs related to inputs/equipment; and costs related to infrastructure/maintenance (Table 3).

There are different methods of costing (i.e. organizing and ordering the distribution of costs) and, as stated above, the perspective and purpose of the study determines the costs to be included.

There is a need to clearly establish which specific activity relates to which costs, or even, which parts of a single cost. Despite the apparent

Direct Cost	**Indirect Cost**
•Resources are directly consumed in order to output production. •e.g: drugs, and medical staff.	•Resources are used for providing support services, allowing other departments to continue production. •e.g: admnistration staff, and laboratory.

Types of Costs

Fixed Cost	**Variable Cost**
•Quantity of resources remain constant, despite number of output produced, at least in the short run. •e.g: x-ray machine, and stethoscope.	•Volume of resources varies with each product. •e.g: needle, and latex gloves.

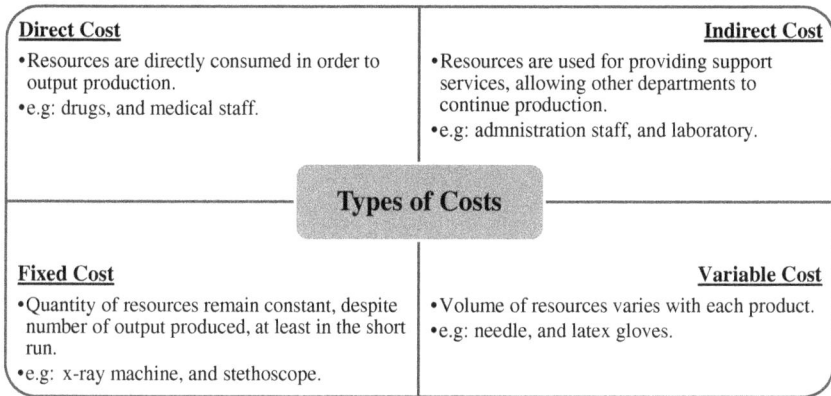

Figure 2.   Costs classification considering purpose and variability of resources used.

Sources: Adapted from Pavignani *et al.* (2009); Drummond *et al.* (2015).

simplicity of this calculation, the greater the diversity of resources used, the greater the complexity involved in defining the real cost. This is the case with the evaluation of health interventions and health policies.

The costing method used must thus be appropriate to the activity or service provided, in accordance with the complexity of its organization and the objective of the analysis. In general, there are two common methods: absorption costing and Activity Based Costing (ABC). The first is the most recommended for cost accounting with regard to complex health services, such as those operating and accommodated across a hospital setting, while ABC is best suited to aiding determination of the costs of a particular activity or intervention (Table 2). Absorption costing is widely used to put a value on the cost of products or services delivered in health care. All costs are absorbed and there is no distinction between fixed and variable costs (Mogyorosy and Smith, 2005).

In the case of both costing methods, costs must be classified as direct or indirect cost, and as fixed or variable cost (Figure 2). Considering costs are the value of resources used to produce something, also known as an output. In health care systems or services, the intended production is health related. Therefore, the expected output would be consults and/or procedures (Pavignani *et al.*, 2009).

As for outcomes measurement, the starting point for the analysis is to select the health condition and intervention or technology. It is then

Costing Analysis	Effectiveness Analysis
Select the practice/activity/service and identify the steps/process of selected activity	Identify which outcomes measurement the selected practice used for diagnosis and to establish treatment, and the expected outcomes
List resources used, be they human resources, equipment or structure/maintenance. Quantify and calculate a value for resources listed	Establish what shall be considered the effectiveness measure, in view of the expected outcomes. There can be more than one outcome for each TCIM and different outcomes for different TCIM
Select a costing method: activity based-costing or absorption costing	Select a method for accompanying the TCIM therapist and individual during treatment. The method can be either retrospective or prospective
Classify the resources needed as variable or fixed costs, and as direct or indirect costs	Design an instrument to keep track of measurements
Reorganize listed resources as established by the chosen costing method	Depending on the treatment period, assign a proportionate value to the outcomes measurement

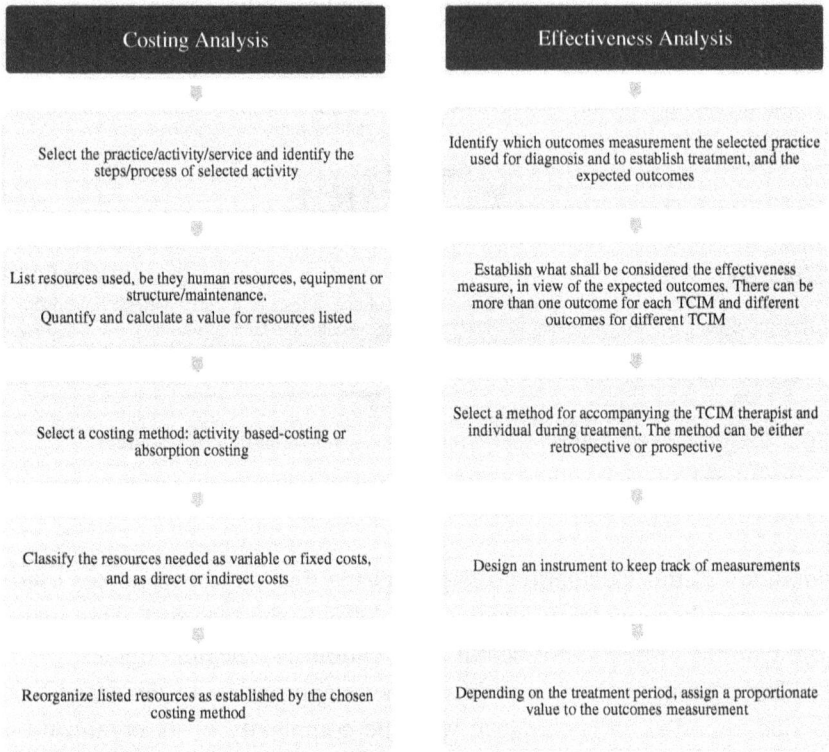

Figure 3. Costing and effectiveness analysis occur concomitantly, following these simplified steps.

necessary to identify the treatment and resources required for its successful implementation. Some health conditions in conventional medicine involve a well-known chain of events and it is possible to identify which variables influence the occurrence or resolution of the disease. Based on this information, health services establish service protocols, reducing the uncertainty surrounding the procedures and resources to be used during care. In the case of TCIM, care protocols need be more flexible, allowing observation of clinical as well as subjective and social outcomes (social interaction, empowerment), since these types of outcomes are measures of the effects of TCIM.

Figure 3 outlines the general steps in conducting a cost-effectiveness analysis.

In short, it was possible to design a number of preliminary general questions for the development of studies in the field of economic assessment of TCIM. First, what type and context of health system is involved? Public or private? Is TCIM part of a specialized service of TCIM or is it provided within a conventional medical service? The context in which TCIM is being used should always be examined with such questions helping to define the perspectives, costs and results of the economic evaluation.

The second question concerns how the TCIM is provided? When one TCIM is performed as part of a specialized service, it is often associated with another or occurs alongside, and in conjunction with, conventional medicine provision (Adams *et al.*, 2013). Users of a TCIM service are consulted in an integrated fashion, and they can therefore be guided in the direction of group activities (such as yoga, meditation and tai chi) as well as receiving specific individual care. Likewise, those who begin with a bodily practice may be encouraged to add an individual practice.

The third question is 'What is the health problem?'. In conventional medicine, it is possible to characterize a specific diagnosis (usually from a medical perspective) and an intervention (pharmaceutical products or surgery). These variables are simpler to evaluate mathematically for conventional medicine compared to TCIM. As part of TCIM and its shared vitalist paradigm (Coulter, 2003), diagnosis takes into account the uniqueness of each individual, the context within which that individual is located and the signs and symptoms by which the vitality of an individual is measured beyond the physical-chemical evidence. For example, from the perspective of Chi circulation in Chinese medicine, the needs of an individual will be identified by the evaluation of the pulse, the tongue and other parts of the body (Luo *et al.*, 2015). Any intervention will be based on this information and will involve not only drug treatment but also interventions specific to this TCIM, such as acupuncture.

The fourth question concerns the ways in which outcomes can be measured. When a patient opts for TCIM, this is usually due to a health problem for which biomedicine has failed to address sufficiently (Hulme and Long, 2005; Sousa and Vieira, 2005). The effectiveness of TCIM should thus include physical-chemical results, but should not be limited to them. The evaluation must also incorporate TCIM-sensitive and specific outcomes measures — such as patient narrative, measurements of happiness/satisfaction and perceived quality of life — which are self-reported and require a different skill-set from that required for health care evaluations.

Finally, therefore, we need to know the kind of knowledge that the problem and the possibilities for measuring outcomes follow in ascertaining the costs. The absorption cost is perhaps the most adequate for this task and can be used both for an integrated service (providing TCIM and conventional medicine) and for a specialized TCIM service.

Conclusion

Based on our recent project experience, the use of mathematical models for economic evaluation in TCIM should be considered with caution and if a standard of care is needed, it will probably be a statistical standard, measured in terms of procedures, activities and resources used for care.

In view of this, the development of cost-effectiveness studies for TCIM still poses a significant theoretical and methodological challenge. There is a need for broader and more in-depth cost-effectiveness studies and research to develop a way of including measures of effectiveness beyond biomedical measurements. Indeed, empirical studies have shown that it is possible to develop cost-effectiveness studies that take into account the specific features of TCIM. Yet, there is also a need to provide training and encouragement for TCIM health professionals and therapists to maintain adequate record of the data needed to monitor the effectiveness of care. Despite the challenges of developing and employing cost-effectiveness analysis to TCIM this is certainly an area that requires further attention and should be considered a core focus for public health and health services research. In many cases, policymakers and other stakeholders invested in health and health care are persuaded by economic, cost-saving evidence alongside evidence of efficacy — it is imperative that TCIM research and researchers work towards providing such evidence where available.

References

Adams, J., Andrews, G., Barnes, J., Broom, A., Magin, P. (eds.), (2012). *Traditional, Complementary and Integrative Medicine: An International Reader*. Palgrave MacMillan, Basingstoke.

Adams, J., Magin, P., Broom, A. (2013). *Primary Health Care and Complementary and Integrative Medicine: Practice and Research*. 10.1142/P875.

Assunção, M. C. T. (2016). Análise de custos de um serviço de práticas integrativas e complementares no município de João Pessoa — PB. Dissertação de Mestrado em Economia da Saúde UFPE-2016. https://repositorio.ufpe.br/handle/123456789/18755.

Bezerra, A. F. B., *et al.* (2016). Relatório de Pesquisa Centro Nacional de Pesquisa- Custo-efetividade das práticas integrativas e complementares na rede de atenção psicossocial: Um estudo multicêntrico. http://cnpq.br/relatorios-de-pesquisa?

Birch, S., Murphy, G. T., MacKenzie, A., Cumming, J. (2015). In place of fear: Aligning health care planning with system objectives to achieve financial sustainability. *Journal of Health Services Research & Policy*, *20*(2), 109–114.

Brasil. Ministério da Saúde (2009). Secretaria de Ciência, Tecnologia e Insumos Estratégicos. Departamento de Ciência e Tecnologia. *Diretrizes Metodológicas: estudos de avaliação econômica de tecnologias em saúde. Brasília*: Ministério da Saúde. http://bvsms.saude.gov.br/bvs/publicacoes/diretrizes_metodologicas_diretriz_avaliacao_economica.pdf.

Brouselle, A., Champagne, F., Contandriopoulos, A. P., Hartz, Z. (org) (2011). *Avaliação: Conceitos e Métodos*. Editora Fiocruz, Rio de Janeiro.

Clement, F. M., Harris, A., Li, J. J., Yong, K., Lee, K. M., Manns, B. J. (2009). Using effectiveness and cost-effectiveness to make drug coverage decisions: A comparison of Britain, Australia, and Canada. *JAMA*, 302, 1437–1443.

Cohen, A. T., Goto, S., Schreiber, K., Torp-Pedersen, C. (2015). Why do we need observational studies of everyday patients in the real-life setting? *European Heart Journal Supplement*s, 17, (Suppl_D), D2–D8. https://doi.org/10.1093/curheartj/suv035.

Coulter, I. (2003). Integration and paradigm clash. In: Tovey, P., Easthope, G. and Adams, J. (eds.). *The Mainstreaming of Complementary and Alternative Medicine: Studies in Social Context*. Routledge, London and New York.

Drummond, M. F., Sculpher, M. J., Claxton, K. Stoddart, G. L., Torrance, G. W. (2015). *Methods for the Economic Evaluation of Health Care Programmes*. 4th Edition, Oxford: Oxford University Press.

Ford, E., Adams, J., Graves, N. (2012). Development of an economic model to assess the cost-effectiveness of hawthorn extract as an adjunct treatment for heart failure in Australia. *BMJ Open*, *2*(5), e001094.

Ford, E., Solomon, D., Adams, J., Graves, N. (2010). The use of economic evaluation in CAM: An introductory framework. *BMC Complementary and Alternative Medicine*, *10*(1), 66.

Gurgel, Jr., Sousa, G. D., Jr., I. M. C., Oliveira, S. R. A., De Assis, F. S., Direrichsen, F. (2017). The National Health Services of Brazil and Northern Europe: Universality, equity, and integrality-time has come for the latter. *International Journal of Health Services*, 47, 002073141773254, 2017.

Herman, P. M., *et al.* (2014). IMPACT — Integrative Medicine PrimAry Care Trial: Protocol for a comparative effectiveness study of the clinical and cost outcomes of an integrative primary care clinic model. *BMC Complementary and Alternative Medicine*, *14*(132), 1–12.

Howard-Wilsher, S., *et al.* (2016). Systematic overview of economic evaluations of health-related rehabilitation. *Disability and Health Journal*, *9*(1), 11–25.

Hulme, C., Long, A. F. (2005). Square pegs and round holes? A review of economic evaluation in complementary and alternative medicine. *Journal of Alternative & Complementary Medicine*, *11*(1), 179–188.

Kim, C.-G., Mun, S.-J., Kim, K.-N., *et al.* (2016). Economic evaluation of manual therapy for musculoskeletal diseases: A protocol for a systematic review and narrative synthesis of evidence. *BMJ Open*, 6, e010556.

Kryscio, R.J., Abner, E. L. (2013). Are Markov and semi-Markov models flexible enough for cognitive panel data? *Journal of Biometrics & Biostatistics*, *4*(1), 10.4172/2155–6180.1000e122.

Luo, J., Xu, H., Liu, B. (2015). Real world research: A complementary method to establish the effectiveness of acupuncture. *BMC Complementary and Alternative Medicine*, *15*(1), 153.

Mogyorosy, Z., Smith, P. (2005). The main methodological issues in costing health care services: A literature review. Centre for Health Economics, Alcuin College, Universidad of York, York, UK. https://www.york.ac.uk/media/che/documents/papers/researchpapers/rp7_Methodological_issues_in_costing_health_care_services.pdf.

Neto, M., Bezerra, A. F. B., Aquino, C. M. F., Sousa, I. M. C., Assunção, M. C. (2016). Avaliação dos custos da unidade de cuidados integrais à saúde Prof. Guilherme Abath. In: Moacyr Rego; Maira Pitta; Tatiane Menezes. (Org.). *Ensaios em Economia da Saúde*, 1st Edition, Livro Rápido, Olinda, pp. 246–264.

Ostermann, T., *et al.* (2011). Health economic evaluation in complementary medicine Development within the last decades concerning local origin and quality. *Complementary Therapies in Medicine, 19*, 289–302.

Pavignani, E., Colombo, S. World Health Organization. (2009). Analysing disrupted health sectors: A modular manual. WHO Press, Geneva.

Reid, R., Steel, A., Wardle, J., Trubody, A., Adams, J. (2016). Complementary medicine use by the Australian population: A critical mixed studies systematic review of utilisation, perceptions and factors associated with use. *BMC Complementary and Alternative Medicine, 16*(1), 176.

Sato, R. C., Zouain, D. M. (2010). Modelos de Markov aplicados a saúde Markov Models in health care. *Einstein, 8*, 376–379.

Sibbritt, D. W., Adams, J. (2010). Back pain amongst 8,910 young Australian women: A longitudinal analysis of the use of conventional providers, complementary and alternative medicine (CAM) practitioners and self-prescribed CAM. *Clinical Rheumatology, 29*(1), 25.

Solomon, D., Adams, J., Graves, N. (2013). Economic evaluation of St. John's wort (*Hypericum perforatum*) for the treatment of mild to moderate depression. *Journal of Affective Disorders, 148*(2), 228–234.

Sousa, I. M. C., Vieira, A. L. S. (2005). Serviços Públicos de saúde e medicina alternativa. *Ciênc. Saúde Coletiva, 10*(Suppl), 255–266.

Thomas, R., Chalkidou, K. (2016). Cost-effectiveness analysis. In Cylus, J., Papanicolas, I., Smith, P.C., (eds.), Health system efficiency: How to make measurement matter for policy and management [Internet]. Copenhagen (Denmark): European Observatory on Health Systems and Policies (Health Policy Series, No. 46.) 6. https://www.ncbi.nlm.nih.gov/books/NBK436886/.

Valla, V. V. (2002). Pobreza, emoção e saúde: uma discussão sobre pentecostalismo e saúde no Brasil. *Revista Brasileira de Educação,* N 19, 63–170. http://www.scielo.br/pdf/rbedu/n19/n19a05.pdf.

Yu Su, S., Muo, C. H., Morisky, D. (2015). Use of Chinese medicine correlates negatively with the consumption of conventional medicine and medical cost in patients with uterine fibroids: A population-based retrospective cohort study in Taiwan. *BMC Complementary and Alternative Medicine, 15*(129), 1–8.

Chapter 4

Traditional, Complementary and Integrative Medicine: Policy, Legal and Regulatory Perspectives*

Jon Wardle, Daniel Gallego-Perez, Vincent Chung and Jon Adams

Introduction

Health policy development is tightly interwoven with the cultural, political and societal climate. In a field such as TCIM, this is further complicated by the professional, political and ideological tensions that often exist between TCIM and conventional medicine. The expansive definition of TCIM also means that extraordinary heterogeneity, variability and inconsistency is often the norm, rather than the exception, for TCIM. Despite these challenges, utilization of TCIM globally is significant and growing (WHO, 2013). Evaluation of policy options requires careful consideration on the cultural, political and social contexts.

The origin of TCIM policy development — at least at a global level as many nations had individual provisions previously — can be traced

---

Note: In this chapter where the original laws are not in English, the quoted phrases are translations by the authors.

back to the Alma Ata Declaration, which arose from the World Health
Organization (WHO) International Conference on Primary Health Care.
This declaration highlighted that '*people have the right and duty to
participate individually and collectively in the planning and implementation of their care, which includes access to traditional medicine*'
(Section VII, Point 7) (WHO, 1978). WHO increasingly recognized the
significant role of TCIM in primary health care, and continued to reaf-
firm its support for TCIM policy development. The *WHO Traditional
Medicine Strategy 2002–2005* specified the anticipated outcomes of
increasing governmental support for TCAM among member states, promoting integration of TCAM into member states' national health care
systems, and increased recording and preservation of indigenous knowledge of TCIM. WHO initiatives under the WHO Traditional Medicine
Strategy have been successful in encouraging countries to develop policies around TCIM. However, not all progress indicators have been taken
up with equal enthusiasm. For example, although 119 member states
have developed regulation for herbal medicines, only 69 have developed
formal national TCIM policies (see Figure 1) — though this may
also reflect the fact that it is often much easier to develop a specific

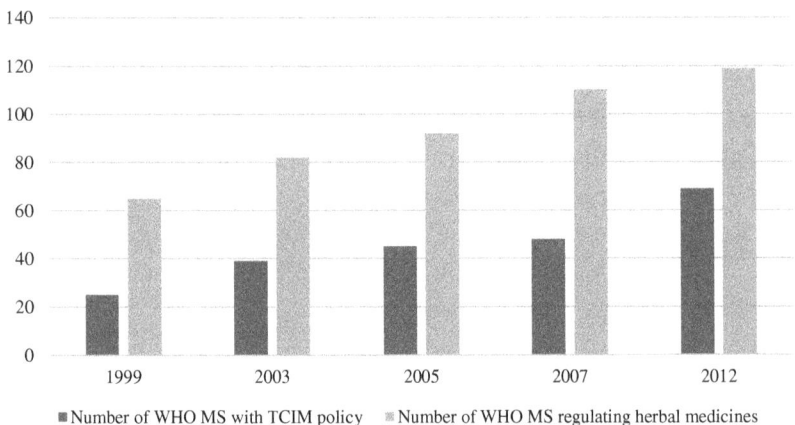

Figure 1.   Monitoring changes in country progress indicators defined by the WHO
Traditional Medicine Strategy (WHO, 2013). WHO — World Health Organization.
MS — Member states.

regulation, such as for herbal medicines, than to develop and implement a national policy.

In addition to the strategic direction offered by the WHO Traditional Medicine Strategy, regional WHO offices are often responsible for implementation of this Strategy at regional or country level. For example, the Pan-American Health Organization (or WHO Regional Office for the Americas — PAHO/AMRO) has led a number of regional and country-level initiatives for the promotion of TCIM. These have included: the 1993 Resolution CD37.R5 (*Salud de los Pueblos Indígenas*), which urges member states to promote changes in health systems and to develop alternative models of health for indigenous populations and research networks; the creation of conceptual frameworks for creating intercultural health care models (PAHO, 2002); the development of regional strategies for promotion of the integration of TCIM into national health systems (PAHO, 2003). More recently, PAHO/AMRO has reinitiated its focus on developing a regional action plan for TCIM and strengthening its technical cooperation, launching the effort in Managua, Nicaragua in 2017 (Weeks, 2017). Another example is the *Regional Strategy for Traditional Medicine in the Western Pacific 2011–2020* promulgated by the WHO Western Pacific Regional Office (WPRO), which aims to promote safe and effective use of TCIM, as well as their inclusion among member states' national health systems (WPRO, 2012) [http://www.wpro.who.int/publications/2012/regionalstrategyfortraditionalmedicine_ 2012 .pdf].

While most countries have made significant progress in implementing the WHO Traditional Medicine Strategy, some continue to experience challenges. The *WHO Traditional Medicine Strategy 2014–2023* identified the following areas as continuing to be challenging: the development and enforcement of TCIM policy and regulations; integration, in particular identifying and evaluating strategies and criteria for integrating TCIM into national and primary health care; safety and quality, notably assessment of products and services, qualification of practitioners, methodology and criteria for evaluating efficacy; an ability to control and regulate TCIM advertising and claims; TCIM research and development; education and training of TCIM practitioners; information and communication, such as sharing information about policies, regulations, service profiles and research data, or obtaining reliable objective information resources for consumers.

To properly address these challenges, the updated WHO Traditional Medicine Strategy recommends the following focus areas: (i) building the knowledge base that will allow TCIM to be managed actively through appropriate national policies that understand and recognize the role and potential of TCIM; (ii) strengthening the quality assurance, safety, proper use and effectiveness of T&CM by regulating products, practices and practitioners through T&CM education and training, skills development, services and therapies and (iii) promoting universal health coverage by integrating T&CM services into health service delivery and self-health care.

Interculturality and Traditional Medicine

The development of the concept of 'interculturality' has brought — as a result of the struggle for recognition of several indigenous groups — an increasing awareness of the need to preserve and promote the knowledge, heritage and practices of indigenous communities and social groups, and has had a great influence on policy development at the national level in many countries. These concepts have become codified by the development of the United Nations Education, Scientific and Cultural Organization (UNESCO) *Convention on the Protection and Promotion of the Diversity of Cultural Expressions*, which extends to health, and recognizes the importance of traditional knowledge as a source of intangible and material wealth, and in particular the knowledge systems of indigenous peoples. The World Intellectual Property, the World Trade Organization and WHO have developed a joint publication discussing intellectual property protection for traditional knowledge, of which TCIM is an integral part. One issue of interculturality in TCIM policy development that is rarely discussed, though is starting to receive attention, is that even when the importance of interculturality is recognized, most modern political and legislative structures are Western in nature. As such, care needs to be taken to ensure TCIM policy development, legislation and regulation do not result in cultural misappropriation or the abuse of indigenous medical intellectual property (Ijaz and Boon, 2018).

While many countries have been eager to recognize and integrate indigenous traditional medicines (TM) around an interculturality framework, most countries have shown more hesitation in implementing policy, legislative and regulatory initiatives around complementary medicine (CM). However, even though TM is relatively well defined within national policy contexts (i.e. the medicine indigenous to a specific culture), its definition becomes problematic at a global level. CM is often simply an indigenous medicine from another country, and TM may become a CM when transported outside its country of origin. The growth of acupuncture and traditional Chinese medicine (TCM) outside of China is the most prominent example of this. Currently, China is promoting the globalization of TCM via the geo-political influence of its Belt and Road's Initiative. Possible insights to how the future of TM globalization will progress may come from an evaluation of the development of TCM among Silk Road countries (Tang *et al.*, 2017). Indian medical systems such as Ayurveda are also increasingly popular outside of India, yet their status as non-indigenous CM means they are not officially sanctioned outside of that country. This also means that well-established TM in some countries may be virtually unknown outside those settings. Integration of Māori Traditional Medicine (Rongoā Māori) is encouraged in the New Zealand health system, for example, but is virtually unknown outside of that country (Ahuriri-Driscoll *et al.*, 2008).

Barriers to TCIM Policy Development and Implementation

The major barriers to TCIM policy development and implementation are structural and political. Structural issues include problems defining TCIM in a way appropriate for inclusion in policy and the lack of regulatory prerequisites for policy development. CM's definition is predominantly based on exclusion (from conventional medicine) rather than on a set of unified professional traits and this results in CM housing many often disparate treatments and modalities. Due to this definitional issue, countries may have to choose to implement policy and legislation that focuses on specific aspects of TCIM (e.g. chiropractic, indigenous medicines or medicinal plants), in which case much of the TCIM sector may fall outside the policies. The other difficulty, is when countries attempt to create broad, generic TCIM legislation, whose 'one-size-fits all' nature may necessitate certain compromises on public safety. An example of these two issues is TCIM health practitioner regulation in Australia. Chinese medicine, chiropractic and osteopathy have been registered in Australia under the National Registration and Accreditation Scheme, which is currently closed to new professions, despite naturopaths also being recommended for inclusion by several government agencies (Wardle *et al.*, 2016). Registration of these systems is based on development of codified professional standards of practice and training. To ensure accountability for unregistered TCIM professions, Australian governments have agreed on a national rollout of an innovative negative licensing model (i.e. a statutory Code of Conduct for all persons purporting to practice health, where breaches may result in disciplinary action), but is not dependent on profession-specific standards. This initiative has been at once astoundingly successful and a dismal failure — while this has resulted in an unprecedented level of accountability for many unregistered TCIM practitioners, for TCIM professions whose potential risk has been shown to warrant registration it has proven to be an ineffective substitute (Wardle, 2014). While 'catch-all' TCIM policy initiatives do offer an improvement where no policies exist, they must be complemented with specific TCIM policy, legislative and regulatory tools that address the needs of the nation in which they are set.

Political barriers to TCIM policy development and implementation largely centre on professional dynamics and ideological tensions between TCIM and conventional medicine. Detractors often posit that policy, legislation or regulation grants TCIM an unwarranted or undeserved legitimacy, with some suggesting we should not 'legitimise the witchdoctors' (Caulfield, 2013). However, these arguments are usually ideological in nature, and there is unequivocal evidence that regulating TCIM offers significant public benefit (Lin and Gillick, 2011). Moreover, when included in regulatory and legislative schemes, TCIM regulation is usually more efficient and more responsive than conventional medicine regulation (Milbank *et al.*, 2017).

Despite the lack of evidence supporting the claim, arguments that TCIM should not be granted legitimation through policy, legislative or regulatory recognition do sometimes carry weight, and can stall TCIM policy development. For example, in the United Kingdom the Department of Health recommended statutory registration of herbalists in order to appropriately protect public safety. However, this recommendation was ignored by the health secretary so as to avoid granting herbalists the 'full trappings of professional recognition which are applied to practitioners of orthodox healthcare', and instead registration was moved to a voluntary scheme that was known to be largely ineffective (Kmietowicz, 2010). Marginalization of TCIM may also be counter-productive, entrenching oppositional stances in TCIM practice that can be problematic for public health (Gort and Coburn, 1988). However, debate on whether specific TCIM practitioner groups, practices or products 'deserve' or 'warrant' registration may no longer be relevant. Arguably, as health care becomes increasingly consumer-driven, the debate as to whether regulation 'legitimises TCIM' is increasingly moot, with lack of policy, legislative and regulatory action serving only to deny minimum standards and accountability in a sector already perceived by the public as legitimate by virtue of their significant utilization.

Conceptual TCIM Policy Models

Holliday (2003) proposes a conceptual model for health policy options based on an in-depth review of TCIM integration in East Asia. This model — based on two key dimensions of mixed health systems (relationship between the State and TCIM and the relationship between biomedicine and TCIM in that state) — offers options on four distinct quadrants: unification (with strong links between vibrant medical traditions with non-discriminatory state practice); equalization; subjugation and marginalization (see Figure 2)

This conceptual model clearly articulates the level of TCIM policy development possible within certain contexts, and identifies potential

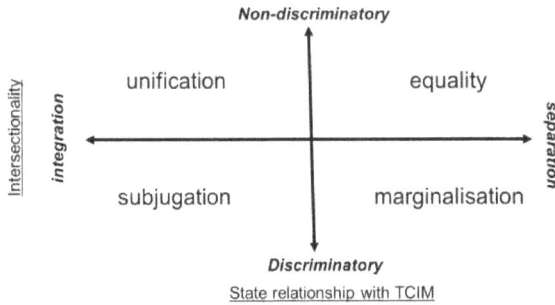

Figure 2.   Options for health policy systems for integration of TCIM (adapted from Holliday, 2003).

barriers to favoured policy approaches. Integration of TCIM, more specifically traditional Chinese medicine, in Hong Kong offers an example here, one which will be examined in more detail in a case study later in this chapter. Holliday's study occurred prior to the implementation of the Chinese Medicine Ordinance and classed Hong Kong in the *marginalization* quadrant, as the TCIM sector was both separated from the conventional health sector by legislation (or more correctly, not recognized at all), and discriminated against in its relationship with biomedicine (via exclusion from health provision). As the Hong Kong government changes its relationship with TCIM, based largely on the Chinese Medicine Ordinance, and moves to increasingly recognize and integrate TCIM, it is likely to reposition in the *equality* sector.

The integration of TCIM into health systems is a separate topic but the success of any integrative model is entirely dependent on the local political system. The model of integration will largely depend on whether the policy and legislative environment is tolerant (allows, but does not actively encourage integration), inclusive (encourages interaction between TCIM and conventional medicine) or allows truly integrative care (equal weight to each medicine supported by political action). This in turn will impact the level of TCIM integration observed at the patient level, and whether such integration is ad-hoc and self-determined, or truly multidisciplinary in nature. Lin *et al.* (2015) developed a model which links

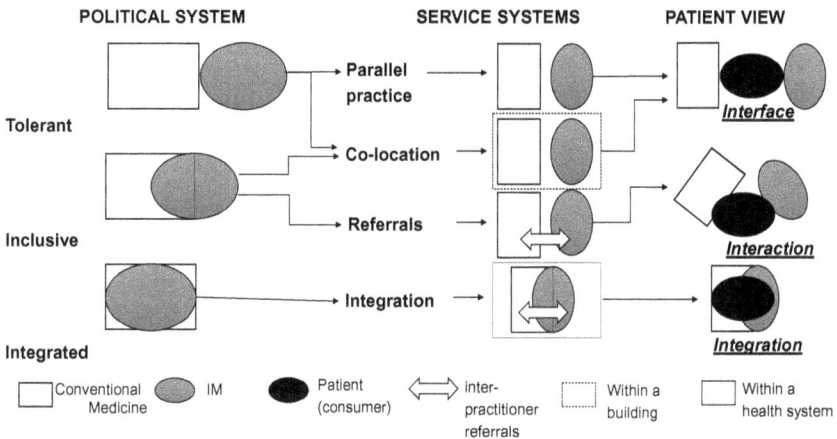

Figure 3.   A conceptual framework of CAM and medical integration: policy, delivery and consumer levels (modified from Lin *et al.*, 2015).

policy, service delivery and consumer perspectives (Figure 3). This model is particularly useful as it highlights how policy environments are likely to affect TCIM integration from the patient perspective.

Differing Approaches to TCIM Policy Development and Implementation — Latin American Case Studies

Although these conceptual models above are useful for analysing and modelling potential policy initiatives, case studies also offer insights into how different types of TCIM policy development can impact TCIM integration and practice. There is a wide range of legislative approaches to TCIM, from constitutional-level legislation to non-existent. Similarly, there are numerous approaches to TCIM regulation, from restriction of practice modalities and practitioners to tolerance of unregistered practitioners. There are also various levels of integration, from national-level integration programs to non-existent initiatives. Latin America offers an interesting case study in TCIM policy development, as it is embedded within a WHO region, which, while currently invigorating activity at the regional level, had largely left nations to interpret the WHO Traditional Medicine Strategy in their own way.

Constitutional Provisions

Some Latin-American nations have entrenched TCIM into the national constitution with many instilling the rights of indigenous peoples into their traditional practices and knowledge in their constitution and a smaller number explicitly and overtly extending this to health practices. For example, Article 2 of the Mexican constitution affirms Mexico as a 'pluricultural nation that guarantees preservation of all elements of the culture and identity of indigenous communities', including TM. Further, it recommends that to ensure effective access to universal health care, the nation must take proper advantage of TM. Although not explicitly inclusive of TCIM practices that are not indigenous to those countries, these provisions are often used to guide more expansive and inclusive TCIM policies and strategies. However, some nations also explicitly recognize *both* TM and CM practices. For example, Article 44 of the Ecuadorian constitution notes that 'the State... recognizes, respects and promotes the development of traditional and alternative medicine, whose practice would be regulated by law'. Some countries do not identify indigenous traditional practices and instead fulfil their commitment to TCIM through constitutional discussion of 'complementary medicines'.

Statutory Law

Other Latin-American nations have chosen to establish the right to access TCIM via statutory instruments. Nicaragua is one of the only countries globally that has a national law mandating the government to promote TCIM practice and research. Nicaragua has enacted legislative instruments that aim to provide access to both its own indigenous traditional systems of medicine while also ensuring access to traditional systems not indigenous to Nicaragua but which remain popular (such as Chinese medicine, naturopathy and homeopathy). Law 759 of 2011 — known as the *Ancestral Traditional Indigenous Medicine Law* — states as its goal to recognize, protect and promote the right of indigenous and afro-descendant communities to their health practices and expressions. Through this law, initiatives such as inter-cultural medical education and treatment of culture-bound syndromes (such as Grisi siknis) are formally enabled. The development of inter-cultural medical education at the *Universidad de las Regiones Autónomas de la Costa Caribe Nicaragüense* (URACCAN), where medical practitioners and nurses are taught both traditional and biomedical medical approaches throughout their education (Cupples and Glynn, 2014), is one example of the changes initiated through this approach. However, Nicaragua has also recognized that non-indigenous TCIM are also popular in the country. Law 774 of 2011 — known as the Natural Medicine, Complementary Therapies & Natural Products Law — states as its goal to institutionalise, promote, protect and regulate the individual or collective use of non-conventional health practices. Under the augur of this law, the country has developed a national institute of TCIM, created a directorate for natural products regulation (Resolution 173-2015), involved existing TCIM practitioners in health care delivery, and formalized training for conventional health practitioners in TCIM.

Governmental Structures

Many Latin-American countries have developed governmental structures to assist in implementing TCIM policies and strategies, with some existing at the highest level of government. For example, the Bolivian government has enacted a *Vice-Ministry of Traditional Medicine and Interculturality*. The Vice Ministry is charged with the promotion of TM, which is seen as emblematic of a historical and sovereign medical system. This is part of a broader national inter-cultural initiative aimed at dismantling colonial structures and, in the case of health policy, developing an intrinsically sovereign national health system that includes the incorporation of traditional Bolivian medicine (Johnson, 2010). To achieve this the Vice- Ministry oversees: TM's active incorporation alongside biomedicine in their health system; the establishment of academic programs for TM study and promotion; the regulation, certification and accreditation of TM, based on appropriate use and proven knowledge of beneficial practices; and the protection of TM as a cultural resource and heritage codified in law (Ministerio de Salud y Deportes, 2006). The Peruvian government has also developed a governmental structure focused on intercultural health, but has instead chosen to pursue this through a national centre under the remit of the Ministry of Health rather than via a separate formal government ministry or department (the *National Centre for Intercultural Health* — CENSI).

In Mexico the government has developed the *Directorate for Traditional Medicine and Intercultural Development*. As opposed to the Bolivian experience — which focuses almost exclusively on indigenous traditional medicine — Mexico is one of the countries where a focus on indigenous TM has also opened the door to other TCIM modalities, largely in recognition of the pluricultural nature of the country. Mexico has used the TM framework within legislation — and the infrastructure this legislation has enabled — to help accommodate TCIM in the health system. The Mexican directorate deals with making sure health care approaches within areas where indigenous communities live take into consideration the practices and traditions of those communities. However, it also takes on responsibility for ensuring access to and standards in TCIM as used in Mexico.

The presence of a formal government ministry or directorate does not necessarily correlate with increased progression towards TCIM integration. Cuba and Brazil are held as the most outstanding examples of integration of TCIM into formal medical systems, albeit for different reasons and via different approaches (Guido *et al.*, 2015). These countries show that bureaucracy alone is not a guarantee of TCIM integration — while developing governmental structures, the formalization of these structures has not been to the same extent as other countries in the region. In Cuba, a special model of integration has been developed since the 1960s to rescue native traditional knowledge as well as that from countries and regions beyond Cuba. TCIM has been one of Cuba's most important resources for dealing with the lack of some pharmaceuticals and is highly integrated within primary health care. However, the most important TCIM-specific government agency in Cuba is not a ministry or directorate, but a program within the Ministry.

Brazil is also in many ways a unique case — although lacking the kind of legislative framework adopted by many other countries in the region it is one of the most advanced in terms of TCIM integration. Brazil has focused on development of a national policy, the *National Policy on Integrative and Complementary Practices in Health*, which has existed in various iterations and traverses the health care system even in the absence of a dedicated TCIM institute or department. The Brazilian approach has been effective in focusing upon practical implementation and application of its TCIM strategy, which has most likely been assisted by the fact that Brazil has (mostly) a single-payer health system. Brazil was one of the first countries to formally acknowledge and implement TCIM as part of its commitment to the Alma-Ata Declaration, and this early start has undoubtedly helped to cement its regional leadership role in TCIM integration (Guido *et al.*, 2015). Nevertheless, the Brazilian experience shows that formalized structures and legislative frameworks in and of themselves may fail to ensure appropriate TCIM policy development and implementation — some countries with far more exhaustive legislative frameworks may not have the bureaucratic infrastructure, resources or political will to implement legislative provisions fully (as is the case in Nicaragua and Ecuador).

Legislation

Legislation differs slightly from statutory law approaches in that they are not over-arching TCIM laws directing broad government action, but instead more focused on issues associated with TCIM. However, the manner in which legislation is implemented can vary significantly across Latin America. Chile does not have the same level of official governmental infrastructure on TCIM as other countries (despite established departments within the Ministry devoted to TCIM), and lacks a national TCIM policy, but its legislative efforts have been well organized, and in most cases largely coordinated and pre-emptive. Chile has the most progressive approaches regarding practice regulation for non-medical TCIM practitioners in Latin-America. In 2005, Decree No. 42 was passed regulating the exercise of TCIM medical practices, and under this framework, national licensure examinations and training standards have been developed for acupuncturists, homeopaths and naturopaths. Unlike most countries in the region, Chile has also developed a publicly available national list of licensed TCIM practitioners. However, the government has not yet committed to practical action for TCIM integration and despite various types of integrative efforts, many have proven unsustainable and dependent on changing national political agendas. Nevertheless, compared with many countries in the region which restrict practice of most non-indigenous TCIM to conventionally trained medical practitioners (e.g. Argentina), the Chilean arrangements are remarkably permissive.

Some countries have relied on 'diffuse legislation' for TCIM policy. This scenario results when numerous TCIM policies and legislative reforms are introduced, but there is no government policy, infrastructure or system-wide integration effort guiding their development. Even in countries with a relatively permissive attitude towards TCIM and its integration — such as Colombia — legislation can be convoluted and complex. As Table 1 indicates, there are multiple TCIM-specific policies and laws in Colombia, and even for specific TCIM (in this case homeopathy and medicinal plants) legislative arrangements can be quite diffuse and complex. It should be noted, however, that guidelines for TCIM integration into the national health care system in that country are currently under development.

The reality for many countries, however, is that there is sparse, minimal or non-existent legislative TCIM provisions. The Dominican Republic and Venezuela, for example, do have minimal TCIM legislative provisions, but these are often administrative in nature (e.g. templates to register a TCIM practice) or are absorbed into other health legislation (e.g. a line about TCIM within other health care legislation). Other countries, such as Guatemala, do not have legislative provision but have integrated TCIM into their national health care model via intercultural health. In most instances where few provisions exist — and certainly in instances where no restrictive provisions exist — these countries appear to be tolerant of non-medical TCIM practices. Similarly, some countries where TCIM practice is both popular and significantly utilized may have no legislative provisions as appears to be the case in countries such as Costa Rica and Paraguay though the later has some incipient indigenous health provisions.

Table 1.   Diffuse legislation for TCIM practice, homeopathy and medicinal plants in Colombia.

Generic TCIM Practice Legislation	Homeopathy Legislation	Medicinal Plants Legislation
Law 12 of 1905 modified by **Law 83 of 1914, Law 67 of 1920, Law 85 of 1922** and **Law 35 of 1929**: Practice of Homeopathy	**Decree 3554 of 2004**: By which regulates the regime of sanitary registry, monitoring and sanitary control of the homeopathic medicines for human use and dictates other dispositions	**Decree 677 of 1995**: Regime of Registers and Licenses, the Quality Control, as well as the Regimen of Sanitary Surveillance of Medicines, Cosmetics, Pharmaceutical Preparations based on Natural Resources
Law 14 of 1962: Medical practice and Homeopathy	**Decree 1737 of 2005**: By which the preparation, distribution, dispensation, commercialization, labelling, labelling and packing of the masterful and officinal homeopathic medicines are regulated and other dispositions are dictated	**Resolution 03131 of 1998**: Adopts the technical annex of the GMP manual for pharmaceutical preparations based on natural resources
Law 100 of 1993: Creates the SGSSS		**Decree 337 of 1998**: Provisions on natural resources used in pharmaceutical preparations
Decree 2753 of 1997: Cultural Diversity and TCIM		**Resolution 243710 of 1999**: Sets guidelines on labels, packaging and labels, the use of sticker and authorization of exhaustion of packaging
Resolution 2927 of 1998: Regulates TCIM practice	**Decree 1861 of 2006**: By which the Decree 3554 of 2004 is modified and added and other dispositions are dictated	**Decree 549 of 2001**: obtaining the Certificate of Compliance with Good Manufacturing Practices by laboratories
Resolution 1396 of 2001: CUPS Coces, includes TCIM	**Decree 4858 of 2007**: By which article 26 of Decree 1861 of 2006 is modified	**Decree 2266 of 2004**: The regimens of sanitary registrations are regulated, and monitoring and sanitary control and publicity, fitoterapéuticos products
Resolution 1043 of 2006: Enabling MATC Services		**Decree 3553 of 2004**: modifies Decree 2266 of 2004
Law 1164 of 2007: Human Health Talent: Includes TCIM	**Resolution 4594 of 2007**: Whereby the Manual of Good Manufacturing Practices for Homeopathic Medicines is issued and other provisions are issued	**Decree 162 of 2004**: modifies article 3 of Decree 549 of 2001

(Continued)

Table 1.   (Continued)

Generic TCIM Practice Legislation	Homeopathy Legislation	Medicinal Plants Legislation
Law 1438 of 2011: TCIM included in the principles of APS	**Resolution 3665 of 2009**: By which the Guide to Verify Compliance with Good Manufacturing Practices for Homeopathic Medicines is adopted and other provisions are issued	**Resolution 004320 of 2004**: Regulates the advertising of over-the-counter phytotherapeutic medicines and products
Agreement 029 of 2011: TCIM in POS		**Resolution 005107 of 2005**: adopts the Verification Instrument of Compliance with Sanitary Conditions for Laboratories that elaborate Phytotherapeutic Products
		Decree 3752 of 2006: it modifies the Decree 2350 of July 26, 2004 and other dispositions are dictated
		Resolution 2834 of 2008: By which the Vademecum of Colombian Medicinal Plants is adopted and guidelines are established to update
		Decree 272 of 2009: modifies the paragraph of article 24 of Decree 3249 of 2006, modified by article 6 of Decree 3863 of 2008
		Decree 4927 of 2009: modifies article 6 of Decree 2266 of 2004, modified by article 3 of Decree 3553 of 2004
		Resolution 000126 of 2009: establishes the essential conditions for the opening, operation, monitoring and sanitary control of health food stores
		Resolution 527 of 2010: modifies the paragraph of article 6 and article 13 of Resolution 126 of 2009

Legal Recognition of Traditional Knowledge in Biomedically Dominated Systems

Case law — also known as judge-made law or sometimes interpreted as being synonymous with common law — is a body of law that is highly influential in development and implementation of policy, legislative and regulatory provisions in common law countries (mostly those with a history of British colonial influence). Common law is beginning to examine the role of traditional knowledge in more and more detail. One of these areas is in health practitioner regulation. The law imposes a duty on health practitioners to exercise reasonable care and skill in the provision of professional advice and treatment. The standard by which such reasonable care and skill has been measured in recent times was against the *Bolam* principle, from the English case *Bolam v Friern Barnet Hospital Management Committee*, which placed primacy of importance on the accepted nature of treatment within the medical profession. This was explained in more detail in the English case *Sidaway v Governors of the Bethlehem Royal Hospital and Maudsley Hospital* as *a doctor is not negligent if her acts in accordance with a practice accepted at the time as proper by a responsible body of medical opinion even though other doctors adopt a different practice. In short, the law imposes the duty of care: but the standard of care is a matter of clinical judgment.*

A variant of this 'peer professional defence' is observed in most common law countries. The primacy of peer-opinion in defence has been progressively modified over time — for example, the Australian case *Rogers v Whitaker* modified the test to make peer-professional opinion rather than conclusive. But what this precedent means is that, provided treatment is provided within a framework of rationality and safety, clinicians are ultimately held to the standards identified as appropriate by peer clinicians rather than judges (or other non-clinicians). This 'peer opinion' standard of care expected of health practitioners appears also to ring true for TCIM, even where there may be little (scientific) evidence and practice in a paradigm divergent from conventional medical thought (Wardle, 2016). That is, even for TCIM, case law is increasingly recognising the validity of traditional bodies of knowledge.

In the English case of *Shakoor v Situ* the judge considered the question of whether the same principles applying to Western medical practitioners applied to practitioners of traditional Chinese medicine. The judgment stated that although the Chinese herbal medicine practitioner was not required to be held to the same standard of care as an orthodox practitioner (i.e. they were to be held to the standards of Chinese medicine), as part of the practitioner's scope of practice 'it will often be necessary to have regard to the fact that the practitioner is practising his art alongside orthodox medicine'. However, the judge also noted that the peer professional opinion was valid in Chinese medicine because, even though it may not be viewed as a legitimate therapy by many, it adequately demonstrated a body of knowledge, noting 'unlike some alternative therapies, [traditional Chinese herbal medicine] has a long and distinguished history; it has an oral tradition extending back some 4,000 years or more and a written tradition extending back some 2,000 years'.

Case law is beginning to examine traditional knowledge in more detail, and misrepresentation of traditional knowledge as increasingly being viewed as equally misleading as misrepresentation of scientific evidence. The area in which case law is most developed in this area appears to be the promotion of homeopathic vaccination alternatives. This has been primarily based on the fact that homeoprophylaxis is inconsistent with established and recognized homeopathic traditions (Vithoulkas, 2016). While the scientific credibility of homeopathic vaccination alternatives has been questioned in Courts (for example *Australian Competition and Consumer Commission v Homeopathy Plus! Australia Pty Limited*), its inconsistency with the homeopathic traditional body of knowledge has been cited in each of these cases as a major determinative factor in deciding against homeopathic vaccination. Traditional evidence as it relates to homeoprophylaxis has also been used in legal cases outside of the health and medical arena — most notably in family law cases around parental disputes on vaccination (e.g. *Kingsford and Kingsford* in the Family Court of Australia). While TCIM cases in the Courts remain relatively rare, the precedent that traditional knowledge is a valid knowledge form that should not just be acknowledged, but also protected, is increasingly apparent in judgments.

These interpretations raise an interesting issue — how do policymakers or lawyers recognize or identify traditional systems of knowledge as legitimate? For a system such as Chinese medicine this is relatively easy, as it has a long history of documentation and, through China's substantial support, is slowly being integrated into international initiatives such as the *International Classification of Diseases* (the 11th edition has recently released an appendix of East Asian diagnoses). However, this body of knowledge may be harder to identify for indigenous medical systems that have been largely passed down via oral tradition. Such lack of clarity often underpins the controversy that inclusion of traditional health language in TCIM policy, legislation and regulation attracts. For example, when the Australian *Therapeutic Goods Administration* implemented a pre-approved list of over 1,000 traditional health claims that could be used for marketing TCIM products, there was outrage from many critics as to the nature of these claims, as many had no definitive or authoritative source that could be readily identified, and were instead based on a scoping exercise, which itself was identified as the best solution specifically due to the lack of formal documentation (Community Affairs Legislation Committee, 2018). The lack of substantial codification of practice and traditional use in TCIM health practitioners may make it difficult for policy makers and lawmakers to identify when claims are truly misleading or deceptive, or when claims are divergent from standard practice for that profession. As such, development of further understanding of TCIM products and practices at a foundational level may be the first step to ensuring appropriate integration of TCIM into policy, legislative and regulatory initiatives.

Conclusion

In recognition of the growing utilization of TCIM and the potential associated risks and benefits, governments are increasingly required to develop policy, legislative and regulatory initiatives focused on TCIM. There is no 'one-size-fits-all' approach to TCIM policy and legislation, and any initiatives will need to fully appreciate social, political or cultural factors that interface with TCIM use. Public health and health services research in TCIM, in particular, can assist with robust TCIM policy, legislative and regulatory developments by providing a rigorous examination and understanding of TCIM use and practice and the societal, political and cultural contexts that influence such behaviours and practices. While well-developed and well-thought out TCIM policy is required to ensure optimal TCIM integration, it should be remembered that policy development and health service delivery are two inter-connected but separate topics that warrant sufficient attention to detail in their development and implementation.

References

Ahuriri-Driscoll, A., *et al.* (2008). *The future of Rongoā Māori: Wellbeing and Sustainability.* Wellington: Ministry of Health (New Zealand).

Caulfield, T. (2013). Don't Legitimise the Witch Doctors. *National Post*, 22 January 2013.

Community Affairs Legislation Committee (2018). *Community Affairs Legislation Committee — Senate Standing — Therapeutic Goods Amendment (2017 Measures No. 1) Bill 2017 [Provisions] and Therapeutic Goods (Charges) Amendment Bill 2017 [Provisions] — Report, dated February 2018*, Australian Senate: Canberra.

Cupples, J., Glynn, K. (2014). Indigenizing and decolonizing higher education on Nicaragua's Atlantic Coast. *Singapore Journal of Tropical Geography, 35*, 56–71.

Gort, E., Coburn, D. (1988). Naturopathy in Canada: Changing relationships to medicine, chiropractic and the State. *Social Science & Medicine, 26*, 1061.

Guido, P., *et al.* (2015). The state of the integrative medicine in Latin America: The long road to include complementary, natural, and traditional practices in formal health systems. *European Journal of Integrative Medicine, 7*, 5–12.

Holliday, I. (2003). Traditional medicines and modern societies: An exploration of integrationist options through East Asian experience. *Journal of Medicine and Philosophy, 28*, 373–389.

Ijaz, N., Boon, H. (2018). Statutory regulation of traditional medicine practitioners and practices: The need for distinct policy making guidelines. *The Journal of Alternative and Complementary Medicine, 24*, 307–313.

Johnson, B. (2010). Decolonization and its paradoxes: The (re) envisioning of health policy in Bolivia. *Latin American Perspectives, 37*, 139–159.

Kmietowicz, Z. (2010). Registering herbalists will improve patients' safety, says health secretary. *BMJ, 340*, c1897.

Lin, V., Canaway, R., Carter, B. (2015). Interface, interaction and integration: How people with chronic disease in Australia manage CAM and conventional medical services. *Health Expectations, 18*(6), 2651–2665.

Lin, V., Gillick, D. (2011). Does workforce regulation have the intended effect? The case of Chinese medicine practitioner registration. *Australian Health Review, 35*, 455–461.

Millbank, J., *et al.* (2017). Complementary health practitioners disciplined for misconduct in Australia 2011–2016. *Journal of Law and Medicine, 24*, 788–802.

Ministerio de Salud y Deportes (Bolivia) (2006). *Plan estrategico: Medicina traditional y salud intercultural, 2006–2010*. La Paz: MSD.

Pan American Health Organization (2002). *Harmonization of Indigenous and Conventional Health Systems in the Americas. Strategies for Incorporating Indigenous Perspectives, Medicines, and Therapies into Primary Health Care.*, PAHO: Washington, DC.

Pan American Health Organization (2003). *Medicinas y Terapias Tradicionales, Complementarias y Alternativas. Evaluación del Plan de Trabajo 2000–2001 y Plan de Trabajo 2002–2003*, PAHO, Washington, DC.

Tang, K., *et al.* (2017). China's Silk Road and global health. *Lancet, 390*(10112), 2595–2601.

Wardle, J. (2014). Holding unregistered health practitioners to account: An analysis of current regulatory and legislative approaches. *Journal of Law and Medicine, 22*, 350–375.

Wardle, J. (2016). Defining deviation: The peer professional defence and its relation to scope expansion and emerging non-medical professions. *Journal of Law and Medicine, 23*, 662–677.

Wardle, J., *et al.* (2016). Is health practitioner regulation keeping pace with the changing practitioner and healthcare landscape? An Australian perspective. *Frontiers in Public Health, 4*, 91.

Weeks, J. (2017). Articulated medicine: Pan American health organization reengages traditional and complementary medicine efforts. *The Journal of Alternative and Complementary Medicine, 23*, 745–746.

Western Pacific Regional Office (WHO) (2012). *Regional Strategy for Traditional Medicine in the Western Pacific 2011–2020*, WPRO: Manila.

World Health Organization (2001). *WHO Traditional Medicine Strategy 2002–2005*, WHO: Geneva.

World Health Organization (2013). *WHO Traditional Medicine Strategy 2014–2023,* WHO: Geneva.

World Health Organization, World Intellectual Property Organization and World Trade Organization (2012). *Promoting Access to Medical Technologies and Innovation — Intersections between public health, intellectual property and trade,* Geneva, WHO–WIPO–WTO.

Chapter 5

Coordination, Collaboration and Capacity Building Through National Practice-Based Research Networks: A New Paradigm of Research in Traditional, Complementary and Integrative Medicine

Jon Adams, Amie Steel, Janet Schloss and Wenbo Peng

Introduction

Health and medical research are often criticized as disconnected from the concerns, perspectives and behaviours of those under study (Rycroft-Malone *et al.*, 2016). Indeed, researchers have themselves at times, wittingly or unwittingly, helped propagate this impression. The long-standing focus upon randomized controlled trials and other experimental designs (in public health and medicine more generally) as the gold standard has done little to promote a more inclusive flavour to the research process (Breckenridge *et al.*, 2018). Similarly, the power dynamics encouraged in a traditional research model with the researcher hailed as 'expert' and the participant treated as nothing more than a 'subject' (non-expert) to be passively involved in fieldwork has also discouraged rich participant engagement often as to avoid what is seen as potential contamination of 'clean', rigorous scientific enquiry. These critiques are no less relevant for TCIM as they are for other health and health care research fields and there have been calls from within the TCIM research community to address these features (Paterson, 2007). Unfortunately, despite a diversity of approach and methodology, the TCIM research field continues to harbour a predominant focus and privileged standing for designs and models that are removed from the grass-roots reality of health care delivery and consumption (Adams, 2007).

A wider review of the health research project highlights a number of possible avenues by which TCIM research may begin to attend to these challenges and recalibrate enquiry in a way that connects directly to practice, policy and stakeholders' experiences and behaviours. For example, as Chapter 6 in this collection identifies, the development of implementation and translation science models and insights may help foster TCIM research activity that has a direct impact upon grass-roots activity and practice (also see Steel *et al.*, 2018). Another possible approach that holds potential in this regard is the development of practice-based research networks (PBRNs). The remainder of this chapter outlines the concept and origins of PBRN designs and highlights how the PBRN model of enquiry can be adopted and adapted to TCIM-related issues. As this chapter argues and shows it is possible to operationalize the PBRN design to address a wide range of TCIM research questions and ultimately help reframe debate and focus around issues of interest to patients and practitioners in daily routine care. We draw directly upon our extensive experience designing and conducting world-first large-scale PBRN projects focused upon TCIM in high-income countries in the hope of inspiring others to draw upon such networks or even design and establish their own PBRN initiatives around TCIM in their own country/region/jurisdiction.

What is a Practice-Based Research Network? Definition, History and General Aims

A practice-based research network (PBRN) is a group of ambulatory practices that affiliate together and collaborate with academic institutions for the purpose of conducting research using data collected from practitioners and patients, and to ultimately improve the quality of patient care (Davis *et al.*, 2012; Graham *et al.*, 2007). PBRNs have been growing in popularity globally since the 1960s (Lindbloom *et al.*, 2004; Thomas *et al.*, 2001) and provide a vehicle through which research questions directly grounded in daily practice can be linked with critical and rigorous research methods (Davis *et al.*, 2012). PBRNs provide an opportunity for important research questions identified by practitioners in grass-roots clinical practice (but otherwise often neglected by researchers) to be repositioned as central to critical, rigorous research enquiry.

Characteristics of a PBRN vary in a number of ways including member composition, affiliation and size. However there are a number of key characteristics which are common among many PBRNs (Davis *et al.*, 2012). Namely, PBRNs include: at least 15 ambulatory practices and/or 15 clinicians devoted to the primary care of patients; a statement of the PBRN's purpose and mission, including an ongoing commitment to research; a community advisory board or similar to solicit advice and feedback from the communities of patients served by the PBRN clinicians; an organizational structure independent of any single study; and communication processes (e.g. newsletters, emails, conference calls, etc.) to keep all stakeholders connected. Ultimately, the process of establishing and maintaining a PBRN requires a great deal of infrastructure and the cost of sustaining this infrastructure is one of the most substantial barriers to successful PBRNs (Green *et al.*, 2005).

Until recent years, PBRNs may have included TCIM practices or practitioners, but they have not focused exclusively upon TCIM. This oversight can be attributed to both infrastructure and cost-related barriers to establishing a PBRN which are amplified within TCIM. The accepted PBRN model described above is premised on a number of factors which may not be congruent with prevailing practitioner culture within TCIM. Firstly, all stakeholders involved in a PBRN are expected to embody an ongoing commitment to research. However, there may be a culture of scepticism towards research within TCIM practitioner communities (Veziari *et al.*, 2017). Some of this scepticism centres on a concern among TCIM clinicians that research cannot appropriately respond to the complexities of TCIM systems of care (Veziari *et al.*, 2017). While the PBRN model is argued to provide a valuable solution to this concern within the broader health care sector (Peterson *et al.*, 2012), the secondary issue of capacity and research literacy among TCIM (Veziari *et al.*, 2017) further hinders researchers communicating the potential for PBRNs to support research which honours the complex, individualized approach to care seen in TCIM. Researchers looking to develop a TCIM PBRN also have to overcome the challenge of poor infrastructure within TCIM professions as TCIM clinicians are often community-based and exist outside of the established health care systems and settings (Steel *et al.*, 2018). This structural separation can mean researchers must rely heavily on professional organizations and opinion leaders to inform, motivate and enrol clinicians in PBRNs. Equally, the independent practice model of many TCIM clinicians reduces the likelihood that PBRN members will have shared electronic health records and so the 'big data' approach common to most primary care PBRN within conventional medicine (Riley-Behringer *et al.*, 2017) is not practical for TCIM PBRNs (Adams *et al.*, 2015).

Currently, there are eight TCIM-focussed PBRNs based primarily in the United States and Australia (Agency for Healthcare Research and Quality, 2018). Research produced through these PBRNs currently focuses on the characteristics of TCIM clinicians and the individuals accessing TCIM services (Hawk *et al.*, 2001; Licciardone *et al.*, 2014; Wolever *et al.*, 2012). Other studies explore the approach to care employed in TCIM practice as well as the clinical outcomes of that care such as safety and effectiveness (Abrams *et al.*, 2013; Degenhardt *et al.*, 2014). In comparison, TCIM research conducted through non-TCIM PBRNs more commonly reports the prevalence of TCIM use in conventional medical settings or doctor-patient communication about TCIM (Sleath *et al.*, 2005; Flannery *et al.*, 2006; Shelley *et al.*, 2009).

Establishing PBRNs for TCIM

A PBRN design has a number of distinct but interrelated opportunities for the TCIM field. First, as explained in the opening of this chapter, this network design helps facilitate research more closely related to the behaviours and practices of those in daily routine care. Second, a PBRN coordinates research effort and resource not only helping avoid duplication but also encouraging follow-up effort to build upon earlier insights. In a field such as TCIM, where research funding remains relatively ad-hoc and harder to come by (Wardle and Adams, 2013) and the ranks of researchers are relatively small, this prospect of co-ordinating research activity is perhaps even more crucial. Third, a PBRN is able to accommodate and encourage a broad range of different studies utilising a wide array of study methods and designs and as such, a PBRN can represent potentially good return on investment (conditional to the quality and quantity of output produced) (Adams *et al.*, 2015; Amorin-Woods *et al.*, 2018). Closely linked to this last point, a PBRN can, if designed appropriately, help establish a 'program' approach to research whereby the focus is not just upon immediate output but also upon fostering a growing, sustainable research culture in TCIM (Adams *et al.*, 2017a). A PBRN can also help engage practitioners in the research world providing them with unique opportunities to collaborate and lead enquiry as well as 'reframe' their thinking and understanding around the research process (perceiving it as complementary to and ultimately aiding their practice and the patients and communities they serve) (Mold and Peterson, 2005). All these benefits have partly motivated the TCIM PBRN initiatives that we introduce and describe below.

The Australian Chiropractic Research Network (ACORN) PBRN

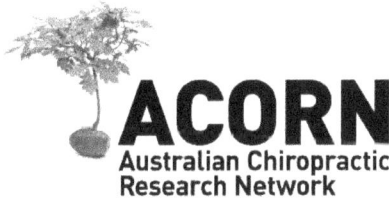

History

The Australian Chiropractic Research Network (ACORN) project was established in 2014 and to date is the first large-scale national voluntary

PBRN exclusively examining chiropractic care in the world (http://www.acorn-arccim.com/). The ACORN PBRN program has been registered with the Agency for Healthcare Research and Quality (AHRQ) PBRN Resource Centre. The Chiropractors' Association of Australia (CAA) funded the ACORN PBRN and senior health researchers at the Australian Research Centre in Complementary and Integrative Medicine (ARCCIM), University of Technology Sydney independently designed, led and conducted this PBRN project. CAA is the largest chiropractic health organization in Australian with both national and state-based infrastructure, which can guarantee to promote the ACORN PBRN to the vast majority of Australian chiropractors and collect extensive data for future research on the chiropractic profession. There are three stages of the ACORN PBRN process, including the design and promotion activities such as branding and practitioner-focused promotional campaign to all potential participants (Stage One), baseline workforce questionnaire distribution with invitation pack and the launch of an Expression of Interest (EOI) form for nested sub-studies proposals (Stage Two), and the implementation of nested sub-studies (Stage Three).

Design

Chiropractors practicing in Australia generally work in the private clinic sector and the majority of them operate independent businesses. It is not feasible to demand these Australian chiropractors to join a pre-allocated patient record management system which will cause significant financial burden and professional argument. A sub-study PBRN approach is considered best fit in a profession where no unified patient record management system exists. Therefore, the ACORN PBRN was built upon such sub-study model. This approach allows the ACORN PBRN to focus upon practitioner-related information collection and consistent outcomes over time. Although the design of the ACORN PBRN cannot be facilitated to directly collect data from patients in the initial stage, under the sub-study model, the ACORN PBRN can actively accommodate nested sub-studies to collect data via patient records (with practitioners' help) at a later phase. Furthermore, the ACORN PBRN is extremely suitable for research capacity building that potential PhD and Masters students can apply for a sub-study of the ACORN PBRN.

Sample and response rate

The ACORN practitioner questionnaire and consent form were sent via group emails containing embedded links directly to the online questionnaire or hard copy from March 2015 to July 2015. At the time of the ACORN recruitment period, there were 4684 registered chiropractors in Australia and 2005 chiropractors completed the practitioner questionnaire (response rate: 43%). Among these 2005 chiropractors, 1680 chiropractors signed up to the ACORN PRBN practitioner database for the recruitment of future sub-studies. In addition, both of these two samples (i.e. the ACORN workforce database and the ACORN PBRN database) were found to be broadly representative of the Australian chiropractic profession in terms of age, gender and practice location, compared to the entire group of registered chiropractors by the Australian Health Practitioner Regulation Agency (AHPRA). The practitioner questionnaire used for the ACORN PBRN consists of 21 items including information on practitioner characteristics (e.g. age, gender and highest level of chiropractic professional qualification), practice characteristics (e.g. average patient care hours/week, practice location and professional referral relationships) and clinical management (e.g. frequency of discussion with patients regarding lifestyle aspects, patients' conditions, and clinical techniques).

Outputs and success to date

The ACORN PBRN has already produced a prolific volume of quality research outputs in just the first 3 years of operation (post-data collection) attracting 10 sub-studies to date involving an impressive 32 international researchers — not only based across Australia (including RMIT Unviersity, Murdoch University, University of Technology Sydney, Macquarie University, University of Sydney) but also at key universities across the globe (including University of Alberta, Canada; Palmer University, US; Hong Kong Polytechnic University, Hong Kong; University of Southern Denmark, Denmark; Karolinska Institute, Sweden). The sub-studies completed to date have examined a wide range of topics from research-capacity, interest and potential in Australian chiropractic through to treatment of headaches and migraine, use of nutritional advice, use of non-thrust mobilization for neck pain, approach to clinical uncertainty among chiropractors, treatment of older adults with neck pain and engagement with chiropractic research by chiropractors.

Moreover, the ACORN PBRN has to date generated nine manuscripts with many published in prestigious Q1 journals in their respective fields (Adams *et al.*, 2015, 2016, 2017a, 2017b, 2018a, 2018b; Moore *et al.*, 2017; Lee *et al.*, 2018; Amorin-Woods *et al.*, 2018). It is important to note from these many ACORN PBRN outputs that while a few are published in chiropractic journals (helping inform the profession of the importance of the PBRN and directly relay findings about daily routine care to the clinicians themselves), others have attracted publication in journals beyond the profession (e.g. *BMJ Open*, *BMC Neurology* and *Australian Journal of Rural Health*). Such a broad dissemination strategy and success is essential to not only ensuring the profession engage with research they are intimately involved in but also to help 'spread the word' and inform significant others (policymakers, industry, health care managers and practitioners of other modalities) beyond the profession of the realities of chiropractic care and the opportunities of utilising chiropractic in the pursuit of better health outcomes.

The Osteopathy Research and Innovation Network (ORION) PBRN

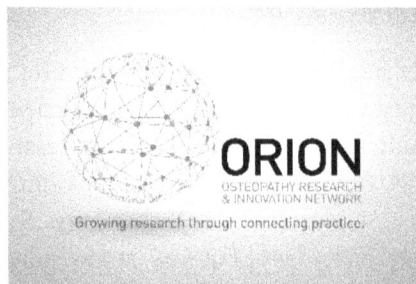

History

The Osteopathy Research and Innovation Network (ORION) project is the first national-scale voluntary PBRN of Australian osteopathy (http://www.

orion-arccim.com/). The ORION PBRN is funded by Osteopathy Australia (OA). OA is the largest national osteopathy professional organization in Australia, representing more than 85% of Australian osteopaths. As such, the ORION PBRN is feasible to establish a national long-term research database to inform future sub-studies on osteopathy, and provide evidence base with respect to patient-focused topics and daily osteopathy care from the perspective of osteopaths. More importantly, the ORION PBRN was designed to advance research capacity focusing upon the osteopathy profession, in particular via facilitating Masters and PhDs' projects. Furthermore, the ORION project is independently designed and conducted by senior researchers at the Australian Research Centre in Complementary and Integrative Medicine (ARCCIM), University of Technology Sydney. This team has established a Project Steering Committee, promoted this PBRN at a variety of osteopathy-relevant professional and academic events to recruitment OA members and non-OA osteopaths, launched the ORION PBRN website, obtained human ethics approval, and finished the data collection of ORION fieldwork in 2016.

Design

Similar to the situation of the chiropractic profession, osteopaths practicing in Australia are generally working in private clinics. Therefore, the ORION PBRN also employed a sub-study design to ensure coordinated ongoing research and capacity building for the osteopathy profession. The ORION PBRN Steering Committee members have designed an Expression of Interest (EOI) form to help osteopaths, researchers and others manage ORION PBRN sub-study application. As described in the ORION website, Masters and PhD students and/or their supervisors are encouraged to conduct osteopathy-focused sub-studies drawing upon the ORION PBRN practitioner database for participant recruitment purposes.

Sample and response rate

There were 2020 practicing osteopaths in Australia at the time of the ORION PBRN recruitment period according to the AHPRA registration record. A total of 992 osteopaths completed the ORION practitioner questionnaire with a response rate of 49.1%. In addition, 801 Australian osteopaths consented to be involved in the ORION PBRN for the further nested ORION sub-studies. In comparison to the AHPRA registry data of osteopaths, no statistically significant difference has been found with the OROIN database as well as the ORION PBRN database in terms of key demographic indicators (i.e. age, gender and practicing location). Therefore, the ORION PBRN sample is nationally representative of the entire Australian osteopathy profession.

An invitation pack consisting of a 27-item online osteopathy practitioner questionnaire (accessed via SurveyGizmo) and consent form was designed and emailed to registered osteopaths in Australia. Any participant completed the questionnaire and signed up the consent form indicating that they agreed to join the ORION PBRN database. With regards to the ORION practitioner questionnaire, participants were asked about their practitioner characteristics such as age, gender and years in private osteopathy practice. They were questioned about their practice characteristics such as the average patient care hours and patient visits per week, sending and receiving professional referrals and use of diagnostic imaging. They were also asked about their clinical management such as the frequency of discussion about lifestyle factors with patients, the frequency of treating patients with various conditions, a range of patient sub-groups and a list of techniques/methods used in patient care. Moreover, this questionnaire include research engagement related items such as the referral rights of osteopaths, the understanding of osteopathy research findings and the relationship between research evidence and clinical practice.

Outputs and success to date

At the time of writing, the ORION PBRN has to date produced an initial baseline workforce manuscript (Adams *et al.*, 2018a) outlining the most comprehensive osteopathy workforce analysis for many years in Australia. Another seven baseline secondary analysis papers are currently in various stages of preparation, submission and journal review. Moreover, with a view to helping grow sustainable osteopathy research in Australia (and in connection with osteopathy researchers beyond Australia), the ORION PBRN has been fortunate enough to date to attract interest from researchers and practitioners across Australia, the UK, Sweden and the US. Three sub-studies are currently in train with one having successfully completed primary data collection, another preparing to collect data and a third at the design and preparation stage. A prime objective of the Osteopathy Australia — UTS:ARCCIM partnership around ORION is to generate interest, coordination, collaboration and capacity among Australian universities that house osteopathy undergraduate programs (RMIT University, Victoria University and Southern Cross University) and it is encouraging to report that both secondary analysis of baseline ORION practitioner data and development of sub-study primary data has already involved engagement from a number of osteopathy researchers representing these institutions. Further collaborations are planned for the clinical interest groups housed at Osteopathy Australia including sports science and paediatrics groups with regard to designing and developing further sub-studies in core areas of daily routine care.

The Practitioner Research and Collaboration Initiative (PRACI) PBRN

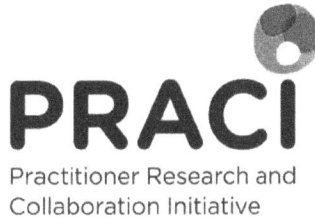

PRACI
Practitioner Research and
Collaboration Initiative

History

In 2014, Endeavour College of Natural Health chose to finance the establishment of a multimodal complementary medicine PBRN as this infrastructure was identified by the institution's leadership as an important and useful instrument to facilitate ongoing research within profession's that align with the College's graduate programs. The logistics of conducting research in disparate professions such as those considered TCIM are challenging, particularly where there is a small number of clinicians, and where the professional infrastructure in place does not support cohesion among the practitioner community. For many complementary medicine professions in Australia, one of the significant outcomes of such fracturing is that most professional associations (often competing for membership in the same profession) do not have sufficient funding to extend beyond basic operational functions. When combined with a low level of research engagement among the professional leadership the ability to build a PBRN for most complementary medicine professions has always been limited. For these reasons, Endeavour funded and led the development of the Practitioner Research and Collaboration Initiative (PRACI) (Steel *et al.*, 2014).

The effective establishment of PRACI required the research team to establish communication, trust and engagement with the wider TCIM practitioner community. Given the fractured nature of many TCIM practitioner communities in Australia, the research team needed to establish relationships with numerous professional bodies and other commercial organizations. The initiative was supported by many of these organizations, although some larger associations such as the Australian Traditional Medicine Society and Australian Natural Therapists Association did not agree to assist with recruiting clinicians for PRACI from their membership base. For this reason, the support of commercial companies with a customer base drawn primarily from CM practitioners were also key to PRACI recruitment and, along with other the practitioner associations, ensured our PRACI members were representative of the wider clinician community (Steel *et al.*, 2017).

Design

PRACI was designed to be as flexible as possible in response to the diversity of individual clinical practice models within and between the target professions. All clinicians who identified as holding a qualification in any one of fourteen TCIM professions (see Table 1) were invited to register with PRACI. Interested clinicians were asked to complete a two-phase baseline survey. The first survey collected data about clinician and practice characteristics including locality, qualifications, areas of special clinical interest and patient throughput. A follow up survey was then

Table 1.   Professions included in the Practitioner Research and Collaboration Initiative.

Acupuncturists	Massage therapists
Aromatherapists	Musculoskeletal therapists Myotherapists
Ayurveda practitioners	Naturopaths
Bowen therapists	Nutritionists (non-dietetic)
Chinese herbalists	Reflexologists
Homeopaths	Western herbalists
Kinesiologists	Yoga teachers

administered to all PRACI members with profession-specific questions based on four different professional categories (i.e. manual therapies, Ayurveda, ingestive medicines, Traditional Chinese medicine). These second phase surveys collected more detailed information about practice patterns and clinical approach based on the different professional categories. The data from both survey phases were then collated to enable researchers to conduct sub-studies that target defined clinician sample populations (e.g. acupuncturists with a special interest in women's health; clinicians in rural settings who see more than ten patients per week) as appropriate to the intended research question.

Recruitment for PRACI occurred in two rounds with the first round in 2015 and a second round in 2017.

Overview of PRACI membership

Following both PRACI recruitment rounds, PRACI membership now includes 124 acupuncturists, 74 aromatherapists, 12 Ayurveda practitioners, 81 Bowen therapists, 66 Chinese herbalists, 71 homeopaths, 46 kinesiologists, 601 massage therapists, 111 musculoskeletal therapists/ myotherapists, 281 naturopaths, 158 nutritionists, 128 reflexologists, 129 Western herbalists and 41 yoga teachers. While some practitioners may be qualified in more than one profession, there are a total of 1054 clinicians registered with PRACI across all fourteen professions making this PBRN the most diverse, nationally-representative complementary health care PBRN in the world.

Outputs and success to date

Since its opening for sub-studies in 2016, 10 sub-studies have been conducted through PRACI. In addition to the four manuscripts reporting aspects of the development of PRACI (Reid and Steel, 2015; Steel *et al.*, 2014, 2017, 2018), PRACI sub-study results have also been published (Fisher *et al.*, 2018; Leech *et al.*, 2018; Yang *et al.*, 2018) and presented at national and international conferences. Most recently, the PRACI PBRN was presented at the North American Primary Care Research Group PBRN Conference in Washington D.C.

ORC-NZ & AMRIT UK

Following the success of PRACI, ACORN and ORION, the PBRN design and model (as designed and implemented by UTS:ARCCIM) has attracted interest from similar professional bodies beyond Australia. At time of writing, UTS:ARCCIM is currently developing two other PBRNS — one with Osteopaths New Zealand (ONZ) and another with the Ayurvedic Practitioners Assoiation (APA), UK. These two PBRNS — Osteopathy Research Connect New Zealand (ORC-NZ) and AMRIT, respectively, — follow similar aims, designs and anticipated outcomes as the ACORN, ORION and PRACI PBRNs. While being significantly smaller in their membership numbers (ranging from approximately 200–500 practitioner members) they are both nevertheless national in their coverage and represent a once-in-a-generation opportunity to advance the research capacity and evidence-base for their respective professions in their particular jurisdictions.

Extending Insights via more TCIM PBRNs

With regards to a number of key aspects and features, the TCIM-focused PBRN scholarship developed to date has been world-leading — producing practitioner databases with some of the largest representation of national professional total populations ever recorded in the field and incorporating cutting-edge techniques and tools to help improve the quality of PBRN designs and outputs.

Yet, PBRN work remains underdeveloped in the TCIM field. As this chapter has identified there is plenty of opportunity for many more TCIM PBRNs to be established and for much more TCIM-focused PBRN work to be undertaken. Obvious gaps in this sub-field of TCIM research well positioned for immediate attention group around different TCIM professions and jurisdictions. While PRACI and the other PBRNs outlined in this chapter focus upon a selected number of professions across certain countries, a vast range of TCIM modalities and their respective health systems have not yet attracted PBRN attention.

Addressing these gaps in PBRN research requires substantial investment of time and support from professional associations, practitioners, patients and researchers — we should be careful not to underestimate the effort and drive necessary to not only establish but also maintain a viable PBRN — challenges further exacerbated amid efforts to conduct nationwide and nationally-representative PBRNs. Nevertheless, despite these difficulties it is clear that PBRNs hold much potential for TCIM helping to serve the research community, practitioner base and patient body in unique ways and with an unswerving dedication to collaboration and fostering overdue connection between the research and practice agenda of TCIM.

References

Abrams, D. I., Dolor, R., Roberts, R., Pechura, C., Dusek, J., Amoils, S., Guarneri, E. (2013). The BraveNet prospective observational study on integrative medicine treatment approaches for pain. *BMC Complementary and Alternative Medicine*, *13*(1), 146.

Adams, J. (ed.), (2007). *Researching Complementary and Alternative Medicine*. Routledge.

Adams, J., Steel, A., Chang, S., Sibbritt, D. (2015). Helping address the national research and research capacity needs of Australian chiropractic: Introducing the Australian Chiropractic Research Network (ACORN) project. *Chiropractic and Manual Therapies*, *23*(1), 12.

Adams, J., Steel, A., Moore, C., Amorin-Woods, L., Sibbritt, D. (2016). Establishing the ACORN national practitioner database: Strategies to recruit practitioners to a national Practice-Based Research Network. *Journal of Manipulative and Physiological Therapeutics*, *39*(8), 594–602.

Adams, J., Peng, W., Steel, A., Lauche, R., Moore, C., Amorin-Woods, L., Sibbritt, D. (2017a). A cross-sectional examination of the profile of chiropractors recruited to the Australian chiropractic research network (ACORN): A sustainable resource for future chiropractic research. *BMJ Open*, *7*(9), e015830.

Adams, J., Lauche, R., Peng, W., Steel, A., Moore, C., Amorin-Woods, L. G., Sibbritt, D. (2017b). A workforce survey of Australian chiropractic: The profile and practice features of a nationally representative sample of 2,005 chiropractors. *BMC Complementary And Alternative Medicine*, *17*(1), 14.

Adams, J., Sibbritt, D., Steel, A., Peng, W. (2018a). A workforce survey of Australian osteopathy: Analysis of a nationally-representative sample of osteopaths from the Osteopathy Research and Innovation Network (ORION) project. *BMC Health Services Research*, *18*(1), 352.

Adams, J., de Luca, K., Swain, M., Funabashi, M., Wong, A., Pagé, I., Sibbritt, D., Peng, W. (2018b). Prevalence and practice characteristics of urban and rural/remote Australian chiropractors: Analysis of a nationally-representative sample of 1,830 chiropractors. *Australian Journal of Rural Health* (In press).

Adams, J., Lauche, R., de Luca, K., Swain, M., Peng, W., Sibbritt, D. (2018c). Prevalence and profile of Australian chiropractors treating athletes or sports people: A cross-sectional study. *Complementary Therapies in Medicine*, *39*, 56–61.

Agency for Healthcare Research and Quality (2018). Practice-based Research Networks: Research in everyday practice. https://pbrn.ahrq.gov/pbrn-registry, Accessed on 17 July 2018.

Amorin-Woods, L. G., Moore, C., Adams, J. (2018). How does a practice-based research network facilitate evidence-informed practice within the chiropractic profession in Australia? A commentary. *Chiropractic Journal of Australia*, *46*(2), 173–185.

Breckenridge, J. P., Gianfrancesco, C., de Zoysa, N., Lawton, J., Rankin, D., Coates, E. (2018). Mobilising knowledge between practitioners and researchers to iteratively refine a complex intervention (DAFNE plus) pre-trial: Protocol for a structured, collaborative working group process. *Pilot and Feasibility Studies*, *4*(1), 120.

Davis, M. M., Keller, S., DeVoe, J. E., Cohen, D. J. (2012). Characteristics and lessons learned from practice-based research networks (PBRNs) in the United States. *Journal of Healthcare Leadership*, *4*, 107.

Degenhardt, B. F., Johnson, J. C., Gross, S. R., Hagan, C., Lund, G., Curry, W. J. (2014). Preliminary findings on the use of osteopathic manipulative treatment: Outcomes during the formation of the practice-based research network,

DO-Touch.NET. *The Journal of the American Osteopathic Association*, *114*(3), 154–170.

Fisher, C., Adams, J., Frawley, J., Hickman, L., Sibbritt, D. (2018). Western herbal medicine consultations for common menstrual problems; practitioner experiences and perceptions of treatment. *Phytotherapy Research*, *32*(3), 531–541.

Flannery, M. A., Love, M. M., Pearce, K. A., Luan, J., Elder, W. G. (2006). Communication about complementary and alternative medicine: Perspectives of primary care clinicians. *Alternative Therapies in Health and Medicine*, *12*(1), 56–63.

Graham, D. G., Spano, M. S., Stewart, T. V., Staton, E. W., Meers, A., Pace, W. D. (2007). Strategies for planning and launching PBRN research studies: A project of the Academy of Family Physicians National Research Network (AAFP NRN). *The Journal of the American Board of Family Medicine*, *20*(2), 220–228.

Green, L. A., White, L. L., Barry, H. C., Nease, D. E., Hudson, B. L. (2005). Infrastructure requirements for practice-based research networks. *The Annals of Family Medicine*, *3*(suppl 1), S5–S11.

Hawk, C., Long, C. R., Boulanger, K. T. (2001). Prevalence of nonmusculoskeletal complaints in chiropractic practice: Report from a practice based research program. *Journal of Manipulative and Physiological Therapeutics*, *24*(3), 157–169.

Lee, M. K., Amorin-Woods, L., Cascioli, V., Adams, J. (2018). The use of nutritional guidance within chiropractic patient management: A survey of 333 chiropractors from the ACORN practice-based research network. *Chiropractic and Manual Therapies*, *26*(1), 7.

Leech, B., Schloss, J., Steel, A. (2018). Investigation into complementary and integrative medicine practitioners' clinical experience of intestinal permeability: A cross-sectional survey. *Complementary Therapies in Clinical Practice*, *31*, 200–209.

Licciardone, J. C., Kearns, C. M., King, H. H., Seffinger, M. A., Crow, W. T., Zajac, P., Devine, W. H., Abu-Sbaih, R. Y., Miller, S. J., Berkowitz, M. R., Dyer, R. (2014). Somatic dysfunction and use of osteopathic manual treatment techniques during ambulatory medical care visits: A CONCORD-PBRN study. *The Journal of the American Osteopathic Association*, *114*(5), 344–354.

Lindbloom, E. J., Ewigman, B. G., Hickner, J. M. (2004). Practice-based research networks: the laboratories of primary care research. *Medical Care*, *42*(4), III-45.

Mold, J. W., Peterson, K. A. (2005). Primary care practice-based research networks: Working at the interface between research and quality improvement. *The Annals of Family Medicine*, *3*(suppl 1), S12–S20.

Moore, C., Adams, J., Leaver, A., Lauche, R., Sibbritt, D. (2017). The treatment of migraine patients within chiropractic: Analysis of a nationally representative survey of 1869 chiropractors. *BMC Complementary and Alternative Medicine*, *17*(1), 519.

Paterson, C. (2007). Involving consumers in CAM research. In Adams, J. (Ed.), *Researching Complementary and Alternative Medicine*. Routledge, London.

Peterson, K. A., Lipman, P. D., Lange, C. J., Cohen, R. A., Durako, S. (2012). Supporting better science in primary care: A description of practice-based research networks (PBRNs) in 2011. *The Journal of the American Board of Family Medicine*, *25*(5), 565–571.

Reid, R., Steel, A. (2015). The importance of the PRACI project for grass roots complementary medicine practice: A call for practitioner involvement. *Australian Journal of Herbal Medicine*, *27*(3), 101.

Riley-Behringer, M., Davis, M. M., Werner, J. J., Fagnan, L. J., Stange, K. C. (2017). The evolving collaborative relationship between Practice-Based Research Networks (PBRNs) and Clinical and Translational Science Awardees (CTSAs). *Journal of Clinical and Translational Science*, *1*(5), 301–309.

Rycroft-Malone, J., Burton, C. R., Bucknall, T., Graham, I. D., Hutchinson, A. M., Stacey, D. (2016). Collaboration and co-production of knowledge in healthcare: Opportunities and challenges. *International Journal of Health Policy and Management*, *5*(4), 221.

Shelley, B. M., Sussman, A. L., Williams, R. L., Segal, A. R., Crabtree, B. F. (2009). 'They don't ask me so I don't tell them': Patient–clinician communication about traditional, complementary, and alternative medicine. *The Annals of Family Medicine*, *7*(2), 139–147.

Sleath, B., Callahan, L., Vellis, R. F. D., Sloane, P. D. (2005). Patients' perceptions of primary care physicians' participatory decision-making style and communication about complementary and alternative medicine for arthritis. *The Journal of Alternative and Complementary Medicine*, *11*(3), 449–453.

Steel, A., Adams, J., Sibbritt, D. (2014). Developing a multi-modality complementary medicine practice-based research network: The PRACI project. *Advances in Integrative Medicine*, *1*(3), 113–118.

Steel, A., Leach, M., Wardle, J., Sibbritt, D., Schloss, J., Diezel, H., Adams, J. (2018). The Australian complementary medicine workforce: A profile of

1,306 practitioners from the PRACI study. *The Journal of Alternative and Complementary Medicine*, *24*(4), 385–394.

Steel, A., Rapport, F., Adams, J. (2018). Towards an implementation science of complementary health care: Some initial considerations for guiding safe, effective clinical decision-making. *Advances in Integrative Medicine*, *5*(1), 5–8.

Steel, A., Sibbritt, D., Schloss, J., Wardle, J., Leach, M., Diezel, H., Adams, J. (2017). An Overview of the Practitioner Research and Collaboration Initiative (PRACI): a practice-based research network for complementary medicine. *BMC Complementary and Alternative Medicine*, *17*(1), 87.

Thomas, P., Griffiths, F., Kai, J., O'dwyer, A. (2001). Networks for research in primary health care. *British Medical Journal*, *322*(7286), 588–590.

Veziari, Y., Leach, M. J., Kumar, S. (2017). Barriers to the conduct and application of research in complementary and alternative medicine: A systematic review. *BMC Complementary and Alternative Medicine*, *17*(1), 166.

Wardle, J., Adams, J. (2013). Are the CAM professions engaging in high-level health and medical research? Trends in publicly funded complementary medicine research grants in Australia. *Complementary Therapies in Medicine*, *21*(6), 746–749.

Wolever, R. Q., Abrams, D. I., Kligler, B., Dusek, J. A., Roberts, R., Frye, J., Edman, J. S., Amoils, S., Pradhan, E., Spar, M., Gaudet, T., Guarneri, E., Homel, P., Amoils, S., Lee, R. A., Berman, B., Monti, D. A., Dolor, R. (2012). Patients seek integrative medicine for preventive approach to optimize health. *Explore: The Journal of Science and Healing*, *8*(6), 348–352.

Yang, L., Peng, W., Adams, J., Sibbritt, D. W. (2018). Treating people with arthritis with traditional Chinese medicine (TCM): An examination of the perception of TCM practitioners. *Acupuncture in Medicine*, acupmed-2017.

Chapter 6

A Holistic Approach to Implementation Science (IS): Broadening the IS Gaze to Traditional, Complementary and Integrative Medicine

Jon Adams, Amie Steel and Rebecca Reid

'If translational research is the answer, what's the question? Who gets to ask it?'

(Wandersman *et al.*, 2012)

Introduction

This is an era where quality health care service delivery is expected to prioritise paradigms that may not always be in alignment with each other, such as evidence-based medicine (EBM) and patient-centred care. It is challenging for most health professionals to navigate these tensions, and traditional, complementary and integrative medicine (TCIM) clinicians are no different. This chapter will overview the recently established field of implementation science (IS) and the role it plays in the delivery of evidence-based medicine across all aspects of health care including

TCIM. It will also identify aspects of TCIM which provide an opportunity for IS to expand and deepen its impact on evidence-based health service delivery.

History and Advancement of Implementation Science

The vision behind the EBM movement as first framed by Guyatt *et al.* (1992) was noble — to create a health care system in which the community receive care informed by best available evidence. The first iteration of the model as laid out by Guyatt and colleagues met with criticism suggesting the focus on research evidence was at the expense of clinical practice reality (Shahar, 1998). In response, the EBM model was adapted to more clearly account for the importance of patient preferences and clinician experience within the application of evidence in a clinical setting (Sackett *et al.*, 1996). Nevertheless, even following such amendments the operationalization of the EBM vision remained significantly problematic. The gap between published research evidence and daily routine care remained significant and any attempt to bridge the divide required dedicated consideration not previously undertaken — the resulting consideration lay the foundations for the field of IS (Dearing and Kee, 2012).

IS can be defined as the study of methods to promote the integration of research findings and evidence into health care policy and practice (Dearing and Kee, 2012). One important component of IS in health is knowledge translation (KT), which concentrates on the synthesis, exchange and application of knowledge by relevant stakeholders (World Health Organization, 2006) including, but not limited to, health practitioners. So, while KT focuses on influencing a change in practice behaviour based on new knowledge, IS offers research methodology to explore, plan, execute and evaluate KT. In the context of KT, there are a number of significant challenges limiting the application of best evidence in clinical decision-making. The IS field has shifted over recent years from a focus upon individual practitioner decision-making (Bero *et al.*, 1998) to a consideration of professional cultures and organizational structures and policies (Gagnon *et al.*, 2014). Meanwhile, it is increasingly acknowledged that a diverse number of factors and contexts have a bearing upon the wider process of KT and implementation. One core area that requires consideration relates directly to the issues of *awareness*, *acceptance* and *adoption* of new knowledge by health care practitioners (Green and Seifert, 2005). Within the context of clinical practice, this means clinicians must have *awareness* of new knowledge before it can be a basis for a change in practice. They must then *accept* this new knowledge as accurate and relevant to their practice and patients before they can agree to *adopt* a new behaviour within their own clinical approach.

Of late, IR in health has broadened its focus to include, for example, health promotion issues (Dobbins and Traynor, 2015) and there is literature that argues for the need to diversify use of perspectives and methods (Wandersman *et al.*, 2012) and consider insights from grassroots stakeholders (Rycroft-Malone *et al.*, 2013). Knowledge mobilization (KM) is an approach within IS which seeks to address the complexities of KT by acknowledging diversity in the types of knowledge which may influence health care and health choices, and ensuring this diversity is respected (Cooper and Levin, 2010). KM acknowledges different stakeholders' values and emphasizes sharing knowledge between parties for better health outcomes overall (Cooper and Levin, 2010). KM recognizes the paternalism inherent in KT whereby the researcher is viewed as generating all knowledge of value and the clinician is a vessel who can receive that knowledge to inform their clinical decisions which their patients will accept and follow without question (Kislov *et al.*, 2014).

However, signifying its origins within the mainstream clinical science paradigm and its overriding concern to translate evidence-based medicine (EBM) into daily routine practice (Hutton *et al.*, 2008; Nilsen, 2015), IS in health remains almost exclusively: driven by clinical medical perspectives and a 'top-down' approach to behaviour change (preoccupied with a limited notion of evidence and efficacy at the expense of patient needs, perspectives and input); emphasising the 'gold standard' trial design and experimental/quasi-experimental design (thereby attempting to control or negate the influence of the cultural/social and denying or side-lining the importance and relevance of qualitative, culturally-sensitive methods); focused on conventional medical settings, which are frequently well-defined and clearly-demarcated sites such as hospitals, thus neglecting investigation of community-based, informal practice and health-seeking; and focused upon health professionals as core or even sole agents of change (diminishing the appreciation of patient agency in health behaviour and decision-making and, again, neglecting patient needs and perspectives).

Opportunities for IS and TCIM

While IS has arisen from the EBM movement and has focused on mainstream health services, researchers have recently begun to extend the lens of IS to include traditional, complementary and integrative medicine (TCIM) (Steel *et al.*, 2018b). In doing so, a number of challenges and opportunities surrounding the IS of TCIM have come to light. For example, the diversity of training, scope and philosophies associated with the professions within the broad church of TCIM presents challenges to IS researchers in that novel IS interventions must be customised to the specific needs of a profession rather than approaching TCIM as a 'uniform entity' (Steel *et al.*, 2018). It is worth noting here that 'traditional', 'complementary' and 'integrative' medicine all share core features and often overlap in many areas, yet are distinct categories unto themselves. For the purposes of this chapter, all three will be discussed together. However as each is distinct there may be some points raised which do not relate directly to all three.

Current research shows TCIM practitioners are an increasingly important component of people's overall approach to managing health complaints (Dubois *et al.*, 2017; Gall *et al.*, 2018; Reid *et al.*, 2016) and that they draw upon a mixture of both professional and lay information sources in their information-seeking (Frawley *et al.*, 2014; Geisler and Cheung, 2015; Murthy *et al.*, 2017). Meanwhile, the clinical evidence for different informal TCIM practitioner procedures varies greatly between conditions of global importance such as cancer (Bao *et al.*, 2014), diabetes (Medagama and Bandara, 2014), and pain management (Close *et al.*, 2014) and many evidence gaps remain. Indeed, there are specific sites of ambiguity as to efficacy, benefit and risk within and across the different TCIM provider treatments and these ambiguities inevitably shape both practitioner and patient experiences and the subsequent decision-making around treatment choice (Dowell *et al.*, 2018; Steel and Adams, 2011a, 2011b).

Yet, beyond the innovative but limited work on this topic to date, we still know very little about the cultural/social terrain of TCIM care, especially with regard to stakeholders' prioritizing, evaluating and authenticating available TCIM clinician treatments. This is despite the potential of TCIM provider use to fundamentally recast roles and experiences for those with chronic disease (holding potential to concurrently both challenge and enable better care and health outcomes) (Adams *et al.*, 2018). Addressing this significant research gap provides a rich sociological platform upon which to build meaningful and successful translation design and strategies for helping guide person-centred, safe and effective care. Given there has been very little research examining the design and testing of translational strategies and tools regarding informal health care and use (beyond a hospital setting) (Steel *et al.*, 2018), the study of IS in TCIM holds real potential to guide community-based practices to advance a broad evidence-base for policy, practice and engagement in the area of TCIM.

In particular, TCIM offers an opportunity to more deeply explore KM. TCIM clinicians acknowledge the value of different types of knowledge to inform their clinical decision-making. Intuition, for example, is described by some clinicians as a useful tool to direct aspects of clinical care (Steel and Adams, 2011b). Equally, the insights and experience of previous clinicians as passed down through oral or written language — here referred to as traditional knowledge — is also held in high regard in TCIM (Jagtenberg *et al.*, 2006). Even the patient's embodied experience of their own health and the life course of their condition is considered valuable by TCIM practitioners as they seek to interpret and treat the individualized presentation of the health complaint (Foley and Steel, 2017b; Wardle and Seely, 2007). Alongside these views on alternative sources of knowledge and wisdom are issues raised by members of TCIM clinical communities about the impact of EBM paradigmatic perspectives on the ability for the retention, respect and ongoing use of these types of knowledge (Jagtenberg *et al.*, 2006; Wardle and Seely, 2007).

In tandem with the rising interest and attempts at applying EBM in all clinical settings, there has been increasing awareness and pressure from within social, political and clinical groups for contemporary health care to become more person-centred (Epstein *et al.*, 2010). As such, recent years have seen slow developments in the way the EBM model is being interpreted and applied (Miles and Loughlin, 2011; Olsson *et al.*, 2013). This is particularly the case in arenas where research end-users such as policymakers and clinicians recognize that while the experimental RCT design still provides important insights to the efficacy of treatments in laboratory settings, there are limitations to using findings from RCTs as a source of knowledge to inform complex person-centred clinical care (Porzsolt *et al.*, 2015; Tunis *et al.*, 2003). These concerns are not limited to TCIM but are equally as relevant to TCIM (Verhoef *et al.*, 2005), and may perhaps be even more so given the TCIM philosophical focus on individualized treatments (Foley and Steel, 2017a).

Within this context, the scholarship of IS within TCIM offers a number of opportunities for both areas of study. The remained of this chapter examines some of these opportunities through the lens of the three pillars of EBM: research evidence; patient perspective; and clinician experience.

Emphasis on New Approaches to Advancing Clinical Research

As a result of its roots in the EBM movement, there has been a hierarchy of research evidence that has been historically applied within IS (Evans, 2003). The randomized clinical trial (RCT) was held as the 'gold standard' of evidence, particularly when the results of multiple RCTs were synthesized through meta-analysis or across multiple sites (Evans, 2003). However, the RCT design has been since described as deficient in providing useful answers to inform clinical decisions within real-life settings (Godwin *et al.*, 2003). The perceived weaknesses of RCTs have been identified both within conventional health care (Brass, 2010; Tunis *et al.*, 2003) and TCIM (Verhoef *et al.*, 2002, 2005).

With this in mind, the clinical research community developed new research designs which acknowledged and accommodated the complexities of clinical practice, particularly within the context of the growing influence of policies supporting the delivery of person-centred care (Tunis *et al.*, 2003). Most notably, pragmatic clinical research designs were established with researchers developing the pragmatic-explanatory continuum indicator summary (PRECIS) tool to offer some rigour to researchers seeking to conduct clinical research which more closely matched the way care was delivered in the real world (Thorpe *et al.*, 2009). Comparative effectiveness research evolved as a facet of pragmatic research whereby an intervention was compared with another available active treatment for the condition of interest rather than an inactive substance (placebo) (Luce *et al.*, 2009; Tunis *et al.*, 2010).

In tandem with these advancements in research design, the TCIM research community began exploring their own changes to the prevailing RCT methodologies to address the perceived limitations of the RCT design (Verhoef *et al.*, 2002). The proposed solution — titled 'Whole Systems Research' (WSR) — was presented as a rigorous method for examining TCIM practice in a manner that respected the underpinning philosophies and principles of TCIM approaches to care (Verhoef *et al.*, 2005). In practice, WSR is a variation of the pragmatic clinical research design developed within conventional health research, but whereas pragmatic clinical research methodology was constructed through the lens of single interventions (e.g. drug trials), the WSR approach allowed for individualized care employing a personalized selections of multimodal treatment options. This point of difference is becoming less noticeable as leading conventional health research institutes emphasize the importance of building patient-centred care into interventions which can be studied through pragmatic and comparative effectiveness trials (Basch *et al.*, 2012). Meanwhile, the rhetoric of WSR within TCIM has not resulted in a substantial amount of WSR research output and it is possible that using different lexicon to describe the same methodology may have created a barrier to attracting funding and support from those outside of TCIM.

The advances in clinical research methodology as outlined in this section have direct impact on IS. There is growing interest and preference within IS research to draw on results from pragmatic clinical studies and to employ pragmatic research designs when evaluating the impact of IS interventions (Glasgow *et al.*, 2012). The health research community have even acknowledged the value of research approaches such as WSR by defining guidelines for robust reporting of complex interventions (Hoffmann *et al.*, 2014). Similarly, government agencies and researchers are providing structured recommendations for the appropriate inclusion of patient representatives in research teams (Institute, P.C.O.R., 2018; National Health Service, 2018; Staniszewska *et al.*, 2011).

Overall, the available clinical research methodology has advanced significantly since the first iteration of the EBM model, in part due to the challenges experienced by IS researchers and clinicians in implementing the findings of experimental RCTs. While TCIM has acknowledged the limitations of RCT design, the TCIM research community has been less effective in adopting and applying these newer clinical research methods and guidelines, perhaps seeking instead to focus on TCIM as its own methodological specialization (Oberg *et al.*, 2015; Verhoef *et al.*, 2005). However, recent work suggests TCIM researchers may be realising and addressing this gap (John, 2018; Steel *et al.*, 2017).

Emphasis on Patient Perspectives

International health policy has seen a growing emphasis on person-centred care — that which consciously adopts the perspectives of individuals and views them as participants as well as beneficiaries of care — in recent years (World Health Organization, 2018). While person-centred care has emerged as a growing concern to those designing, providing and evaluating health care and systems (McCormack and McCance, 2016), the patient's needs and experiences have, as yet, failed to truly translate into EBM and IS. The impact of the policy-driven push for delivery of person-centred care is also seen in research initiatives within and beyond IS. In fact, there is a growing emphasis, and in some countries a requirement, to include patient representatives during the full life cycle of a research project (from design through to implementation and interpretation of findings) (Shippee *et al.*, 2015). This approach it is argued ensures evidence-based health care is culturally and socially relevant to the individuals who will be using the treatment (Haywood *et al.*, 2015). Indeed, the IS field in health has failed to place rich, in-depth understandings of patient experience, needs and perspectives central to developing and evaluating different translational strategies and tools. As a result, IS researchers still relegate the role of the patient and community-based action to a secondary concern; interpret evidence for decision-making and practice in narrow clinical research terms (following EBM) congruent with biomedicine/biomedical practitioners; and neglect or, at best, play down the conceptual consideration and empirical investigation of the social and cultural as fringe 'add-ons' (Shoveller *et al.*, 2016).

In contrast to the challenges experienced by IS researchers attempting to accommodate patient perspectives, one of the defining characteristics of much TCIM is the person-centred principles underpinning care (Foley and Steel, 2017a). This characteristic of TCIM has been described as a 'pull factor' in that it attracts individuals to use TCIM (Foley and Steel, 2017b). In fact, much of TCIM use in the community is largely patient-led, with individuals actively choosing TCIM (Wye *et al.*, 2009) and reporting experiencing a sense of empowerment as a result of their TCIM use (Foley and Steel, 2017b). A recent study of TCIM users across a number of TCIM professions confirmed that clinicians deliver care which patients experience as person-centred and empowering (Foley and Steel, 2017c). Other research has also explored TCIM clinicians' perceptions of clinical evidence and found patient's own experience of their condition was an important source of knowledge which was used by the practitioner to inform clinical decision-making (Steel and Adams, 2011a, 2011b).

Within the context of IS and KM, TCIM may provide an opportunity for researchers to better understand and explore different perceptions of evidence and knowledge from the patients perspective. Through TCIM, IS researchers may be able to extend the current emphasis on patient-reported outcome measures to find novel ways to mobilize the embodied knowledge of patients and use that knowledge to inform not only clinical decision-making but also future clinical research. As already mentioned, this process may have begun through participatory research design. However, TCIM clinical consultation approaches could be employed through the lens of IS to extend current practices by respectfully acknowledging patient perspectives as a legitimate source of knowledge and evidence.

Emphasis on Clinician Experience

In alignment with the importance of understanding patient's experience within the EBM model and IS research, is the value of clinical expertise and experience from TCIM clinicians in grassroots practice. Within EBM, clinician experiences and expertise display as equal elements alongside patient preferences and research evidence (Haynes *et al.*, 2002) and constitute a crucial pillar within the EBM framework. Essentially, clinical experience is deeply rooted in the clinical knowledge, clinical skills and expert opinions of clinicians (Wieten, 2018), which is continually informed by the progression of research findings and through the process of assessing clinical observations (Wyer and Silva, 2009). While clinicians are well adept in their professional area of expertise and hold a wealth of learnt and tacit knowledge implemented in clinical practice, the wisdom that clinicians develop through integration of traditional and scientific knowledge with observation of patients is an underutilized resource within an EBM-driven model of IS. This is particularly the case within IS where the predominant focus has been translation of evidence-based findings into clinical decision-making.

While the transfer of new research into clinical practice, or evidence-informed practice, is undoubtedly an important outcome of IS, there is also an opportunity for IS methods to be used to translate clinical insights into future research, or practice-informed evidence. For this bi-directional translation to occur effectively, researchers need to employ, and in some cases develop, appropriate research designs that capture clinical wisdom and insights. In some instances, IS researchers may choose to simply engage clinicians actively in an iterative research engagement cycle during the piloting of a clinical study to ensure the final proposed intervention is informed by the direct clinical experience (Breckenridge *et al.*, 2018).

In other circumstances, IS researchers may be better placed to employ rigorous research methods designed to capture novel clinical insights in order to inform future clinical research. Such research designs may simply include surveys of clinicians' experience of managing a specific health condition and document clinical observations of the effect of treatment, value of tests, or relationship between the condition of interest and concomitant conditions (Leech *et al.*, 2018b). Delphi methods may also be employed to develop consensus among clinicians on important topics associated with their area of expertise (Hawk *et al.*, 2012; Hill *et al.*, 2016; Leaver *et al.*, 2013). Such approaches to employing IS for advancing practice-informed research has particular value in TCIM where clinicians often draw on deductive reasoning to link contemporary research with traditional knowledge to explore new possible treatment approaches (Steel and Adams, 2011a). Equally, the holistic, multisystem viewpoint of many TCIM professions may provide valuable insights into the aetiology or pathophysiology of health problems which only receive superficial examination within biomedicine (Leech *et al.*, 2018a). These are only two examples of several research designs appropriate for ensuring clinical insights and experience are captured and IS methods are effectively employed to mobilize clinical knowledge and wisdom.

A further complication within the IS landscape of TCIM is the significant influence of traditional evidence. Traditional evidence is considered a foundational aspect to TCIM, and is often relied upon in clinical practice to inform clinical decisions (Leach and Gillham, 2011). However, its use in scientific research is undervalued. Traditional knowledge is often lost, disregarded, or receives limited attention from researchers restricting its inclusion in robust, rigorous research. Considering its foundational position in TCIM, traditional knowledge can contribute to informing research and clinical practice through a cyclic process involving research being conducted by or with clinicians, and employing IS to manifest the outcomes of such research back into clinical practice. Engaging with clinicians and their traditional knowledge as a legitimate source of evidence can assist in formalising a rigorous process to assess the many facets of traditional evidence. Undertaking research which incorporates or centres on traditional knowledge sources in such a manner will ensure that findings are easily translatable and implemented into clinical practice at the grassroots level with direct and valued input from clinicians.

In addition, the texts where TCIM traditional knowledge may be documented is commonly overlooked by researchers or at best relegated to an interesting artefact which provides context to the contemporary research designs being used. Yet, these same texts are an important source of information within TCIM practice and educational curriculum (Steel and Adams, 2011a; Steel *et al.*, 2018). Traditional texts contain a vast volume of knowledge that has been developed by those considered to be founders of TCIM, and has been a continued source of reference by clinicians in their assessment of treatment interventions thus informing clinical knowledge and practice (Steel and Adams, 2011b). However, its importance in research is overlooked. IS researchers are well placed to work with TCIM clinicians to develop robust processes of critical appraisal to support appropriate use of traditional texts as legitimate sources of evidence. Equally, through the incorporation of traditional texts in future research projects, IS researchers are well placed to assist TCIM clinicians in the appropriate preservation of much of the wisdom that arises from traditional knowledge sources. IS also has the capacity, by employing the methodologies of de-implementation, to help TCIM clinicians identify traditional treatments that are less effective and/or are no longer relevant in contemporary health service contexts.

Conclusion

IS and TCIM have much to gain and learn from the other. To date, focusing primarily on conventional health care, IS has been somewhat contained in both focus and approach. Yet, TCIM provides an opportunity for IS to expand and deepen its engagement with other health care practices and as a consequence question and refine the pillars of the EBM model from which IS has arisen. IS also affords TCIM an opportunity to apply rigorous research methods to fundamental features of TCIM, thereby strengthening the role of TCIM clinical practice within contemporary health care settings. Both the engagement with IS among TCIM researchers and an interest in TCIM among those conducting IS are in their very early days, restricted at present to just a small number of studies and handful of researchers. Nevertheless, the relationship between IS and TCIM is one that cannot be ignored and if TCIM research is to increase (some may claim establish) its relevance and impact upon daily routine practice and health behaviour the adoption and adaptation of IS insights, models and techniques should be a priority for further scholarship.

References

Adams, J., Prior, J., Sibbritt, D., Connon, I. (2018). The use of self-care practices and products by women with chronic illness: A case study of older women with osteoarthritis and osteoporosis. In *Women's Health and Complementary and Integrative Medicine.* Routledge, New York, pp. 89–105.

Bao, Y., Kong, X., Yang, L., Liu, R., Shi, Z., Li, W., Hou, W. (2014). Complementary and alternative medicine for cancer pain: An overview of systematic reviews. *Evidence-Based Complementary and Alternative Medicine, 2014,* 1–9.

Basch, E., Aronson, N., Berg, A., Flum, D., Gabriel, S., Goodman, S. N., Meltzer, D. (2012). Methodological standards and patient-centeredness in comparative effectiveness research: The PCORI perspective. *Journal of the American Medical Association, 307*(15), 1636–1640.

Bero, L. A., Grilli, R., Grimshaw, J. M., Harvey, E., Oxman, A. D., Thomson, M. A. (1998). Closing the gap between research and practice: An overview of systematic reviews of interventions to promote the implementation of research findings. *BMJ, 317*(7156), 465–468.

Brass, E. (2010). The gap between clinical trials and clinical practice: The use of pragmatic clinical trials to inform regulatory decision making. *Clinical Pharmacology & Therapeutics, 87*(3), 351–355.

Breckenridge, J. P., Gianfrancesco, C., de Zoysa, N., Lawton, J., Rankin, D., Coates, E. (2018). Mobilising knowledge between practitioners and researchers to iteratively refine a complex intervention (DAFNE plus) pre-trial: Protocol for a structured, collaborative working group process. *Pilot and Feasibility Studies, 4*(1), 120.

Close, C., Sinclair, M., Liddle, S. D., Madden, E., McCullough, J. E., Hughes, C. (2014). A systematic review investigating the effectiveness of Complementary and Alternative Medicine (CAM) for the management of low back and/or pelvic pain (LBPP) in pregnancy. *Journal of Advanced Nursing, 70*(8), 1702–1716.

Cooper, A., Levin, B. (2010). Some Canadian contributions to understanding knowledge mobilisation. *Evidence & Policy: A Journal of Research, Debate and Practice, 6*(3), 351–369.

Dearing, J., Kee, K. (2012). Historical roots of dissemination and implementation science. In Brownson, R., Colditz, G. and Proctor, E. (eds.) *Dissemination and Implementation Research in Health: Translating Science to Practice,* Vol. 55, Oxford University Press, New York, pp. 47–61.

Dobbins, M., Traynor, R. (2015). *Engaging Public Health Decision Makers in Partnership Research.* Paper presented at the Implementation Science, *10*(1), A80.

Dowell, J., Williams, B., Snadden, D. (2018). *Patient-centered Prescribing: Seeking Concordance in Practice.* CRC Press, Florida.

Dubois, J., Scala, E., Faouzi, M., Decosterd, I., Burnand, B., Rodondi, P.-Y. (2017). Chronic low back pain patients' use of, level of knowledge of and perceived benefits of complementary medicine: A cross-sectional study at an academic pain center. *BMC Complementary and Alternative Medicine, 17*(1), 193.

Epstein, R. M., Fiscella, K., Lesser, C. S., Stange, K. C. (2010). Why the nation needs a policy push on patient-centered health care. *Health affairs, 29*(8), 1489–1495.

Evans, D. (2003). Hierarchy of evidence: A framework for ranking evidence evaluating healthcare interventions. *Journal of Clinical Nursing, 12*(1), 77–84.

Foley, H., Steel, A. (2017a). The nexus between patient-centered care and complementary medicine: Allies in the era of chronic disease? *The Journal of Alternative and Complementary Medicine, 23*(3), 158–163.

Foley, H., Steel, A. (2017b). Patient perceptions of clinical care in complementary medicine: A systematic review of the consultation experience. *Patient Education and Counseling, 100*(2), 212–223. doi:http://dx.doi.org/10.1016/j.pec.2016.09.015.

Foley, H., Steel, A. (2017c). Patient perceptions of patient-centred care, empathy and empowerment in complementary medicine clinical practice: A cross-sectional study. *Advances in Integrative Medicine, 4*(1), 22–30.

Frawley, J., Adams, J., Broom, A., Steel, A., Gallois, C., Sibbritt, D. (2014). Majority of women are influenced by nonprofessional information sources when deciding to consult a complementary and alternative medicine practitioner during pregnancy. *The Journal of Alternative and Complementary Medicine, 20*(7), 571–577.

Gagnon, M.-P., Attieh, R., Ghandour, E. K., Légaré, F., Ouimet, M., Estabrooks, C. A., Grimshaw, J. (2014). A systematic review of instruments to assess organizational readiness for knowledge translation in health care. *PloS One, 9*(12), e114338.

Gall, A., Leske, S., Adams, J., Matthews, V., Anderson, K., Lawler, S., Garvey, G. (2018). Traditional and complementary medicine use among indigenous cancer patients in Australia, Canada, New Zealand, and the United States: A systematic review. *Integrative Cancer Therapies*, 1534735418775821.

Geisler, C. C., Cheung, C. K. (2015). Complementary/alternative therapies use in older women with arthritis: Information sources and factors influencing dialog with health care providers. *Geriatric Nursing, 36*(1), 15–20.

Glasgow, R. E., Vinson, C., Chambers, D., Khoury, M. J., Kaplan, R. M., Hunter, C. (2012). National Institutes of Health approaches to dissemination and implementation science: current and future directions. *American Journal of Public Health, 102*(7), 1274–1281.

Godwin, M., Ruhland, L., Casson, I., MacDonald, S., Delva, D., Birtwhistle, R., Seguin, R. (2003). Pragmatic controlled clinical trials in primary care: the struggle between external and internal validity. *BMC Medical Research Methodology, 3*(1), 28.

Green, L. A., Seifert, C. M. (2005). Translation of research into practice: Why we can't "just do it". *The Journal of the American Board of Family Practice, 18*(6), 541–545.

Guyatt, G., Cairns, J., Churchill, D., Cook, D., Haynes, B., Hirsh, J., Irvine, J., Levine, M., Nishikawa, J., Sackett, D. (1992). Evidence-based medicine: A new approach to teaching the practice of medicine. *JAMA, 268*(17), 2420–2425.

Hawk, C., Schneider, M., Evans Jr., M. W., Redwood, D. (2012). Consensus process to develop a best-practice document on the role of chiropractic care in health promotion, disease prevention, and wellness. *Journal of Manipulative and Physiological Therapeutics, 35*(7), 556–567.

Haynes, R. B., Devereaux, P. J., Guyatt, G. H. (2002). Clinical expertise in the era of evidence-based medicine and patient choice. *Evidence Based Medicine, 7*(2), 36–38. doi:10.1136/ebm.7.2.36.

Haywood, K., Brett, J., Salek, S., Marlett, N., Penman, C., Shklarov, S., Staniszewska, S. (2015). Patient and public engagement in health-related quality of life and patient-reported outcomes research: What is important and why should we care? Findings from the first ISOQOL patient engagement symposium. *Quality of Life Research, 24*(5), 1069–1076.

Hill, J., Hodsdon, W., Schor, J., McKinney, N., Rubin, D., Seely, D., Lamson, D. (2016). Naturopathic oncology modified Delphi panel. *Integrative Cancer Therapies, 15*(1), 69–79.

Hoffmann, T. C., Glasziou, P. P., Boutron, I., Milne, R., Perera, R., Moher, D., Johnston, M. (2014). Better reporting of interventions: Template for intervention description and replication (TIDieR) checklist and guide. *BMJ, 348*, g1687.

Hutton, J. L., Eccles, M. P., Grimshaw, J. M. (2008). Ethical issues in implementation research: A discussion of the problems in achieving informed consent. *Implementation Science, 3*(1), 52.

Institute, P.-C. O. R. (2018). Initiative to Support Patient Involvement in Research (INSPIRE). https://www.pcori.org/research-results/2014/initiative-support-patient-involvement-research-inspire.

Jagtenberg, T., Evans, S., Grant, A., Howden, I., Lewis, M., Singer, J. (2006). Evidence-based medicine and naturopathy. *Journal of Alternative & Complementary Medicine*, *12*(3), 323–328.

John, W. (2018). Multimodal approaches in integrative health: Whole persons, whole practices, whole systems. *The Journal of Alternative and Complementary Medicine*, *24*(3), 193–195. doi:10.1089/acm.2018.29045.jjw.

Kislov, R., Waterman, H., Harvey, G., Boaden, R. (2014). Rethinking capacity building for knowledge mobilisation: Developing multilevel capabilities in healthcare organisations. *Implementation Science*, *9*(1), 166. doi:10.1186/s13012-014-0166-0.

Leach, M. J., Gillham, D. (2011). Are complementary medicine practitioners implementing evidence based practice? *Complementary Therapies in Medicine*, *19*(3), 128–136. doi:https://doi.org/10.1016/j.ctim.2011.04.002.

Leaver, C. A., Miller-Davis, C., Wallen, G. R. (2013). Naturopathic management of females with cervical atypia: a Delphi process to explore current practice. *Integrative Medicine Insights*, *8*, IMI. S11088.

Leech, B., Schloss, J., Steel, A. (2018a). Health services research as a framework for expanding a whole systems research agenda in complementary and integrative medicine: The example of intestinal permeability. *European Journal of Integrative Medicine*, *17*, 22–25.

Leech, B., Schloss, J., Steel, A. (2018b). Investigation into complementary and integrative medicine practitioners' clinical experience of intestinal permeability: A cross-sectional survey. *Complementary Therapies in Clinical Practice*, *31*, 200–209.

Luce, B. R., Kramer, J. M., Goodman, S. N., Connor, J. T., Tunis, S., Whicher, D., Schwartz, J. S. (2009). Rethinking randomized clinical trials for comparative effectiveness research: The need for transformational change. *Annals of internal medicine*, *151*(3), 206–209.

McCormack, B., McCance, T. (2016). *Person-centred Practice in Nursing and Health Care: Theory and Practice*. John Wiley & Sons, New York.

Medagama, A. B., Bandara, R. (2014). The use of Complementary and Alternative Medicines (CAMs) in the treatment of diabetes mellitus: Is continued use safe and effective? *Nutrition Journal*, *13*(1), 102.

Miles, A., Loughlin, M. (2011). Models in the balance: Evidence-based medicine versus evidence-informed individualized care. *Journal of Evaluation in Clinical Practice*, *17*(4), 531–536.

Murthy, V., Adams, J., Broom, A., Kirby, E., Refshauge, K. M., Sibbritt, D. (2017). The influence of communication and information sources upon decision-making around complementary and alternative medicine use for back pain among Australian women aged 60–65 years. *Health & Social Care in the Community*, 25(1), 114–122.

National Health Service. (2018). INVOLVE,. Available at: http://www.invo.org.uk/.

Nilsen, P. (2015). Making sense of implementation theories, models and frameworks. *Implementation Science*, 10(1), 53.

Oberg, E. B., Bradley, R., Cooley, K., Fritz, H., Goldenberg, J., Seely, D., Calabrese, C. (2015). Estimated effects of whole-system naturopathic medicine in select chronic disease conditions: A systematic review. *Alternative and Integrative Medicine*, 4(2), 1–12.

Olsson, L. E., Jakobsson Ung, E., Swedberg, K., Ekman, I. (2013). Efficacy of person-centred care as an intervention in controlled trials–a systematic review. *Journal of Clinical Nursing*, 22(3-4), 456–465.

Porzsolt, F., Rocha, N. G., Toledo-Arruda, A. C., Thomaz, T. G., Moraes, C., Bessa-Guerra, T. R., . . . Weiss, C. (2015). Efficacy and effectiveness trials have different goals, use different tools, and generate different messages. *Pragmatic and Observational Research*, 6, 47.

Reid, R., Steel, A., Wardle, J., Trubody, A., Adams, J. (2016). Complementary medicine use by the Australian population: A critical mixed studies systematic review of utilisation, perceptions and factors associated with use. *BMC Complementary and Alternative Medicine*, 16(1), 176.

Rycroft-Malone, J., Seers, K., Chandler, J., Hawkes, C. A., Crichton, N., Allen, C., Bullock, I., Strunin, L. (2013). The role of evidence, context, and facilitation in an implementation trial: Implications for the development of the PARIHS framework. *Implementation Science,* 8(1), 28.

Sackett, D. L., Rosenberg, W. M., Gray, J. M., Haynes, R. B., Richardson, W. S. (1996). Evidence based medicine: What it is and what it isn't. British Medical Journal Publishing Group, 312(7023), 71–72.

Shahar, E. (1998). Evidence-based medicine: A new paradigm or the Emperor's new clothes? *Journal of Evaluation in Clinical Practice*, 4(4), 277–282.

Shippee, N. D., Domecq Garces, J. P., Prutsky Lopez, G. J., Wang, Z., Elraiyah, T. A., Nabhan, M., Firwana, B. (2015). Patient and service user engagement in research: a systematic review and synthesized framework. *Health Expectations*, 18(5), 1151–1166.

Shoveller, J., Viehbeck, S., Di Ruggiero, E., Greyson, D., Thomson, K., Knight, R. (2016). A critical examination of representations of context within research on population health interventions. *Critical Public Health*, 26(5), 487–500.

Staniszewska, S., Brett, J., Mockford, C., Barber, R. (2011). The GRIPP checklist: Strengthening the quality of patient and public involvement reporting in research. *International Journal of Technology Assessment in Health Care*, *27*(4), 391–399.

Steel, A., Adams, J. (2011a). The application and value of information sources in clinical practice: An examination of the perspective of naturopaths. *Health Information & Libraries Journal*, *28*(2), 110–118.

Steel, A., Adams, J. (2011b). Approaches to clinical decision-making: A qualitative study of naturopaths. *Complementary Therapies in Clinical Practice*, *17*(2), 81–84.

Steel, A., Peng, W., Gray, A., Adams, J. (2018a). The role and influence of traditional and scientific knowledge in naturopathic education: A qualitative study *The Journal of Alternative & Complementary Medicine, In Press*. doi. org/10.1089/acm.2018.0293.

Steel, A., Rapport, F., Adams, J. (2018b). Towards an implementation science of complementary health care: Some initial considerations for guiding safe, effective clinical decision-making. *Advances in Integrative Medicine, 2014*, 1–9.

Steel, A., Sundberg, T., Reid, R., Ward, L., Bishop, F. L., Leach, M., Cramer, H., Wardle, J., Adams, J. (2017). Osteopathic manipulative treatment: a systematic review and critical appraisal of comparative effectiveness and health economics research. *Musculoskeletal Science and Practice, 27*, 165–175.

Thorpe, K. E., Zwarenstein, M., Oxman, A. D., Treweek, S., Furberg, C. D., Altman, D. G., Magid, D. J. (2009). A pragmatic–explanatory continuum indicator summary (PRECIS): A tool to help trial designers. *Journal of Clinical Epidemiology, 62*(5), 464–475.

Tunis, S. R., Benner, J., McClellan, M. (2010). Comparative effectiveness research: policy context, methods development and research infrastructure. *Statistics in Medicine, 29*(19), 1963–1976.

Tunis, S. R., Stryer, D. B., Clancy, C. M. (2003). Practical clinical trials: Increasing the value of clinical research for decision making in clinical and health policy. *JAMA, 290*(12), 1624–1632.

Verhoef, M. J., Casebeer, A. L., Hilsden, R. J. (2002). Assessing efficacy of complementary medicine: Adding qualitative research methods to the "Gold Standard". *The Journal of Alternative & Complementary Medicine, 8*(3), 275–281.

Verhoef, M. J., Lewith, G., Ritenbaugh, C., Boon, H., Fleishman, S., Leis, A. (2005). Complementary and alternative medicine whole systems research: Beyond identification of inadequacies of the RCT. *Complementary Therapies in Medicine, 13*(3), 206–212.

Wandersman, A., Chien, V. H., Katz, J. (2012). Toward an evidence-based system for innovation support for implementing innovations with quality: Tools, training, technical assistance, and quality assurance/quality improvement. *American Journal of Community Psychology*, *50*(3–4), 445–459.

Wardle, J., Seely, D. (2007). The challenges of traditional, complementary and integrative medicine research: A practitioner perspective. In J. Adams (ed.), *Traditional, Complementary and Integrative Medicine: An International Reader.* New York, Palgrave MacMillan, pp. 266–282.

Wieten, S. (2018). Expertise in evidence-based medicine: A tale of three models. *Philosophy, Ethics, and Humanities in Medicine: PEHM*, *13*, 2. doi:10.1186/s13010-018-0055-2.

World Health Organization. (2006). *Bridging the "Know–Do" Gap*. Paper presented at the Meeting on Knowledge Translation in Global Health.

World Health Organization. (2018). *WHO Framework on Integrated People-centred Health Services*. Available at: http://www.who.int/servicedeliverysafety/areas/people-centred-care/en/.

Wye, L., Shaw, A., and Sharp, D. (2009). Patient choice and evidence based decisions: The case of complementary therapies. *Health Expectations*, *12*(3), 321–330.

Wyer, P. C., Silva, S. A. (2009). Where is the wisdom? I–A conceptual history of evidence-based medicine. *Journal of Evaluation in Clinical Practice*, *15*(6), 891–898.

Chapter 7

Capacity Building in TCIM: A Focus Upon Public Health and Health Services Research

Jon Adams, Amie Steel, Wenbo Peng, David Sibbritt,
Jon Wardle and Program Fellows*

Introduction

As the current book collection attests, the public health (PH) and health services research (HSR) of TCIM is gaining ground. However, it is imperative we not only facilitate interest but also ensure capacity and sustainability in this significant area of health and health care research (Adams *et al.*, 2012). While a generation of public health and health services

---

*International CM Research Leadership Program Fellows: Felicity Bishop, Caragh Brosnan, Vincent Chung, Holger Cramer, Helen Hall, Romy Lauche, Matthew Leach, Brenda Leung, Nikki Munk, Tobias Sundberg, Lesley Ward, Tony Zhang, Yan Zhang;
International Naturopathy Research Leadership Program Fellows: Ryan Bradley, Kieran Cooley, Joshua Goldenberg, Joanna Harnett, Jason Hawrelak, Erica McIntyre, Rebecca Reid, Janet Schloss, Claudine Van de Venter, Naveen Visweswaraiah;
Chiropractic Academy for Research Leadership (CARL) Fellows and Mentors: Alex Breen, Greg Kawchuk, Katie de Luca, Diana De Carvalho, Andreas Eklund, Matthew Fernandez, Martha Funabashi, Jan Hartvigsen, Michelle Holmes, Melker Johansson, Craig Moore, Isabelle Page, Katie Pohlman, Michael Swain, Arnold Wong.

researchers have shown interest in this topic there remains only a small number of individuals (relatively insubstantial in number when compared to conventional medical research ranks) and even fewer teams dedicated to the PH and HSR of TCIM.

It is well established that research disciplines and fields require strategic forward planning and capacity growth and development in order to attract and retain suitable academics and reach a critical mass where enquiry is sustainable and can serve the needs of practitioners, patients, communities, policymakers and other stakeholders (Cooke, 2005). Nevertheless, it still stands that analysis of the networks, mentoring, leadership and career development opportunities for budding researchers and scholars in the PH and HSR of TCIM does not instil optimism for the quality and future of the field.

This chapter outlines a number of challenges currently facing the PH/HSR of TCIM with regard to capacity building and growth and overviews a number of contemporary initiatives directly aimed at addressing these circumstances. The focus of this chapter is upon research and we highlight a number of recently established international research capacity building endeavours which aim to grow and deepen rigorous PH and HSR in TCIM.

The Challenges and Opportunities for Capacity and Growth in the PH/HSR of TCIM

It is of importance to note that from within the ranks of researchers interested in TCIM many are not located in a rich TCIM-focused environment. While TCIM centres in Universities do exist, and in some cases such as with the Academic Consortium for Integrative Medicine and Health in the US, there are networks of TCIM scholarship, these remain relatively small in number and size when compared to the infrastructure that has grown around conventional medical research. Many who author/co-author publications on TCIM do so from within a range of other related but different fields including ageing and ageing care research; rural health research; nursing, midwifery and other allied health research; anthropology and sociology research; psychology research and to a much lesser extent medicine/medical science research. This important context has in part helped shape the TCIM research community providing both opportunities and challenges.

One potential benefit of the TCIM research field attracting an eclectic mix of researchers from across a vast range of fields is that it encourages and promotes a multidisciplinary perspective and brings a vast range of methodological approaches and fieldwork techniques to the study of the topic. Unfortunately, while many pockets of such multidisciplinary activity around PH and HSR of TCIM exist, the ability of somewhat socially and geographically disconnected scholars (many of whom remain early to mid-career and are still attempting to establish and grow national and international profiles and networks) to initiate and maintain group work and output is severely limited. As a result, many of the individuals who are currently focused upon TCIM research are often inadvertently encouraged to maintain disciplinary boundaries and not always exposed to multidisciplinary thinking.

In most part, whether such a limitation is maintained or not is determined by the perspective, needs and focus of institutional colleagues and perhaps even more importantly, supervisors/line-managers. A relatively junior academic positioned in a nursing faculty for example and who registers interest in TCIM research may be aided or hindered in this endeavour because colleagues/management may or may not deem TCIM a core focus for 'nursing' scholarship or may simply prioritise other issues as helping meet institutional key performance indicators (for example in relation to the quality and impact of journals for publication or likelihood of attracting external funds for research).

The ad-hoc, disjointed environment around TCIM research and researchers also raises recruitment and retention challenges — academics who wish to pursue TCIM-focused work may well have to justify such activity without wider backing or support. This in itself is a major obstacle to growing the ranks of TCIM research. Yet, even when academics may begin to establish a track record in TCIM there is always a risk they may be tempted or driven to a competing field of health research – this may be due to wider opportunities or increased reward elsewhere or simply due to a possible feeling of 'isolation' in pursuing TCIM research amid what is an ever increasingly competitive academic environment.

This contemporary landscape can have dire consequences for projecting a broad research vision that reflects blue-sky thinking and coordinates activity as well as helping to grow capacity and encouraging mentorship and leadership training. As a result, the TCIM field (and PH and HSR enquiry therein) faces a number of significant challenges that may at best represent roadblocks to successful development and at worst could signal an existential threat to the field more broadly.

Addressing the Capacity, Mentorship and Leadership Challenge in TCIM

As mentioned earlier, it is the case that a few exceptions to the environment outlined above do exist. For example, the US Academic Consortium for Integrative Medicine and Health provides a network of activity and collaboration (albeit largely focused upon those who are medically-qualified) and a very small number of Centres/Institutes focused exclusively upon TCIM exist in Australia, across Europe and elsewhere.

However, moving our attention more specifically to PH and HSR in TCIM the landscape is perhaps even more challenging and problematic. Currently, only one TCIM research centre in the world — the Australian Research Centre in Complementary and Integrative Medicine (ARCCIM) — is focused exclusively or predominantly upon a PH and HSR agenda. The ARCCIM, based at the University of Technology Sydney, houses a wide range of academics steeped in rigorous PH and HSR methodology and research design. For example, the ARCCIM Director, Distinguished Professor Jon Adams is a Distinguished Professor of Public Health and the ARCCIM Deputy Director, Professor David Sibbritt, is a Professor of Epidemiology and Biostatistics and the wider team includes senior, mid-career and early career researchers trained in epidemiology, biostatistics, qualitative research, mixed-method design, health economic evaluation, psychology, sociology, health law and policy and implementation and translation science.

ARCCIM's PH and HSR program involves over 60 academics in Australia and internationally and includes over 40 active international research projects with many attracting government Category 1 funding (National Health and Medical Research Council, Australian Research

Council, Department of Health) as well as industry support and partnership. The ARCCIM also has strong links and collaborations with a number of public health associations and institutions around the world including the Brazilian Collective Health Association (ABRASCO), American Public Health Association (APHA), Public Health Association of Australia (PHAA), Chinese Preventive Medicine Association (CPMA), Indonesian Public Health Association (IAKMI), Pan-American Health Organization (PAHO), Public Health Association of South Africa (PHASA) and is involved in work for/with the Australian Federal Governments Therapeutic Goods Administration CM Committee and Ministries of Health in a number of countries including Nicaragua and Indonesia. As the remaining sections of this chapter outline, the ARCCIM team have recently built upon this success to introduce the first systematic international platform of mentorship, leadership and capacity building in TCIM with a heavy focus upon PH and HSR.

TCIM Research Capacity and Leadership Programs: History and Contemporary Initiatives

Before overviewing current TCIM Leadership Program initiatives it is first necessary to introduce a long-standing Program in a different health field that has been a world-first and which has directly shaped and fed into the TCIM programs developed by ARCCIM.

The Oxford International Primary Care Research Leadership Program (herein titled the Oxford Leadership Program) — originally set up as part of the Brisbane Initiative (BI), an international collaboration of heads of primary care departments at a meeting in Brisbane in 2002 and which operates under the aegis of the World Organization of Family Doctors (WONCA) — is hosted by the Nuffield Department of Primary Care Health Sciences at the University of Oxford (www.oxfordleadershippro-gramme.co.uk). To date, the Oxford Leadership Program has competi-tively appointed over 70 Fellows (early career to senior academics) who operate in 11 Cohorts and attend an annual 4 day residential at the University of Oxford. The focus of the program and residentials is to provide a number of structured events/speakers/activities, life coaching (optional) as well as facilitate space and time for Cohort Fellows to organise and prioritise in-cohort activities/sessions they feel will be most valuable and beneficial to their academic growth and career development.

Inspired by his experience as an appointed Senior Fellow and also more recently a Senior Mentor on the Oxford Leadership Program, Distinguished Professor Jon Adams sought partners to establish a similar program in the TCIM field. Indeed, since 2014 a suite of programs have now been developed — all international, all built upon a shared model and based upon a similar set of goals. All the programs have been developed, designed and led by the ARCCIM in collaboration with industry and community-based partners and supporters beyond academia (Massage and Myotherapy Australia, the Jacka Foundation of Natural Therapies, the Blackmores Institute, The Blackmores Foundation, Australian Self-Medication Industry, World Chiropractic Foundation and the European Centre for Chiropractic Research Excellence) as well as with competitive funding from the Canadian Institutes of Health Research.

International CM research leadership and capacity building program

In 2014, UTS:ARCCIM founded the International CM Research Leadership and Capacity Building Program (herein titled CM Research Leadership Program), the first leadership program world-wide with the aim of: identifying and supporting CM research leaders of the future trained in rigorous research design and ethical research practice; advancing practice and policy-relevant CM research; identifying and promoting future research strengths and agendas for CM research in Australia and internationally; and promoting collaboration and strengthening links across the national and international CM research field. Twelve initial Fellows were competitively appointed to the CM Research Leadership Program — a thirteenth Fellow joined the Program via the generous support of the Massage and Myotherapy Australia and was appointed as the 'Massage and Myotherapy Australia International Research Leadership Fellow'. The CM Research Leadership Program Fellows are: Associate

Professor Felicity Bishop, University of Southampton, UK; Dr Caragh Brosnan, University of Newcastle, Australia; Dr Vincent Chung, Chinese University of Hong Kong; Dr Holger Cramer, University of Duisburg-Essen, Germany; Dr Helen Hall, Monash University, Australia; Dr Romy Lauche, University of Technology Sydney, Australia; Dr Matthew Leach, University of South Australia; Dr Brenda Leung, University Lethridge, Canada; Dr Tobias Sundberg, Karolinska Institute, Sweden; Dr Lesley Ward, University of Oxford, UK; Dr Tony Zhang, RMIT University, Australia; and Associate Professor Yan Zhang, Texas Tech University, US.

International naturopathy research leadership and capacity building program

Quickly following the establishment of the CM Research Leadership Program, UTS: ARCCIM founded the International Naturopathy Research Leadership Program in 2016. Following the same model as the previous program, this new initiative appointed 11 Fellows following competitive international expressions of interest. The current Fellows on the Program are: Dr Ryan Bradley, National College of Natural Medicine and the Helfgott Research Institute, US; Dr Kieran Colley, Canadian College of Naturopathic Medicine, Canada; Dr Joshua Goldenberg, Bastyr University Research Institute, US; Dr Joanna Harnett, University of Sydney, Australia; Dr Jason Hawrelak, University of Tasmania, Australia; Dr Erica McIntyre, University of Technology Sydney, Australia; Ms Rebecca Reid, Endeavour College of Health and University of Technology Sydney, Australia; Dr Claudine Van de Venter, University of Cape Town, South Africa; Dr Naveen Visweswaraiah, S-VYASA Yoga University, India; and Dr Janet Schloss, Endeavour College of Natural Health, Australia.

Among other successes from this Naturopathy Research Leadership Program has been a Special Issue dedicated to the leadership and mentoring of the naturopathic field to be published in *The Journal of Alternative and Complementary Medicine* in late 2018/early 2019.

Chiropractic Academy for Research Leadership (CARL)

Following the success of the two established UTS:ARCCIM Leadership Programs and given the need to develop research capacity and leadership within chiropractic, a group of senior health researchers (Professor Adams, UTS; Professor Hartvigsen; University of Southern Denmark; and Professor Kawchuk, University of Alberta) having research interests of relevance to chiropractic, planned and founded the world-first international chiropractic research leadership initiative — the Chiropractic Academy of Research Leadership (CARL) to commence in 2017.

The first cohort of the CARL program consists of 13 early career leaders from 5 professions in 7 countries who represent diverse areas of interests of high relevance for chiropractic (Adam *et al.*, 2018). The CARL Fellows are: Dr Alexander Breen, AECC University College, UK; Dr Diana Memorial University of Newfoundland, Canada; Andreas Eklund, Karolinska Institute; Matthew Fernandez, Macquarie University, Australia; Martha Funabashi, Canadian Memorial Chiropractic College, Canada; Michelle Holmes, AECC University College, UK; Melker Johansson, University of Southern Denmark, Denmark; Katie de Luca, Macquarie University, Australia; Craig Moore, University of Technology Sydney, Australia; Isabele Page, Universite du Quebec a Trois-Rivieres, Canada; Katherine Pohlman, Parker University, US; Michael Swain, Macquarie University, Australia; Arnold Wong, Hong Kong Polytechnic University, Hong Kong.

Leadership Program Outputs and Successes to Date

The three international leadership programs outlined above have all being running for different periods of time to date. Nevertheless, across all three has been produced over 150 peer-reviewed manuscripts and Fellows have collaborated on 11 new TCIM projects and grants to date. Among other successes from this Naturopathy Research Leadership Program has been a Special Issue dedicated to the leadership and mentoring of the naturopathic field to be published in *The Journal of Alternative and Complementary Medicine* in late 2018/early 2019. Beyond such metric-driven outputs (certainly important in our contemporary academic environment) and perhaps equally if not more important have been the less tangible successes of the programs. Each program has to date helped a select but diverse of early to mid-career academics coordinate and collaborate their efforts, connect and build trust as well as provide well-needed confidence and momentum to their activities. Not only do these programs help each and every Fellow in their own academic career development but, more importantly, the Programs are establishing a 'critical mass' of research capacity that will hopefully provide reward and future additional growth in these important health care areas on the international stage.

Concluding Discussion

Where to from here? How do we continue to encourage growth and depth in TCIM research? The research leadership programs developed to date and outlined above are obviously not comprehensive and there is certainly further opportunity for others to model similar initiatives focused upon other modalities (ie TCM), perhaps specific methodologies or sub-fields/disciplines (ie health psychology) and/or geography and location (ie there is much potential for a research leadership program for TM scholars across sub-Saharan Africa or South America).

Obviously, there is a much broader context and environment in which all fields of scholarship have to exist and much of the continuing resistance to TCIM requires a change of approach from others beyond the TCIM academic field. For example, mainstream funders remain cautious, regarding supporting quality TCIM grant applications (Wardle and Adams, 2013). However, we cannot simply wait for mainstream critical PH and HSR and as the established leadership initiatives above have already proven there are extremely encouraging signs that industry and philanthropists are beginning to rise to the demands of leadership, mentorship and capacity building.

As this book illustrates there is plenty of opportunity and material left to investigate on TCIM and the topic/issue is only going to become more worthy, significant and critical for empirical investigation as health systems become increasingly taxed under the pressure of an ageing population and growing burden of chronic illness. The challenge for the TCIM research field is not only to help grow the evidence-base to guide practice and policy decisions but also to foster a critical mass of scholars capable of appropriately addressing the intellectual, political and logistical challenges that will face scholarship in TCIM for many years yet to come. While such a vision will take much political will on behalf of all collaborating stakeholders there is reason to remain optimistic with the recent mentorship and leadership initiatives providing an excellent range of templates for others to draw upon and extend both in terms of TCIM modality and location/background of network members.

References

Adams, J., Andrews, G., Barnes, J., Broom, A., and Magin, P. (eds.), (2012). *Traditional, Complementary and Integrative Medicine: An International Reader.* Macmillan International Higher Education, Basingstoke, Hampshire.

Adams, J., Kawchuk, G., Breen, A., De Carvalho, D., Eklund, A., Fernandez, M., Funabashi M., Holmes, M., Johansson, M., de Luca, K., Moore, C., Page, I., K., Swain, M., Wong, A., Hartvigsen, J. (2018). Leadership and capacity building in international chiropractic research: Introducing the chiropractic academy for research leadership (CARL). *Chiropractic & Manual Therapies*, 26(1), 5.

Cooke, J. (2005). A framework to evaluate research capacity building in health care. *BMC Family practice*, 6(1), 44.

Wardle, J., Adams, J. (2013). Are the CAM professions engaging in high-level health and medical research? Trends in publicly funded complementary medicine research grants in Australia. *Complementary Therapies in Medicine*, 21(6), 746–749.

Section Two
Substantive Topics and Key Issues

Chapter 8

Traditional Medicine and Traditional Birth Attendant Use During Pregnancy and Birthing in Low to Middle-Income Countries

Bradley Leech, Jon Adams and Amie Steel

Introduction

Traditional medicine (TM) is increasingly being used among women during pregnancy and birthing throughout low to middle-income countries (LMICs). Rural and remote regions of LMICs have limited access to health services including skilled birth attendants (SBAs). Many of these rural and remote regions rely on traditional birth attendants (TBAs) to support expectant mothers through pregnancy and birthing. TBAs are trusted and valued members of the community who are frequently the source of information about TM use during pregnancy and childbirth. This chapter will provide an overview of pregnancy and childbirth in LMICs, illustrating many of the obstacles women encounter during pregnancy then it will describe the role TBAs play with a focus on TM use. Lastly a research agenda is discussed situating the current level of knowledge and illustrating gaps in the research.

131

Pregnancy and Childbirth in Low to Middle-Income Countries

In contemporary LMICs pregnancy and childbirth remain a life-threatening event for many woman and newborns. In contrast to high-income countries, the journey of pregnancy and birthing in LMICs is characterized by a wide range of possible complication and even death, many of which are preventable (MacDonald, 2017). Such complications and challenges are exacerbated by the limited number of health care professionals available to many local communities — for example in the Machakos District of Kenya the doctor-patient ration is reported to be 1:62,325 (Kaingu *et al.*, 2011). As a result, a large percentage of births in LMICs occur outside of health facilities and are related to an increased risk of mortality and morbidity (Bukar and Jauro, 2013).

While there has been a 3.3% decline in maternal mortality from 2005 to 2013 throughout 109 LMICs (Verguet *et al.*, 2014), an estimated 153 maternal deaths per 100,000 live births still occur (Bauserman *et al.*, 2015). There are many factors increasing the risk of maternal death in LMICs including a lower education level, a lack of antenatal care, experiencing a caesarean section delivery, experiencing haemorrhaging and the woman having hypertensive disorders (Bauserman *et al.*, 2015). In fact, both haemorrhaging and hypertensive disorders contribute to one-third of maternal deaths in LMICs with ruptured uterus and sepsis being the most lethal obstetric complications (Bailey *et al.*, 2017). Most complications in LMICS occur during delivery with some countries such as Morocco experiencing morbidity rates as high as 38.1% (Elkhoudri *et al.*, 2016).

Globally, 99% of the 4 million neonatal deaths that occur yearly, happen in LMICs with the direct causes being an infection (mainly pneumonia and diarrhoea) (36%), preterm birth (28%) and asphyxia (23%) (Lawn *et al.*, 2005). A large percentage of neonate deaths occur >37 weeks gestation with the majority occurring within 24 hours of delivery (Belizan *et al.*, 2012). The 2017 *Levels and Trends in Child Mortality* annual report (Hug *et al.*, 2017) highlighted many key areas in child survival in LMICs. Firstly, there has been a sharp decline in the under-five mortality rate from

93 deaths per 1000 live births in 1990 to 41 deaths per 1000 live births in 2016 (a 56% decline over this period). However, this remains high compared to 5.3 deaths per 1,000 live births in high-income countries. Approximately 7000 babies in LMICs died in the first 28 days of life every day during 2016. Newborn death rates are highest in Southern Asia (39%) and sub-Saharan Africa (38%) with the five countries accounting for half of all newborn deaths being India (24%), Pakistan (10%), Nigeria (9%), the Democratic Republic of the Congo (4%) and Ethiopia (3%) accounting for half of all newborn deaths worldwide. It has been estimated that if trends continue in the 50 countries which fail to meet the Sustainable Development Goal of child survival, almost 60 million children under the age of 5, especially newborns, will die between 2017 and 2030 (Hug *et al.*, 2017).

What do We Know About Traditional Medicine Use During Pregnancy and Birthing?

The World Health Organization (WHO) has estimated that 80% of individuals residing in rural areas of LMICs use TM for health needs, including during pregnancy and birthing (World Health Organization, 2002). Herbal medicine is the most frequently used TM in LMICs by women during pregnancy with an estimated prevalence range of 20–79.9% (Shewamene *et al.*, 2017). This prevalence is suggested to be lowest in urban areas where SBAs are more accessible and highest in rural areas as access to health care is limited. The largest portion of women who use TM are low-income earners with no formal education (Shewamene *et al.*, 2017). These women source information on TM from mainly TBAs followed by traditional healers and elderly women within the community (Shewamene *et al.*, 2017).

Traditional Birth Attendants

TBAs have long been an essential part of pregnancy and birthing throughout LMICs as they are a major support network for expectant mothers throughout gestation. TBAs are viewed as a trusted and valued member of the community who are generally elderly women that have personally experienced childbirth and support mothers with home deliveries. Typically TBAs have no forming training in midwifery and acquire their knowledge through family members who were previous TBAs, allowing knowledge to be passed down through generations. TBAs are independent of the health care system, receiving no financial or medical support from the government (World Health Organization, 2004). However, in some instances TBAs may receive basic training to help identify mothers and newborns 'at risk' of complications and they are encouraged to refer at risk mothers and newborns to the nearest health facility if accessible (World Health Organization, 2004).

TBAs are valuable and accessible members of the community providing physical and psychological care pre-, intra- and postpartum (Byrne *et al.*, 2016). Many women in LMICs perceive TBAs as the primary person responsible for supporting them throughout their pregnancy (Ngunyulu *et al.*, 2015). In many rural and remote regions, TBAs are the exclusive care option for expectant mothers due to the distance to the nearest birthing facility. It has been suggested that more than half of home deliveries in LMICs are attended by TBAs (Bukar and Jauro, 2013).

TBAs and community elders have been found to use upwards of 35 medical plants for supporting pregnant women with some reports suggesting use of up to 55 different medical plants in their management of pregnancy complications (Alade *et al.*, 2018; Kaingu *et al.*, 2011). Such herbs are prescribed by TBAs for use throughout gestation with most herbal medicines recommended during delivering to avoid complications (Lech and Mngadi, 2005). TBAs have also been identified as advising women with regard to other related issues. For instance, TBAs will sometimes advise on delivery position (with squatting being the preferred position promoted by TBAs) (Lech and Mngadi, 2005). TBAs use a variety of techniques to remove placenta if retained such as abdomen/uterus massage (23.4–47%), manual extraction (15–24.6%), and advising the mother to blow an empty bottle (18.2%) (Bucher *et al.*, 2016; Lech and Mngadi, 2005). TBAs also advise women on dietary and nutritional recommendations for foetus growth, energy during labour and postpartum food intake (Byrne *et al.*, 2016).

TBAs appear to treat many common ailments associated with pregnancy (Alade *et al.*, 2018). However, they have also been found to lack basic hygiene practices resulting in increased risk of infectious disease. This is of significant concern as infectious diseases are the single greatest direct cause of neonatal deaths in LMICs (Lawn *et al.*, 2005). Another area where TBAs appear to use inappropriate or outdated practices is with regard to obstetric complications and newborn care (Bucher *et al.*, 2016). These practices vary demanding on many geographical and cultural attributes with one study reporting 34% of TBAs as employing some form of potentially harmful product such as cow dung, red ochre, soil or ash to cover the cord stump (Lech and Mngadi, 2005).

Skilled birth attendants (SBAs) are qualified as either a midwife, nurse, or doctor and are able to manage all areas of pregnancy and childbirth (Munabi-Babigumira *et al.*, 2017). In some LMICs such as Kenya, there has been a rise in the number of births attended by an SBA in recent years (Kenya National Bureau of Statistics — KNBS *et al.*, 2010, 2015). Although SBAs are qualified in many areas relating to childbirth they still encounter many challenges affecting their ability to provide optimal patient care (Munabi-Babigumira *et al.*, 2017). A major challenge is convincing expecting mothers to deliver at the health facility rather than having a home birth (Byrne *et al.*, 2016). SBAs often perceive the strength of TBAs to be emotional support for mothers and an asset to the community and health care system (Byrne *et al.*, 2016).

It has recently been proposed that the role of TBAs requires redefinition in response to an increasing number of modern health facilities becoming available, especially in developing regions. One study suggests that TBAs may be a vital aspect of supporting facility-based delivery by referring or accommodating women in labour to attend a health facility (Pyone *et al.*, 2014). The collaboration of care by TBAs and SBAs is a viable proposition for LMICs (Byrne *et al.*, 2016). While TBAs support and encourage mothers to visit a health facility for immunization and postnatal care (Lech and Mngadi, 2005), there remains controversy surrounding *when* TBAs should refer expecting mothers to seek assistance via a health facility (Bucher *et al.*, 2016).

The WHO has supported and encouraged the integration of TBAs into the health care system over the last two decades (Stanton, 2008). However, many challenges have been identified and are required to be addressed for optimal patient care (Wilunda *et al.*, 2017). Integrative care between TBAs and the health care system has been implemented in Timor-Leste, with a high degree of success (Ribeiro, 2014). In particular, since incorporating TBAs into the national health care system a reduction of maternal mortality has been observed from 660 per 100,000 live births in 2003 to 557 per 100,000 live births in 2010. Such integrative care has also seen an increase in referrals by TBAs to SBAs and has also increased the access to health care in rural communities (Ribeiro, 2014).

Determinants of Traditional Medicine Use in Pregnancy and Birthing

Women in LMICs have a cultural trust towards TM given the long history of use, accessibility and affordability. Many women in LMICs perceive TM as more effective than Western medicine in treating complications and ailments associated with pregnancy (Shewamene *et al.*, 2017) and women are more inclined to use TM compared to Western medicine due to cost considerations (Shewamene *et al.*, 2017). It has been suggested that a major factor determining women's TM use in LMICs is related to limited access to Western medicine (Shewamene *et al.*, 2017). Traditional healers and TBAs are usually accessible in rural areas where Western medical facilities are not. Furthermore, some TM such as herbal medicine can be grown in the community and is often gathered from the bush or sourced from traditional healers (Nyeko *et al.*, 2016).

Reasons for TM Use During Pregnancy and Birthing

TM is used throughout pregnancy from preconception and contraception to inducing labour and postnatal care (Table 1). The majority of the TM used by women is to: treat common ailments associated with pregnancy such as nausea, morning sickness and abdominal pain; assist with labour;

Table 1.   Action of traditional medicine use.

Preconception

Spermicidal	(Alade *et al.*, 2018)
Contraception	(Alade *et al.*, 2018)
Fertility (76.2%)	(Kaadaaga *et al.*, 2014)

Pregnancy

Abortifacient	(Alade *et al.*, 2018; Rasch *et al.*, 2014)
Nausea (21.7–31.8%)	(Bayisa *et al.*, 2014; Laelago *et al.*, 2016; Nyeko *et al.*, 2016)
Morning sickness (21.1%)	(Bayisa *et al.*, 2014)
Vomiting (15.3–21.7%)	(Bayisa *et al.*, 2014; Laelago *et al.*, 2016; Nyeko *et al.*, 2016)
Nutrition	(Mureyi *et al.*, 2012)
Cough (15.0–31.0%)	(Bayisa *et al.*, 2014)
Abdominal pain (9.1–42.5%)	(Bayisa *et al.*, 2014; Laelago *et al.*, 2016; Nyeko *et al.*, 2016)
Malaria (2.83–3.1%)	(Bayisa *et al.*, 2014; Laelago *et al.*, 2016)
Cold (71.7%)	(Laelago *et al.*, 2016)
Protection against evil spirits	(Mureyi *et al.*, 2012)

Birthing/Delivery

Labour inducing (28.3%)	(Alade *et al.*, 2018; Mureyi *et al.*, 2012; Nyeko *et al.*, 2016)
Pain during labour	(Elkhoudri *et al.*, 2016)
Facilitate childbirth (13.3%)	(Elkhoudri *et al.*, 2016)
Widening birth canal	(Mureyi *et al.*, 2012)
Preventing perineal tearing	(Mureyi *et al.*, 2012)
Placenta retention	(Ticktin and Dalle, 2005)

Postnatal/Postpartum

Lactation (9.4%)	(Elkhoudri *et al.*, 2016)
General health (6.1%)	(Elkhoudri *et al.*, 2016)

and prevent perineal tearing, prolonged labour and placental retention TM use in some parts of sub-Saharan Africa incorporates religion and the belief in God, with TM, used to '*protect against evil spirits*' during pregnancy (Mureyi *et al.*, 2012).

TM Used During Pregnancy and Birthing

A recent systematic review has examined the use of TM for maternal and reproductive health complaints as well as for well-being among African women (Shewamene *et al.*, 2017). The herbal medicine frequently used by these women includes ginger, garlic, aniseed, fenugreek, green tea, eucalyptus, peppermint rue, madder, garden cress, cinnamon, bitter leaf, neem leaves, palm kernel, bitter kola and jute leaves. These herbal medicine ingredients are prepared and administered in various ways. The most popular methods to prepare herbs for the use during pregnancy is crude/whole plant (43.2%) and infusion/extract (23.2–42.3%) followed by maceration (19.2–23.2%), decoction (10.5–17.3%) and powder/crushed (19.2%) (Alade *et al.*, 2018; Bayisa *et al.*, 2014; Elkhoudri *et al.*, 2016). Typically these preparations are taken orally (22–84.9%), applied topically (10.1%) or applied intra-vaginally (13.0–33.0%) (Alade *et al.*, 2018; Laelago *et al.*, 2016; Rasch *et al.*, 2014). Many of the TMs used for pregnancy and birthing in LMICs, especially herbal medicine, are reported in the literature for their use in pregnancy and also other conditions not related to pregnancy or birthing (Alade *et al.*, 2018).

TM incorporates a large number of internal, physical and psychological therapies. The main TM therapy used by women during pregnancy in LMICs is herbal medicine. However, other TM used during pregnancy and birthing have limited research exploring their application and especially their effectiveness (Mureyi *et al.*, 2012). Preliminary evidence indicates that practices used by women during pregnancy and birthing in LMICs vary from the conventionally accepted method such as manual exercise, steam baths and castor oil to unorthodox treatments including elephant dung and soil from a burrowing mole (Mureyi *et al.*, 2012).

TM Use During Pregnancy and Birthing: A Summary

Herbal medicine remains the most widely used TM category during pregnancy and birthing in LMICs (Shewamene *et al.*, 2017). A substantial proportion of such herbal medicine use is employed throughout pregnancy especially during delivery to avoid complications (Lech and Mngadi, 2005).

TBAs have long been an essential part of pregnancy and birthing in LMICs with women viewing TBAs as trusted and valued members of the community. Whereas SBAs provide a service which addresses many of the shortcomings encountered by TBAs, women's trust in SBAs is limited (World Health Organization, 2004). Both TBAs and SBAs appear to hold much potential in helping ensure safe, assessable and affordable pregnancy for women in LMICs.

Research Agenda

The use of TM during pregnancy and birthing in LMICs remains a significant area for further research attention. Previous research agendas have highlighted and focused on mortality and morbidity during pregnancy and birthing (Dean *et al.*, 2013; Lackritz *et al.*, 2013; Souza *et al.*, 2014). However, there has been a lack of in-depth discussion regarding possible strategies to incorporate and advance the use of TM during pregnancy and birthing (where safe and feasible).

One important focus requiring further research attention and resources is the rich details around the current and potential role and responsibilities of TBAs in the care of pregnant women in LMICs. In order to optimise care for such women it will be necessary to draw upon research insights regarding all relevant providers, TBAs included. On a broader level, there are also policy, regulation and health system issues that require investigation — the rationale, strategy and process of potentially integrating (mainstreaming) TBAs into the local and national health system require attention.

Previous research has highlighted a number of areas where unintentional harm may come to either the expecting mother or newborn under the care of a TBA (Bucher *et al.*, 2016). Nevertheless, it seems probable to suggest that despite these risks women in LMICs will continue to manage their pregnancy and birthing outside the formal health system and associated health facilities, access (or lack of) alone appears likely to dictate such circumstances. Ensuring TBAs are appropriately trained and equipped for their defined role in the community is important. Recent research suggests that training and utilising TBAs to support facility-based delivery is a role which may be both feasible and acceptable (Pyone *et al.*, 2014).

The WHO reported in 2002 on the role of TBAs suggesting they may be best suited to providing companionship, health promotion and assistance during pregnancy and birth (World Health Organization, 2004). Later in 2004 the WHO in collaboration with the International Confederation of Midwives (ICM) and the International Federation of Gynaecology and Obstetrics (FIGO) further elaborated on how TBAs may work alongside SBAs (World Health Organization, 2004). However, the consideration of the application of herbal medicine and how this may be incorporated into the care of women during pregnancy appears to have been overlooked in both reports. Collectively, it appears that TBAs remain a vital resource in providing support for pregnancy and childbirth in LMICs. However, it is interesting to note that contemporary programs and initiatives appear to be promoting a role for TBAs in the referral of mothers to locally available health facilities for delivery rather than promoting their role as directly assisting mothers with home deliveries (Wilunda *et al.*, 2017).

The challenges of integrating TBAs into the health care system have previously been identified (Wilunda *et al.*, 2017) — regarding communication issues with health facilities, accessibility (distance to the nearest health facility), insecurity/safety, ill-equipped personnel and medical supplies, constraints within the health system and a lack of incentives/income. These challenges ought to be investigated further to understand the implications for patient care and to help inform future strategies and tools for improvement.

Many countries have implemented various interventions to support a change in focus from a TBA-led to a SBA-led delivery (Miller and Smith, 2017). A multifaceted approach involving training of TBAs and the sensitization of health care providers along with communities and women has been suggested as one means to help overcome many of the barriers experienced during the implementation of TBAs in their new role of providing companionship, health promotion and assistance during pregnancy and birth (Miller and Smith, 2017; World Health Organization, 2004).

Recent years appear to have ushered in somewhat of a critical transition whereby TBAs are facing possible extinction and being replaced by SBTs. Such a transition may result in SBTs attending birthing and reducing potential hygiene complications associated with childbirth. However, if less TBAs assist with childbirth, some aspects of traditional knowledge regarding birthing may be lost, resulting in knowledge gaps. As such, documenting the practices and knowledge of TBAs is perhaps more significant now than ever before and this should be the focus of future investigation.

The safety and effectiveness of herbal medicine use during pregnancy is critical to investigate considering TBAs are the major resource regarding the use and application of herbal medicine. Additionally, exploratory research can help describe and capture other practices TBAs use beyond herbal medicine such as manual and psychological therapies. Utilising a health services research framework to investigate the practice habits of TBAs is necessary. In particular, under what circumstances do TBAs prescribe or women use these practices? After identifying the practices most commonly used, exploring the safety and effectiveness is warranted. The information obtained will further strengthen the evidence on the application of herbal medicine use in pregnancy and birthing.

Majority of women in LMICs who use TM during pregnancy do not disclose the use of TM to their physicians (Shewamene *et al.*, 2017) and the reasons for the lack of disclosure have not been widely explored. Attempting to understand such an issue, which in those cases where medical pluralism is accessed, holds potential for both direct and indirect risks, is certainly a priority area for future investigation.

Conclusion

It appears clear that TM and TBAs constitute substantial services for pregnancy in LMICs and researchers focused on this stage of a women life would do well to consider these traditional practices and those providing them as highly significant to their investigations. Such in-depth investigation has much potential to not only shed light on this important area of health- and support seeking among pregnant and birthing women but to also help contextualise and optimise all maternity care in LMICs.

References

Alade, G., Oladele, A., Okpako, E., Ajibesin, K., Awotona, O. (2018). A survey of plants used for family planning in Bayelsa State, southern Nigeria. *Journal of Intercultural Ethnopharmacology*, 7(1), 25–44.

Bailey, P. E., Andualem, W., Brun, M., Freedman, L., Gbangbade, S., Kante, M., Singh, K. (2017). Institutional maternal and perinatal deaths: A review of 40 low and middle income countries. *BMC Pregnancy Childbirth, 17*(1), 295.

Bauserman, M., Lokangaka, A., Thorsten, V., Tshefu, A., Goudar, S. S., Esamai, F., Bose, C. L. (2015). Risk factors for maternal death and trends in maternal mortality in low- and middle-income countries: A prospective longitudinal cohort analysis. *Reprod Health, 12*(Suppl 2), S5.

Bayisa, B., Tatiparthi, R., Mulisa, E. (2014). Use of herbal medicine among pregnant women on antenatal care at nekemte hospital, Western Ethiopia. *Jundishapur Journal of Natural Pharmaceutical Products, 9*(4), e17368.

Belizan, J. M., McClure, E. M., Goudar, S. S., Pasha, O., Esamai, F., Patel, A., Goldenberg, R. L. (2012). Neonatal death in low- to middle-income countries: A global network study. *American Journal of Perinatology, 29*(8), 649–656.

Bucher, S., Konana, O., Liechty, E., Garces, A., Gisore, P., Marete, I., Esamai, F. (2016). Self-reported practices among traditional birth attendants surveyed in western Kenya: A descriptive study. *BMC Pregnancy Childbirth, 16*(1), 219.

Bukar, M., Jauro, Y. S. (2013). Home births and postnatal practices in Madagali, north-eastern Nigeria. *Nigerian Journal of Clinical Practice, 16*(2), 232–237.

Byrne, A., Caulfield, T., Onyo, P., Nyagero, J., Morgan, A., Nduba, J., Kermode, M. (2016). Community and provider perceptions of traditional and skilled birth attendants providing maternal health care for pastoralist communities in Kenya: A qualitative study. *BMC Pregnancy Childbirth, 16*, 43.

Dean, S., Rudan, I., Althabe, F., Webb Girard, A., Howson, C., Langer, A., Bhutta, Z. A. (2013). Setting research priorities for preconception care in low- and middle-income countries: Aiming to reduce maternal and child mortality and morbidity. *PLoS Medicine, 10*(9), e1001508.

Elkhoudri, N., Baali, A., Amor, H. (2016). Maternal morbidity and the use of medicinal herbs in the city of Marrakech, Morocco. *Indian Journal of Traditional Knowledge, 15*(1), 79–85.

Hug, L., Sharrow, D., You, D. (2017). *Levels and Trends in Child Mortality: Report 2017 (English)*. Retrieved from Washington, DC: World Bank Group. http://documents.worldbank.org/curated/en/358381508420391876/Levels-and-trends-in-child-mortality-report-2017.

Kaadaaga, H. F., Ajeani, J., Ononge, S., Alele, P. E., Nakasujja, N., Manabe, Y. C., Kakaire, O. (2014). Prevalence and factors associated with use of herbal medicine among women attending an infertility clinic in Uganda. *BMC Complementary and Alternative Medicine, 14*, 27.

Kaingu, C. K., Oduma, J. A., Kanui, T. I. (2011). Practices of traditional birth attendants in Machakos District, kenya. *Journal of Ethnopharmacology, 137*(1), 495–502.

Kenya National Bureau of Statistics — KNBS, National AIDS Control Council/ Kenya, National AIDS/STD Control Programme/Kenya, Health, M. o. P., Sanitation/Kenya, and Kenya Medical Research Institute. (2010). *Kenya Demographic and Health Survey 2008–2009.* Retrieved from Calverton, Maryland, USA: http://dhsprogram.com/pubs/pdf/FR229/FR229.pdf.

Kenya National Bureau of Statistics, Ministry of Health/Kenya, National AIDS Control Council/Kenya, Kenya Medical Research Institute, Population, N. C. f., and Development/Kenya. (2015). *Kenya Demographic and Health Survey 2014.* Retrieved from Rockville, MD, USA: http://dhsprogram.com/ pubs/pdf/FR308/FR308.pdf.

Lackritz, E. M., Wilson, C. B., Guttmacher, A. E., Howse, J. L., Engmann, C. M., Rubens, C. E., Simpson, J. L. (2013). A solution pathway for preterm birth: Accelerating a priority research agenda. *The Lancet Global Health, 1*(6), e328–e330.

Laelago, T., Yohannes, T., Lemango, F. (2016). Prevalence of herbal medicine use and associated factors among pregnant women attending antenatal care at public health facilities in Hossana Town, southern Ethiopia: Facility based cross sectional study. *Archives of Public Health, 74*, 7.

Lawn, J. E., Cousens, S., Zupan, J. (2005). 4 million neonatal deaths: When? Where? Why? *The Lancet, 365*(9462), 891–900.

Lech, M. M., Mngadi, T. P. (2005). Swaziland's Traditional Birth Attendants Survey. *African Journal Reproductive Health, 9*(3), 137–147.

MacDonald, M. (2017). Why ethnography matters in global health: The case of the traditional birth attendant. *Journal of Global Health, 7*(2), 020302.

Miller, T., Smith, H. (2017). Establishing partnership with traditional birth attendants for improved maternal and newborn health: A review of factors influencing implementation. *BMC Pregnancy Childbirth, 17*(1), 365.

Munabi-Babigumira, S., Glenton, C., Lewin, S., Fretheim, A., Nabudere, H. (2017). Factors that influence the provision of intrapartum and postnatal care by skilled birth attendants in low- and middle-income countries: A qualitative evidence synthesis. *Cochrane Database of Systematic Reviews, 11*, CD011558.

Mureyi, D. D., Monera, T. G., Maponga, C. C. (2012). Prevalence and patterns of prenatal use of traditional medicine among women at selected harare clinics: A cross-sectional study. *BMC Complementary and Alternative Medicine*, *12*, 164.

Ngunyulu, R. N., Mulaudzi, F. M., Peu, M. D. (2015). Comparison between indigenous and Western postnatal care practices in Mopani District, Limpopo Province, South Africa. *Curationis*, *38*(1), 1–9.

Nyeko, R., Tumwesigye, N. M., Halage, A. A. (2016). Prevalence and factors associated with use of herbal medicines during pregnancy among women attending postnatal clinics in Gulu district, Northern Uganda. *BMC Pregnancy Childbirth*, *16*(1), 296.

Pyone, T., Adaji, S., Madaj, B., Woldetsadik, T., van den Broek, N. (2014). Changing the role of the traditional birth attendant in Somaliland. *International Journal of Gynecology & Obstetricspublishes*, *127*(1), 41–46.

Rasch, V., Sorensen, P. H., Wang, A. R., Tibazarwa, F., Jager, A. K. (2014). Unsafe abortion in rural Tanzania — the use of traditional medicine from a patient and a provider perspective. *BMC Pregnancy Childbirth*, *14*, 419.

Ribeiro S. D. (2014). Traditional birth attendance (TBA) in a health system: What are the roles, benefits and challenges: A case study of incorporated TBA in Timor-Leste. *Asia Pacific Family Medicine*, *13*(1), 12.

Shewamene, Z., Dune, T., Smith, C. A. (2017). The use of traditional medicine in maternity care among African women in Africa and the diaspora: A systematic review. *BMC Complementary and Alternative Medicine*, *17*(1), 382.

Souza, J. P., Widmer, M., Gülmezoglu, A. M., Lawrie, T. A., Adejuyigbe, E. A., Carroli, G., Crowther, C., Currie, S. M., Dowswell, T., Hofmeyr, J., Lavendar, T. (2014). Maternal and perinatal health research priorities beyond 2015: An international survey and prioritization exercise. *Reproductive Health*, *11*, 61.

Stanton, C. (2008). Steps towards achieving skilled attendance at birth. *Bulletin World Health Organization*, *86*(4), 242–242a.

Ticktin, T., Dalle, S. P. (2005). Medicinal plant use in the practice of midwifery in rural Honduras. *Journal of Ethnopharmacol*, *96*(1–2), 233–248.

Verguet, S., Norheim, O. F., Olson, Z. D., Yamey, G., Jamison, D. T. (2014). Annual rates of decline in child, maternal, HIV, and tuberculosis mortality across 109 countries of low and middle income from 1990 to 2013: An assessment of the feasibility of post-2015 goals. *The Lancet Global Health*, *2*(12), e698–e709.

Wilunda, C., Dall'Oglio, G., Scangatta, C., Segafredo, G., Lukhele, B. W., Takahashi, R., Putoto, G., Manenti, F., Betràn, A. P. (2017). Changing the role of traditional birth attendants in Yirol West County, South Sudan. *PLoS One*, *12*(11), e0185726.

World Health Organization. (2002). WHO Traditional Medicine Strategy 2002–2005. Retrieved from http://www.who.int/iris/handle/10665/67163.

World Health Organization. (2004). Making Pregnancy Safer: The Critical Role of the Skilled Attendant. A Joint Statement by WHO, ICM, and FIGO.

Chapter 9

Traditional Medicine in Cancer Care

Janet Schloss and Amie Steel

Introduction

In 2015, 8.8 million people worldwide died from cancer equating to 1 in 6 cancer-related deaths globally (World Health Organization, 2018). Cancer has created a significant burden on country and global economies and the lack of data has impacted the writing and development of cancer policies (World Health Organization, 2018). The economic burden of cancer is significant and continues to increase with current estimates suggesting a burden of approximately US$1.16 trillion (Stewart and Wild, 2014). A substantial proportion of health care services, funding and research addresses cancer prevention and treatment throughout the world, either directly or indirectly (Prager *et al.*, 2018). Thirty to fifty percent of cancers are believed to be preventable by modifying lifestyle factors such as avoiding tobacco, reducing alcohol intake, maintaining a healthy body weight, exercising regularly and addressing infection-related risk factors (World Health Organization, 2018). However, once cancer develops more intensive interventions are needed and may encompass further surgery, chemotherapy, radiotherapy, immunotherapy, pharmacological treatment and other required treatments (Mihai *et al.*, 2014; Inada *et al.*, 2015).

Approximately 70% of cancer deaths occur in low to middle income countries mainly due to late-stage presentation and inaccessible diagnosis and treatments (World Health Organization, 2018). In 2017, approximately only 26% of low-income countries reported having pathology services generally available (World Health Organization, 2018) and given many populations in these countries have limited access to modern medical testing and diagnostic techniques, it is not too surprising that traditional medicine (TM) use is much higher in low to middle countries when compared to high income countries (World Health Organization, 2013).

TM knowledge can be difficult to define as it encompasses such diversity. However, in relation to cancer, it represents indigenous knowledge of the use of traditional systems of medical diagnosis alongside the use of medicinal plants, diets or other lifestyle or traditional treatments (Abbott, 2014; Gall and Adams, 2018). The last two decades have seen a renewed interest in the use of traditional and complementary medicine globally particularly in the developing world (Abbott, 2014). According to the World Health Organization (WHO) data, 70% of the Indian population and 90% of Ethiopia depend on TM for their primary health care, 70% of the population in Chile and 40% of Columbians use TM while 40% of all health care delivered in China is TM (World Health Organization, 2013). This chapter will explore TM from different regions around the world within the context of cancer care.

Africa

The population in Africa relies heavily on TM in both middle and low-income countries (Ly, 2018). Due to Africa's large and diverse cultural nature, TM is still practised by traditional healers and used and sometimes misused by patients (Abdullahi, 2011). TM use across Africa is strongly connected to the social, cultural and spiritual life of communities as well as being more affordable and accessible than conventional medical care for some people (Ly, 2018). In Africa, the accessibility of traditional healers compared to doctors is 1:500 people to 1:40,000 people, respectively (World Health Organization, 2013).

The TM used in Africa is primarily phytotherapy — or plant medicine — which has been maintained for generations in families and passed down within families and ethnic groups. The plants employed within these medicines are generally sourced from the natural environments of the local population and most of the benefits, preparations, use and extractions of these plants have been identified, developed and refined through empirical knowledge (Moyo *et al.*, 2015). There are also a large number of religious and/or mystic practices/rituals used across Africa. A substantial number of cancer patients in Africa resort to these rituals which can include exorcism, offering (sacrifices), fumigation, prayers, invocation, reading sacred texts, visiting places of worship or use of holy water. A number of these patients will also be using the TM medicinal plants and/or conventional treatment (Ly, 2018).

In most African countries, the treatment of cancer remains difficult due to the small number of specialists, the lack of technical equipment and the centralization of large health facilities in capital cities (Beck *et al.*, 2018; Sullivan *et al.*, 2015). In addition, there is an insufficient supply of chemotherapy agents within Africa and even where chemotherapy is available the cost of medicines and/or medical care is prohibitive for a majority of the population (Grosse Frie *et al.*, 2018). Equally, the focus on acute care in many African health systems means that cancer prevention and management of sequelae for cancer survivors are often underserviced by conventional medicine (Sullivan *et al.*, 2015). Subsequently, traditional healers may be called upon to respond to the health needs of the population and provide care to individuals in low income and rural or remote communities (Asuzu *et al.*, 2017).

Individuals with diagnosed cancer will use, if possible, both TM and conventional oncology approaches (Jones *et al.*, 2018). However, such medical pluralism is generally only available to those residing in capital cities (de Souza *et al.*, 2016). As conventional oncology care in Africa focuses specifically on cancer treatment, where this is unsuccessful TM serves as palliative care and accompanies patients with terminal illness until end of life as well as providing support at a spiritual level, in line with local cultural beliefs (Ly, 2018). Patients who are in rural or remote areas of Africa will commonly use TM as their first-line treatment for cancer-related symptoms (Jones *et al.*, 2018) partly due to TM being the only care available in the local area. However, variability in TM practitioner training in cancer care can also mean patients utilising TM may experience delays in both cancer diagnosis and access to conventional medical care (Sullivan *et al.*, 2015). Delayed hospital admittance for cancer patients in Africa is associated with numerous risks including an increased risk of mortality, high levels of pain and suffering due to disease progression, higher treatment costs and a reduced chance of recovery (Asuzu *et al.*, 2017).

The Americas

The nature of TM use for cancer in the Americas varies based on different cultures and population characteristics, informed somewhat by historical and contemporary patterns of immigration. The American indigenous communities have developed and used their own TM healing systems over thousands of years (Koithan and Farrell, 2010). A study of Guatemalan children with cancer reported up to 90% of children were prescribed a form of TM during their cancer treatment — most commonly dietary changes, herbal supplements and prayer (Ladas *et al.*, 2014). Family, friends and religious leaders such as priests were reported as the more common source of information about TM in this study. Researchers have also explored the traditional application of herbal medicines in Peru and found that traditional healers reported 14 different combinations of herbal medicines for cancer management (Bussmann *et al.*, 2010). While the details of the specific plant species employed in these herbal formulas are not described in the study, the researchers did indicate that there was consistency in some of the herbs used across formulations suggesting the healers may be selecting plants based on their diagnosis of the underlying cause of the disease.

Within North America, TM use also reflects the influence of Western European immigration alongside local indigenous culture. For example, although naturopathy originates in Germany it is a well-established TM in North America and has evolved locally in response to the eclectic medicine movement of the 19th century (Baer, 1992). Professional formation of naturopathic oncology has taken place in North America over recent decades and a small but not inconsequential number of individuals with cancer consult with a naturopath to manage their cancer-related symptoms (American Board of Naturopathic Oncology, 2018; Oncology Association of Naturopathic Physicians, 2018; John *et al.*, 2016). Health services research suggests naturopathic physicians in the US and Canada use some common substances such as nutritional supplements, exercise prescription, mind-body medicine and dietary changes within individualized treatment plans (Seely *et al.*, 2018) as well as emphasising the psychological and emotional status of their patients and an awareness of contraindications with conventional treatments within their therapeutic approach (Seely *et al.*, 2018).

Some of the most common TM still being employed for cancer treatment has originated from North America include: Hoxsey's treatment, Gerson therapy (Gerson, 1978), Essiac tea (Kaegi, 1998), laetrile (vitamin B17) treatment (Milazzo and Horneber, 2015) and rife machine (ALSUntangled group, 2014). Many other complementary therapies have been developed and are still in use throughout the Americas. However, their development and use are not linked with traditional systems of medicine. To date, indigenous healers in the US are permitted to treat their own people, and all other TM operates separately to modern medicine in non-medical clinics (Portocarrero *et al.*, 2015) — medical clinics or hospitals that have incorporated TM are all located south of the US, mostly in Mexico (Vickers, 2004).

South Asia

A number of countries within the South Asian region have well-established systems of TM as recognized by the World Health Organization. Within India TM is recognized and integrated into the Department of Health as the Ministry of AYUSH — Ayurveda, Yoga, Homeopathy, Naturopathy, Unani and Sidda. Patients presenting with cancer are offered three treatment options within the Indian health care system. First, is the option of conventional medicine use including chemotherapy, radiation therapy and/or surgery. The second option is the use of a wide range of complementary therapies (including TM options) and the third treatment approach offered is some form of combination of both conventional and complementary/traditional medicine (Halpern, 2016b). These choices are pivotal due to demographics. Access to allopathic doctors for the rural community in India is limited, with AYUSH doctors predominately offering the majority of services (Chandra and Patwardhan, 2018). A census in 2011 showed the distribution of the rural-urban Indian population was 68.8 to 31.2%, respectively, (India Government, 2011). As such, nearly 70% of all Indians may not have access to conventional cancer care and thus may be reliant upon TM for diagnosis and treatment. However, the density of AYUSH doctors in urban areas has been found to be 7 times higher when compared to rural areas (with an estimated 0.2 AYUSH doctors available per 10,000 population in rural areas) (Chandra and Patwardhan, 2018). One third of all cancer patients in India have used TM, and this use is linked to a delay in seeking help from conventional medicine (Broom *et al.*, 2009).

Ayurvedic medicine, which originates from India, is one of the oldest documented traditional systems of medicine still widely used today with approximately 29% of medical doctors and 36% of hospital patients reporting use of Ayurveda in India (Roy and Ghosh 2015). Classical Ayurvedic textbooks have several references to cancer although the terms used vary to the Western classifications: *Gulma* (palpable, hard mass in the abdomen); *Granthi* (tumour, lump or nodule visible on the surface); *Arbuda*: cancerous malignancy; and *Dwirabuda* (malignancy has metastasized to other parts of the body) (Halpern, 2016a). In addition, the Ayurvedic practitioners also understand cancer at a constitutional (or doshic) level — recognising it as a condition of *Vata-Kapha* origin. From an Ayurvedic perspective, cancer treatment involves removal of the tumor (if possible), prescription of herbal treatments and dietary modification, and spiritual treatment. Some herbal medicines used in the Ayurvedic cancer treatment — such as *Boswellia serrata* (Shallaki) (Roy *et al.*, 2016), *Curcuma longa* (Haridara) (Rouhollahi *et al.*, 2015) and *Plumbago zeylanica* (Chitraka) (Oyedapo, 1996) — have emerging research evidence suggesting potential clinical benefit for cancer and cancer symptoms, but the majority of others have not yet undergone rigorous scientific evaluation (Garodia *et al.*, 2007).

Yoga is a mind-body intervention that shares historical and philosophical roots with Ayurveda and is characterized by postures (asana), breathing (pranayama) and associated attitudinal, spiritual and dietary/lifestyle practices (Bhavanani, 2016). Within India, there is a much higher rate of yoga practice reported among medical doctors (21%) compared to hospital patients (8%) (Roy, 2015). While the value of yoga alongside contemporary cancer care has received research attention around the world (Agarwal and Maroko-Afex, 2018; Danhauer *et al.*, 2017), the yoga practice being considered and integrated into conventional oncology health services is largely focusing on postural yoga practice. Proponents of yoga as a traditional system of medicine in India argue that this unidimensional approach to integration limits the overall beneficial effects cancer patients may receive from yoga (Nagendra, 2017). Despite these limitations, yoga practice has been found to improve the physical and psychological symptoms associated with cancer, as well as overall quality of life and markers of immunity in cancer patients (Agarwal and Maroko-Afex, 2018).

Unani medicine is an Arabic-Persian TM that was first introduced to the Indo-Pakistan region around a 1,000 years ago and is now considered indigenous to the area (Dunn, 1976) (Che *et al.*, 2017). Like many TM systems, Unani recognizes the mental, emotional, spiritual and physical causes of illness or health and encourages individuals to take responsibility for their own wellbeing (Lloyd, 2009). In Unani, cancer is seen as the disease of black bile humor (Ansari, 2015) and awareness of Sartan — the Unani term for cancer — can be traced back to ancient times (131–AD) (Aslam *et al.*, 1981). The Unani philosophy positions cancer as the end stage of the degeneration of the metabolic efficiency of the body, and is attributed to the combustion and imbalance of certain humors (Ansari, 2015; Aslam *et al.*, 1981). Cancer is also seen by Unani as not one disease, but several hundred different symptoms affecting virtually any organ. It is thought to be caused by an inadequate diet and other imbalances in various aspects of a person's life. The Unani practitioner's philosophy recognizes the natural healing process as being critical to achieving best possible health and that diseases themselves are natural and it is the practitioner's responsibility to help use nature to heal (Ansari, 2015). The Unani treatment for cancer involves 'simples' — plants, animals and minerals — and formulations which have been tabulated with recipes, methods of preparation, doses (if applicable) and modes of administration (Aslam *et al.*, 1981).

One study in 2005 analyzed patient assessment and satisfaction with TM, globalised complementary and alternative medicine (CAM) and allopathic medicine for cancer in Pakistan (Tovey *et al.*, 2005). As a lower/middle income country (USAID, 2012) Pakistan has a long history of TM which is intrinsically linked with religious and spiritual beliefs (Malik, 1997). Anecdotal evidence still suggests that TM healers remain the primary health service providers for many in Pakistan. In addition, access and usage of TM may be influenced by social class and level of education (Malik and Kahn, 2000). From a survey of 362 cancer patients in Pakistan conducted in 2005, 84% used one or more forms of TM in combination with modern or conventional medicine with 59.7% using more than 1 type of CAM/TM (Tovey *et al.*, 2005).

Europe

TM for cancer treatment in Europe should not be overlooked. As a recognized traditional system of medicine, naturopathy has its roots in Germany and is defined by the principles underpinning practice but is also commonly characterized by the use of specific treatments such as herbal medicine, nutrition and diet therapy, lifestyle advice and hydrotherapy. Within the context of naturopathy, a number of traditional medicines have been developed and used for cancer in Europe such as hyperthermia (Gas, 2011) and mistletoe (*Viscum album*) (Ostermann *et al.*, 2009).

Hyperthermia as a treatment for cancer dates back to around 3000 BC and comes from two Greek words *hyper* (rise) and *therme* (heat) (Gas, 2011). There is contemporary work attempting to identify new techniques that will help ensure hyperthermia is simpler, safer and a more effective treatment for cancer patients (Gas, 2011). Today, hyperthermia is an emerging effective treatment in oncology, particularly in Europe. Even with its long history, it remains in its infancy and further research, designs and understanding is required. New opportunities, particularly with nanotechnology and magnetic fluid hyperthermia treatments which have been observed lately show a lot of promise and have helped this TM become firmly imbedded in modern medicine (Gas, 2011).

Mistletoe treatment for cancer, has a similar background and progression as hyperthermia. Over 100 clinical trials have now been conducted with some suggesting it may have benefit (Zanker, 2015) and a recent systematic review confirmed an extended survival period for cancer patients who were being treated with mistletoe extract (*Iscador*) (Ostermann *et al.*, 2009).

Western Pacific

Research into Traditional Chinese medicine (TCM) has become increasingly popular with efforts to scientifically investigate the efficacy of TCM in cancer (Wang *et al.*, 2012). Examples of these investigations have been the development of certain chemotherapy agents (camptothecin, vincristine) which are known and used traditionally in TCM as poisonous herbs (Wang *et al.*, 2012).

Studies are currently being conducted on other TCM herbs, particularly those known in TCM as poisonous Chinese herbal medicine (PCHM) for potential anti-cancer agents/drugs in the medical fraternity (Wang *et al.*, 2012). In addition to TCM herbal medicine developing into chemotherapy, Chinese herbal medicine formulas have also be used alongside conventional therapy or as stand-alone treatments for cancer (Efferth *et al.*, 2015). Considering a large number of people with cancer are treated with these formulas, randomized clinical trials on these preparation are limited (Efferth, 2015). Acupuncture treatment and cancer has been more of a focus particularly in response to the side effects associated with conventional medical cancer treatment (Fraczek *et al.*, 2016).

Traditional Japanese herbal medicine (Kampo medicine) In Japan, the current standard treatment for cancer is a multidisciplinary treatment approach combining chemotherapy, surgery and radiation with TM (including Traditional Japanese herbal medicine — Kampo medicine) and CAM adapted as supportive measures (Yamakawa *et al.*, 2013).

Recently, 148 Kampo extract formulations have been approved for cancer medical care (Yamakawa *et al.*, 2013). This allows Kampo medical practitioners to be able to use TM ethically with western medicine. The majority of Kampo medicine for cancer is used for supportive care, particularly alleviating side effects from treatment such as chemotherapy-induced peripheral neuropathy (CIPN) (Nishioka *et al.*, 2011). Indeed, Kampo medicine is practised by medical practitioners trained in the fundamental diagnosis of Western medicine and a number of clinical trials on Kampo medicine have been conducted (Yamakawa *et al.*, 2013).

Future Prospects

The WHO have recognized the importance of TM producing the latest *WHO Traditional Medicine Strategy 2014–2023* (World Health Organization, 2013) and considering the economic burden of cancer on the world economy and the lack of access to conventional medical cancer treatments in many low to middle income countries, this strategy is imperative. As seen, there are many diverse TM that have been used and in some cases, are still being used for cancer treatment. Identifying the most appropriate TM for each country that could be integrated into cancer care and treatment, writing policies and educating all health practitioners could be the way of the future. What is important is that all such developments follow a rigorous, scientific evaluation and are underpinned by quality evidence — wherever possible and, most importantly, justified the integration and use of TM may hold much promise for all those seeking to optimise care and support for cancer patients. As with all areas of health care and provision, it is vital that we ensure appropriate approaches to treatment and care are accommodated and that direct and indirect risks to patient care are avoided — in the case of cancer care this is especially important given the potential vulnerability of patients who may be open to many treatment options (Schloss *et al.*, 2018) and as such at risk of undertaking unproven and/or problematic care.

Conclusion

Cancer remains a group of diseases with no cure and varying degrees of treatment success with conventional medicine. The renewed interest in the use of TM globally, particularly for cancer (Abbott, 2014) is indicative of the possible combination of conventional medicine with TM for improved outcomes and quality of life among cancer patients. Indeed, there is great potential in extending future research focus into the public health, health services research and clinical investigation of TM within cancer care as a means of identifying both the challenges and potential opportunities related to concurrent and/or integrative use alongside conventional medical care.

References

Abbott, R. (2014). Documenting Traditional Medical Knowledge. *World Intellectual Property Organization.*

Abdullahi, A. A. (2011). Trends and challenges of traditional medicine in Africa. *African Journal of Traditional, Complementary and Alternative Medicines*, 8(5 Suppl), 115–123.

Agarwal R. P., M.-A. A. (2018). Yoga into cancer care: A review of the evidence-based research. *International Journal of Yoga.*, 11(1), 3–29.

ALSUntangled group. (2014). ALSUntangled no. 23: The Rife machine and retroviruses. *Amyotrophic Lateral Sclerosis and Frontotemporal Degeneration*, 15(1–2), 157–159.

American Board of Naturopathic Oncology. (2018). FABNO. Accessed on 16 July 2018.

Ansari ZA. (2015). Cancer Therapeutics in the Unani System of medicine. *Paper presented at the 9th Indo Global Summit on Cancer Therapy*, Hyderabad, India.

Aslam, M., Bano, H., Vohora, S. B. (1981). Sartan (cancer) and its treatment in Unani Medicine. *American Journal of Chinese Medicine*, 9(2), 95–107.

Asuzu, C. C., Elumelu-Kupoluyi, T., Asuzu, M. C., Campbell, O. B., Akin-Odanye, E. O., Lounsbury, D. (2017). A pilot study of cancer patients' use of traditional healers in the Radiotherapy Department, University College Hospital, Ibadan, Nigeria. *Psychooncology*, 26(3), 369–376.

Baer, H. A. (1992). The potential rejuvenation of American naturopathy as a consequence of the holistic health movement. *Medical Anthropology*, 13(4), 369–383.

Beck, E. J., Shields, J. M., Tanna, G., Henning, G., de Vega, I., Andrews, G., Low-Beer, D. (2018). Developing and implementing national health identifiers in resource limited countries: why, what, who, when and how? *Global Health Action*, 11(1), 1440782.

Bhavanani, A. B. (2016). Health and Well Being: A Yogic Perpective. Accessed on July 16, 2018.

Broom A, N. K., Tovey P, Shirali R, Thakur R, Seth T, Chhetri6 P. (2009). Indian cancer patients' use of traditional, complementary and alternative medicine (TCAM) and delays in presentation to hospital. *Oman Medical Journal*, 24(2), 99–102.

Bussmann, R. W., Glenn, A., Meyer, K., Kuhlman, A., Townesmith, A. (2010). Herbal mixtures in traditional medicine in Northern Peru. *Journal of Ethnobiology and Ethnomedicine*, 6, 10.

Chandra, S., Patwardhan, K. (2018). Allopathic, AYUSH and informal medical practitioners in rural India — a prescription for change. *Journal of Ayurveda and Integrative Medicine*, *9*(2), 143–150.

Che CT, A.-M. (2017). Traditional medicine. *Pharmacognosy*, 2.23.

Danhauer, S. C., Addington, E. L., Sohl, S. J., Chaoul, A., Cohen, L. (2017). Review of yoga therapy during cancer treatment. *Support Care Cancer*, *25*(4), 1357–1372.

de Souza, J. A., Hunt, B., Asirwa, F. C., Adebamowo, C., Lopes, G. (2016). Global health equity: Cancer care outcome disparities in high-, middle-, and low-income countries. *Journal of Clinical Oncology*, *34*(1), 6–13.

Dunn, F. L. (1976). Traditional Asian medicine and cosmopolitan medicine as adaptive systems. *Asian medical systems: A comparative study*, 133–158, DOI.org/10.1093/ecam/neq067.

Efferth T. L. P., BadireenathKonkimalla, V. S. B. (2015). Review: From traditional Chinese medicine to rational cancer therapy. *Trends in Molecular Medicine*, *13*(8), 353–361.

Fraczek, P., Kilian-Kita, A., Puskulluoglu, M., Krzemieniecki, K. (2016). Acupuncture as anticancer treatment? *Contemporary Oncology*, *20*(6), 453–457.

Gall, A., Leske, S., Adams, J., Matthews, V., Anderson, K., Lawler, S., Garvey, G. (2018). Traditional and complementary medicine use among indigenous cancer patients in Australia, Canada, New Zealand, and the United States: A systematic review. *Integrative Cancer Therapies*, *17*(3), 568–581.

Garcia, M. K., McQuade, J., Haddad, R., Patel, S., Lee, R., Yang, P., Cohen, L. (2013). Systematic review of acupuncture in cancer care: A synthesis of the evidence. *Journal of Clinical Oncology*, *31*(7), 952–960.

Garodia, P., Ichikawa, H., Malani, N., Sethi, G., Aggarwal, B. B. (2007). From ancient medicine to modern medicine: Ayurvedic concepts of health and their role in inflammation and cancer. *Journal of the Society for Integrative Oncology*, *5*(1), 25–37.

Gas, P. (2011). Essential facts on the history of hyperthermia and their connections with electromedicine. *Przegląd Elektrotechniczny*. *30*, 30-059.

Gerson M. (1978). The cure of advanced cancer by diet therapy: A summary of thirty years of clinical experimentation. *Physiological Chemistry and Physics*, *10*(5), 449–464.

Grosse F. K., Samoura, H., Diop, S., Kamate, B., Traore, C. B., Malle, B., Kantelhardt, E. J. (2018). Why do women with breast cancer get diagnosed and treated late in sub-saharan Africa? Perspectives from women and patients in Bamako, Mali. *Breast Care (Basel), 13*(1), 39–43.

Halpern, M. (2016a). Managing cancer Part 2: Gulma, Granthi, and Arbuda. *Managing Cancer.* www.ayurvedacollege.com/arcticles/drhalpern/clinical/cancer/2.

Halpern M. (2016b). Managing cancer Part 3: Herbs. *Managing Cancer.* www.ayurvedacollege.com/arcticles/drhalpern/clinical/cancer/2.

Inada, R., Nagasaka, T., Toshima, T., Mori, Y., Kondo, Y., Kishimoto, H., Fujiwara, T. (2015). Aggressive multimodality treatment for advanced rectal cancer. *Acta Medical Okayama, 69*(2), 113–118.

India Government. (2011). Rural urban distribution of population. *Census of India.* Accessed on 27 June, 2018.

John, G. M., Hershman, D. L., Falci, L., Shi, Z., Tsai, W. Y., Greenlee, H. (2016). Complementary and alternative medicine use among US cancer survivors. *Journal of Cancer Survivorship, 10*(5), 850–864.

Jones, D., Cohen, L., Rieber, A. G., Urbauer, D., Fellman, B., Fisch, M. J., Nazario, A. (2018). Complementary and alternative medicine use in minority and medically underserved oncology patients: Assessment and implications. *Integrative Cancer Therapies, 17*(2), 371–379.

Kaegi, E. (1998). Unconventional therapies for cancer: 1. Essiac. The task force on alternative therapies of the canadian breast cancer research initiative. *Canadian Medical Association Journal, 158*(7), 897–902.

Koithan, M., Farrell, C. (2010). Indigenous native American healing traditions. *Journal for Nurse Practitioners, 6*(6), 477–478.

Ladas, E. J., Rivas, S., Ndao, D., Damoulakis, D., Bao, Y. Y., Cheng, B., Antillon, F. (2014). Use of traditional and complementary/alternative medicine (TCAM) in children with cancer in Guatemala. *Pediatric Blood and Cancer, 61*(4), 687–692.

Liu, J., Wang, S., Zhang, Y., Fan, H. T., Lin, H. S. (2015). Traditional Chinese medicine and cancer: History, present situation, and development. *Thoracic Cancer, 6*(5), 561–569.

Lloyd, I. (2009). Traditional and Complementary systems of Medicine. *The Energetics of Health,* 13–27.

Ly, A. K. D. (2006). *About Cancer in Africa: From Epidemiology to Biomedical Applications and Perspectives.* Paper presented at the Boulogne Billancourt, Paris, France.

Ly, A. (2016). Global health, cancer challenges adn control in African settings. *Cancer Therapy & Oncology International Journal, 2*(3), 1–4.

Ly, A. (2018). Traditional medicines and cancer therapies in African landscape. *Journal of Tumor Medicine & Prevention*, *3*(1), 555601.

Malik, I, Q. A. (1997). Communication with cancer patients, experience in Pakistan. In Surbone, A. and Zwitter, M. (eds.), *Communication With the Cancer Patient: Information and the Truth. Annals of the New York Academy of Sciences*, *809*, 300–308.

Malik I. K. N., Kahn W. (2000). Use of unconventional methods of therapy by cancer patients in Pakistan. *European Journal of Epidemiology*, *16*, 155–160.

Mihai, D., Voiculescu, S., Cristian, D., Constantinescu, F., Popa, E., Burcos, T. (2014). Multimodal treatment of aggressive forms of breast cancer. *Journal of Medicine and Life*, *7*(3), 415–420.

Milazzo, S., Horneber, M. (2015). Laetrile treatment for cancer. *Cochrane Database of Systematic Reviews*, (4), Cd005476.

Moyo, M., Aremu, A. O., Van Staden, J. (2015). Medicinal plants: An invaluable, dwindling resource in sub-Saharan Africa. *Journal of Ethnopharmacology*, *174*, 595–606.

Nagendra, H. R. (2017). Integrating yoga in cancer care: Scope and challenges. *Indian Journal of Palliative Care*, *23*(3), 223–224.

Nestler G. (2002). Traditional Chinese medicine. *Medical Clinics*, *86*(1), 63–73.

Nishioka, M., Shimada, M., Kurita, N., Iwata, T., Morimoto, S., Yoshikawa, K., Higasuijima, J., Miyatani, T., Kono, T. (2011). The Kampo medicine, Goshajinkigan, prevents neuropathy in patients treated by FOLFOX regimen. *International Journal of Clinical Oncology*, *16*(4), 322–327.

Oncology Association of Naturopathic Physicians (2018). *Oncology Association of Naturopathic Physicans.* Accessed on 16 July 2018.

Ostermann, T., Raak, C., Bussing, A. (2009). Survival of cancer patients treated with mistletoe extract (Iscador): A systematic literature review. *BMC Cancer*, *9*, 451.

Oyedapo, O. O. (1996). Studies on bioactivity of the root extract of *Plumbago zeylanica*. *International Journal of Pharmacognosy, 34*(5), 365–369.

Portocarrero, J., Palma-Pinedo, H., Pesantes, M. A., Seminario, G., Lema, C. (2015). [Traditional andean healers in the context of change: The case of Churcampa in Peru]. *Revista Peruana de Medicina Experimental y Salud Pública*, *32*(3), 492–498.

Prager, G. W., Braga, S., Bystricky, B., Qvortrup, C., Criscitiello, C., Esin, E., lbawi, A. (2018). Global cancer control: Responding to the growing burden, rising costs and inequalities in access. *ESMO Open*, *3*(2), e000285.

Rouhollahi, E., Zorofchian Moghadamtousi, S., Paydar, M., Fadaeinasab, M., Zahedifard, M., Hajrezaie, M., Mohamed, Z. (2015). Inhibitory effect of *Curcuma purpurascens* BI. rhizome on HT-29 colon cancer cells through mitochondrial-dependent apoptosis pathway. *BMC Complementary and Alternative Medicine*, *15*, 15.015-0534-0536.

Roy V, G. M., Ghosh, R. K. (2015). Perception, attitude and usage of complementary and alternative medicine among doctors and patients in a tertiary care hospital in India. *Indian Journal of Pharmacology*. *47*(2), 137–142.

Roy, V., Gupta, M., Ghosh, R. K. (2015). Perception, attitude and usage of complementary and alternative medicine among doctors and patients in a tertiary care hospital in India. *Indian Journal of Pharmacology*, *47*(2), 137–142.

Roy, N. K., Deka, A., Bordoloi, D., Mishra, S., Kumar, A. P., Sethi, G., Kunnumakkara, A. B. (2016). The potential role of boswellic acids in cancer prevention and treatment. *Cancer Letters*, *377*(1), 74–86.

Schloss J., Alschuler, L. McDonnell, E. (2018). Women's cancers and complementary and integrative medicine: A focus upon prevention, disease management and survivorship. In Adams, S. A., Broom, A., and Frawley, J, (eds.), *Women's Health an Complementary and Integrative Medicine*. Routledge, London.

Seely, D., Ennis, J. K., McDonell, E., Zhao, L. (2018). Naturopathic oncology care for thoracic cancers: A practice survey. *Integrative Cancer Therapies*, 1534735418759420.

Stewart, B. W., Wild, C. P. (2014). World Cancer Report 2014. *International Agency for Research on Cancer*, Lyon, France.

Sudhakar, A. (2009). History of cancer, ancient and modern treatment methods. *Journal of Cancer Science and Therapy*, *1*(2), 1–4.

Sullivan, R., Alatise, O. I., Anderson, B. O., Audisio, R., Autier, P., Aggarwal, A., and Purushotham, A. (2015). Global cancer surgery: Delivering safe, affordable, and timely cancer surgery. *Lancet Oncology*, *16*(11), 1193–1224.

Tang, J. L., Liu, B. Y., Ma, K. W. (2008). Traditional Chinese medicine. *Lancet*, *372*(9654), 1938–1940.

Tovey, P., Broom, A., Chatwin, J., Hafeez, M., Ahmad, S. (2005). Patient assessment of effectiveness and satisfaction with traditional medicine, globalized complementary and alternative medicines, and allopathic medicines for cancer in Pakistan. *Integrative Cancer Therapies*, *4*(3), 242–248.

USAID. (2012). *List of Developing Countries*. https://www.usaid.gov/sites/default/files/documents/1876/310maa.pdf.

Vickers, A. (2004). Alternative cancer cures: "unproven" or "disproven"? *CA: A Cancer Journal for Clinicians, 54*(2), 110–118.

Wang, S., Wu, X., Tan, M., Gong, J., Tan, W., Bian, B., Wang, Y. (2012). Fighting fire with fire: Poisonous Chinese herbal medicine for cancer therapy. *Journal of Ethnopharmacology, 140*(1), 33–45.

Watanabe, K., Matsuura, K., Gao, P., Hottenbacher, L., Tokunaga, H., Nishimura, K., Witt, C. M. (2011). Traditional Japanese Kampo medicine: Clinical research between modernity and traditional medicine-the state of research and methodological suggestions for the future. *Evidence-Based Complementary and Alternative Medicine,* 513842, DOI.org/10.1093/ecam/neq067.

World Health Organization (2013). Traditional Medicine Strategy: 2014–2023. *Essential Medicines and Health Products.* Accessed on 26 June 2018.

World Health Organization (2018). Cancer. Accessed on 26 June 2018.

Yamakawa, J., Motoo, Y., Moriya, J., Ogawa, M., Uenishi, H., Akazawa, S., Kobayashi, J. (2013). Significance of Kampo, traditional Japanese medicine, in supportive care of cancer patients. *Evidence-Based Complementary and Alternative Medicine,* 746486.

Zanker K.S. (2015). Mistletoe through cultural and medical history: The all-healing plant proves to be a cancer-specific remedy. *Journal of Biomedical and Translational Research., 4,* 1–10.

Zhou, J., Xie, G., Yan, X. (2004). *Traditional Chinese Medicine: Molecular Structures, Natural Sources and Applications,* 2nd Edition, Wiley & Sons.

Chapter 10

Traditional, Complementary and Integrative Medicine as Self-Care in Chronic Illness: A Focus Upon Stroke and Older Adults

Jon Adams, Wenbo Peng, Jason Prior, Roger Dunston,
Erica McIntyre, Irena Connon, David Sibbritt, Alex Broom,
Patricia Davidson and Bradley Leech

Introduction

Traditional, complementary and integrative medicine (TCIM) has been found to be widely used for treating post-stroke related conditions, and has attracted increasing research interest from health care practitioners, researchers and policymakers. In this chapter, we explore TCIM self-care (amid the wider pool of TCIM) use among older post-stroke patients as a topic for further research focus. The chapter in part draws upon the details of a relevant case study in progress in Australia and closes with a consideration of a number of possible areas for future research attention.

Chronic Illness and Conventional Health Care Services

Chronic diseases constitute a major public health problem worldwide and related health care expenses are now a significant health-care utilization concern (Papanicolas *et al.*, 2018). The number of Australians aged 60 years plus will double in the next 30 years (AIHW, 2011). Chronic illness rates increase significantly with age (AIHW, 2012). The already inordinate burden of chronic illness in ageing (including cardiovascular disease) is set to expand dramatically, accounting for nearly half of all deaths and disability in Australia by 2020 (Savage, 2009). Chronic illness during ageing has profound impact on an individual's family/community and quality of life (Shaul, 2012) with extensive economic, psychological household burden (Jan, 2012). Yet, conventional health services — both practitioner-delivered and non-CAM forms of self-management (e.g. diet, exercise) — have largely failed to meet the complex needs of older adults (Willison *et al.*, 2012). As a result, people are seeking community-based 'alternatives' for coping with ageing and associated illnesses (Willison *et al.*, 2012) and addressing this research gap is imperative to providing a fuller understanding of community-based responses to chronic illness and to addressing the challenges faced by older adults, their families and communities.

The Context of Stroke

Stroke is a common chronic disease occurring when a blood vessel supplying blood and oxygen to the brain either becomes blocked and which restricts blood flow to brain cells (ischemic stroke) or bleeds into the tissue deep within the brain (hemorrhagic stroke) (American Stroke Assocation, 2016). The most frequent symptoms of stroke include sudden weakness, paralysis of parts of the body (e.g. face, arms or legs), and speech problems (e.g. trouble speaking and difficulty with swallowing) (Australian Stroke Foundation, 2018). Stroke exerts significant burden upon a sufferers' quality of life leading to substantial physical, psychological and social challenges (Cerniauskaite *et al.*, 2012). Stroke is also a major cause of mortality among a majority of high-income countries (Langhorne *et al.*, 2011) with the prevalence of stroke increasing significantly (by 27%) within the last 10 years (Feigin *et al.*, 2014). According to the data released by the Australian Institute of Health and Welfare, there were 37,000 hospitalizations for acute stroke care and 28,000 hospitalizations for stroke rehabilitation care in 2013–2014, with the majority of stroke patients aged over 65 years (National Stroke Foundation, 2015). Indeed, the aging population has been identified as one of the main reasons for the rise of stroke incidence (Mukherjee and Patil, 2011).

A range of conditions and individuals' habits can raise the risk of suffering from stroke (National Heart, Lung and Blood Institute, 2015). There are three groups of stroke risk factors — non-modifiable risk factors (e.g. age, gender and family history of stroke), medical risk factors (e.g. transient ischaemic attack, atrial fibrillation and diabetes) and modifiable risk factors (Australian Stroke Foundation, 2017b). It is important to note that as many as 80% of new or subsequent strokes of all types could be prevented if such modifiable risk factors are controlled (O'Donnell *et al.*, 2016). An international case-control study has reported the ten most common modifiable risk factors of stroke regardless of the patients' socio-demographic characteristics, including high blood pressure (hypertension), smoking or alcohol dependence and improper lifestyle pattern (e.g. diet and physical activity). Notably, some of the modifiable risk factors of stroke are strongly interrelated and individuals with stroke may have more than two risk factors (Straus *et al.*, 2002). Acute stroke survivors have an 11.1% risk of recurrent stroke after 1 year, a 26.4% risk after 5 years and a 39.2% risk after 10 years (Hankey, 2014). Predictors of long-term recurrent stroke include prevalent vascular risk factors, previous symptomatic vascular disease, unstable vascular disease, embolic sources and causes and possibly cerebral microbleeds (Hankey, 2014). Recurrent stroke which makes up 25–30% of all strokes highlights the ineffective secondary prevention methods implemented in the community (Hankey, 2014).

All acute stroke patients need immediate attention and should be admitted to hospital as soon as possible (Australian Stroke Foundation, 2017a). The medical management for acute stroke include, but are not limited to, reperfusion therapy, neurointervention, antithrombotic therapy, hemicraniectomy, glycaemic therapy and surgery (Australian Stroke Foundation, 2017a). As the medical/surgical treatment of stroke has obtained impressive development in the last decade, a large proportion of patients with stroke now survive the initial disease (Langhorne *et al.*, 2011). In Australia, a total of 475,000 people were living with stroke in 2017 and the number of stroke sufferers is estimated to be one million by 2050 (Deloitte Access Economics, 2018). The time period required for full recovery from stroke varies across patients and some stroke sufferers may have long-term or lifelong disabilities (National Heart, Lung and Blood Institute, 2015).

Upon hospital discharge, 12.8% of post-stroke patients are reported to be dependent on others (carers/family) for basic living activities (Pinedo *et al.*, 2014). Moreover, 29% of stroke survivors 6 months post-stroke are reported to experience severe disabilities while living in the community, representing a major health burden (Rouillard *et al.*, 2012). As such, rehabilitation is a major component and priority of post-stroke patient care (Jones *et al.*, 2013) and research shows self-management or self-care conducted by informal carers provide main bulk of ongoing care for stroke survivors (National Stroke Foundation, 2015). The 2017 clinical guidelines for stroke management also recommends that home-based rehabilitation may be a favored model for delivering rehabilitation in the community (Australian Stroke Foundation, 2017a). However, although a number of self-care pro-grams have been implemented in many diseases and conditions (e.g. arthritis and diabetes), post-stroke self-care has not received coordi-nated attention (Jones *et al.*, 2013). In fact, there is often no uniform nationwide post-stroke rehabilitation service available in many high-income countries (Guidetti *et al.*, 2014). Although there are a limited number of stroke self-management programs, initial findings suggest promising results (Jones, 2013) and supporting the rehabilitation of stroke survivors through targeted programs has been suggested as a key aspect of improving community mobility (Rouillard *et al.*, 2012). It has been suggested that exercise and education programs may improve the health-related quality of life of community-dwelling stroke survivors (White *et al.*, 2013). However, community-dwelling stroke survivors who have undertaken an intensive inpatient rehabilitation program still appear to experience a lack of independence 6 months post stroke (Rouillard *et al.*, 2012).

Interventions for long-term secondary stroke prevention currently involve a combination of pharmacological and lifestyle behaviours (Hankey, 2014). Integrative medicine/health care involving a combination of conventional rehabilitation and acupuncture/Chinese herbal medicine has been shown to improve overall stroke rehabilitation outcomes (Fang *et al.*, 2016). Self-care can include a wide range of health care practitioners and different treatment methods to help improve patients' physical and psychological problems (Jones *et al.*, 2013) and such self-care rehabilitation of post-stroke patients may involve TCIM approaches alone or in addition to conventional treatments (Hart, 2010). The first-line conventional medications prescribed to post-stroke patients are anticoagulants or blood thinners. Nevertheless, caution on behalf of stroke survivors as a result of risks relating to these commonly-used medications can lead to the use of TCIM for symptom relief (Miller *et al.*, 2004). Unfortunately, despite all these interesting early findings, no work to date has systematically examined the use of TCIM (alone or within a wider context of care and treatments) among a cohort of stroke survivors and this is undoubtedly a rich area for further study and possibly improved post-stroke health outcomes.

The Utilization of TCIM (Self-Care) as a Component of Post Stroke Rehabilitation

The range of TCIM therapies and products used for post-stroke rehabilitation is varied including both self-care and non-self-care modalities. To clarify, this particular distinction is based upon an appreciation that some TCIM is exclusively or predominantly practitioner-led. Whether via a medically trained provider or otherwise, this form of TCIM is initiated and guided via expert help and requires consultation (numerous consultations in many cases) with a health professional. In contrast, TCIM self-care refers to those practices, behaviours and technologies that are exclusively or predominantly patient-led or community-led (i.e. not requiring significant and/or ongoing practitioner directives). As previous writing has identified, the reframing of some TCIM as self-care is more than just a change in categorization, it also has significant implications for our empirical and conceptual considerations and orientations (Adams *et al.*, 2018). The importance of TCIM self-care for approaching chronic illness includes refocusing attention upon: (1) the disconnect between these forms of TCIM and conventional medical care and provision; (2) TCIM approaches that are often philosophically divergent from conventional medical approaches; (3) treatments and practices that are well and truly beyond the control of the state or related health practitioners and (4) activities that may in many cases hold much potential and opportunity for helping those with stroke and other chronic illness cope with living with their symptoms. What is fundamental about TCIM self-care is that it is predominantly covert in nature, initiated and undertaken by individuals and community-based actors beyond the gaze of the conventional medical fraternity (Adams *et al.*, 2018) and this can mean the users of these self-care practices are perhaps even more prone to direct and indirect risks than others employing the services of TCIM practitioners (Adams *et al.*, 2014).

Acupuncture is reported to be the most frequently used TCIM treatment, followed by herbal medicine, Chinese (herbal) medicine, mind and body practices (e.g. yoga and meditation), manual therapies (e.g. chiropractic and remedial massage therapy) and other TCIM modalities (Feigin, 2007; Shah *et al.*, 2008; Wu *et al.*, 2008). Tai Chi appears to be an effective intervention to reduce fall rate among stroke survivors (Taylor-Piliae *et al.*, 2014). Stroke patients report seeking help from TCIM treatments not only for relief from both physical and mental health symptoms (Hart, 2010). Furthermore, stroke patients have indicated secondary stroke prevention as an area where they desire further information (Walsh *et al.*, 2015). Several reviews have been published on the benefits of TCIM in the management of post-stroke (Lennon *et al.*, 2013; Zhang *et al.*, 2014). However, the current evidence is unable to support the clinical effect of overall TCIM or single TCIM self-care and non self-care with regard to post-stroke recovery, mainly due to the poor research study design and complex active components of herbs (Feigin, 2007; Zhang *et al.*, 2014).

Where to From Here? A Proposed Case Study of TCIM Self-Care Among Older Stroke Patients in Australia

In line with the details described above, despite a lack of solid evidence-based TCIM treatments including both self-care and non-self-care interventions, TCIM appears to be one component of health seeking among older post-stroke patients in high-income countries highlighting a substantial gap in scholarship around stroke rehabilitation care. As a means of exploring the opportunities and future research gaps and opportunities around TCIM (self-care) use for stroke, this chapter now introduces an active project (ongoing at time of writing) which will provide the world-first, in-depth investigation of this specific topic. This chapter will also outline a number of areas for future investigation around this important topic.

The project in progress is a sub-study of a larger, well-established study — the 45 and Up Study — an ongoing long-term cohort health study focusing upon individuals aged 45 and over who live in New South Wales (NSW), Australia (Banks *et al.*, 2008). The Sax Institute established and manages the 45 and Up Study, in collaboration with a number of key partners such as Cancer Council NSW, NSW Division of the National Heart Foundation of Australia; NSW Government Family and Community Services and the Australian Red Cross Blood Service.

Residents in NSW were randomly sampled from the Medicare Australia enrolment database, which is the national health care system operated by the Department of Human Services to fund primary health care of Australian citizens, permanent residents, some temporary residents and refugees. To date, the 45 and Up Study is the largest long-term cohort study of health services research ever implemented in Australia with more than one in 10 NSW men and women aged older than 45 years (more than a quarter of a million) having participated in the baseline study (Sax Institute, 2009). The baseline recruitment of the 45 and Up Study commenced in 2006 and was completed in 2009. For the baseline questionnaire, participants were asked about their demographic characteristics, health behaviours, health status, medical history, known chronic diseases and associated treatments. Every five years, this same questionnaire is repeated.

The current authors and colleagues designed a sub-study which received competitive funding from the Australian Research Council (ARC) and draws upon the 45 and Up Study in order to recruit participants. This sub-study remains in progress at time of writing and explores the use of TCIM self-care among older Australians with stroke. A total of 1,300 participants of the 45 and Up Study have indicated that they have diagnosed as having stroke. All these post-stroke participants were mailed a consent form and a specific questionnaire to provide more information on their TCIM self-care for stroke relief for the recruitment of this 45 and Up Sub-study, with 576 returning a completed questionnaire (response rate: 44.3%). In the questionnaire for this sub-study, participants were questioned regarding their social-demographic characteristics, lifestyle behaviours, health care use and expenses and a range of health indicators including their sleep behaviour and quality of life.

Post-stroke patients in the 45 and Up Sub-study were also required to stipulate the time when they were first diagnosed with stroke, rate their disability degree via the modified Rankin Scale (Wilson *et al.*, 2002) and mark their fatigue level via the modified Fatigue Impact Scale — 5-item version (D'souza, 2016), respectively. This sub-study aims to identify older stroke patients' [*self-care*] management of stroke-related symptoms alongside their utilization of conventional medical treatments. To be specific, concerning health care utilization, these post-stroke participants were required to indicate whether they had consulted any conventional medical doctor (options: general practitioners, hospital doctors, cardiologists and neurologists), any allied health provider (options: speech pathologists, nurses, pharmacists, physiotherapists, occupational therapists, counsellors, psychologists and dietitians) and/or any TCIM practitioner (options: acupuncturists, Chinese medicine practitioners, naturopath/herbalists, chiropractors, osteopaths, massage therapists, yoga instructors, meditation instructors, nutritionists, homoeopaths and an 'other' TCIM practitioner option) in the last 12 months as part of their stroke care. Also, the post-stroke participants were further asked about their use of a broad range of TCIM products in the previous year for the management of stroke, including herbal medicines, caffeine-related products or drinks,

CoQ10, folic acid, ginkgo, garlic, homeopathic remedies, multivitamins/minerals, vitamin B12, vitamin C, vitamin D, vitamin E, multivitamin B, omega 3, physical activities, St John's wort, Tai Chi without instructor, yoga without instructor, meditation without instructor and mindfulness. The names of all prescribed medications taken for treating stroke during the last 12 months were also collected via the questionnaire. With regards to health care costs, post-stroke participants reported their out-of-pocket expenses including with regard to TCIM practitioner consultations, TCIM self-care product use and conventional medicine use in the last 12 months.

While this work remains in progress (and specific results and findings are yet to be available) it is important to consider this study within the wider framework of TCIM research around stroke among older adults. There are many research possibilities that can be explored around this topic and, drawing directly upon the sub-study outlined, we here discuss a number that may hold particular merit and help further understand critical issues around the wider picture of health-seeking among those with stroke.

Research Agenda in TCIM Self-Care Among Older Stroke Survivors

Post-stroke constitutes a significantly important period in the journey of stroke sufferers which also has a heavy burden upon health care systems. There is increasing recognition that rehabilitation care is very important for the recovery of post-stroke survivors, and self-care is often used by these stroke survivors or their carers (Frost *et al.*, 2015). TCIM self-care is not only used for treating physical behaviour changes but also employed for supporting emotional issues among those living post-stroke (Jones *et al.*, 2013). A qualitative study has reported the top four self-care needs of stroke patients, referring to preventing falls, staying active, managing emotional changes and maintaining sufficient nutrition (Pierce *et al.*, 2004). Despite emerging TCIM self-care research, studies of this topic designed exclusively for older stroke survivors remain scarce and the appropriate approach of TCIM self-care programs unclear (Lennon *et al.*, 2013). Importantly, most self-care interventions including TCIM self-care methods are multicomponent in nature (Lennon *et al.*, 2013) — a TCIM self-care program is highly likely to be employed alongside usual conventional medical care or other treatment(s). As such, further in-depth studies in the field of post-stroke patient care are required to further understand the circumstances and features of TCIM self-care regarding stroke survivorship and test the effect and feasibility of TCIM self-care in this health area. Below we select just three areas of enquiry (among many possible areas) that can help advance our knowledge of TCIM self-care with regard to stroke rehabilitation.

Longitudinal analyses of TCIM self-care for post-stroke

A longitudinal study design can help identify the ongoing experience and effect of interventions focusing upon use of treatments and a range of changes affecting stroke survivors over time (Caruana *et al.*, 2015). It is important that enquiry on this topic go beyond purely cross-sectional analysis in order to explore changes in experience, motivation and outcomes regarding TCIM self-care from early stages post-stroke onwards. As already identified a number of physical indicators and behaviours of individuals post-stroke are likely to fluctuate over time at different periods post stroke event (Tse *et al.*, 2017) and it is not unreasonable to assume the same with regard to TCIM self-care. Among other questions that can be answered via a longitudinal analysis are: Do patients post-stroke tend to utilize more or less TCIM self-care the longer the period since stroke event? Does such utilization change in its composition and features? And to what extent is such TCIM self-care use over time relayed to or enquired about by conventional medical providers?

Examination of decision-making process and communication of stroke survivors using TCIM self-care

Given widespread TCIM self-care utilization for chronic diseases including stroke in high-income countries and the current lack of available evidence for these treatments, it is essential to identify how stroke survivors' experience, perceive and evaluate such use. Decision-making around TCIM self-care is a complex process and individuals may experience different symptoms and sequelae at the rehabilitation stage (Hart, 2010). In-depth exploration of the nature of such self-care use is therefore needed to help clinicians understand the motivation of stroke patient use, how to better instruct their patients regarding TCIM self-care practice, and how to improve or embrace such community-based care into their clinical stroke care (Riegel *et al.*, 2017). Additionally, a proportion of older post-stroke patients suffer from psychological problems which are generally difficult to fix and may impact on an individuals' capacity to self-care (Jones *et al.*, 2013). As such, older patients post-stroke should be encouraged to communicate with their formal or informal carers and it is necessary for conventional medical providers to actively enquire with their patients with stroke regarding both TCIM self-care and TCIM non-self-care use. Initially, studies of various designs focusing upon the communication and disclosure between stroke survivors and health care providers are required to help minimize direct and indirect safety issues related to concurrent care which can in many cases take place in a communication-vacuum (Wardle and Adams, 2014).

Cost-effective evaluation of TCIM self-care use for the management of stroke

Long-term conventional medical treatment and rehabilitation costs and indirect expenses from self-care impose significant economic burden on post-stroke patients (Demaerschalk *et al.*, 2010). The heavy burden of direct and indirect costs associated with stroke care highlight an urgent need for cost-effective analysis of *all* treatment/care options (including TCIM self-care) with a view to helping reduce health system expenditure for stroke-related health services (Demaerschalk *et al.*, 2010; Hughes *et al.*, 2015). The covert nature of TCIM self-care renders such investigation both potentially challenging and rewarding but, ultimately, there is much opportunity in exploring the possible cost-saving from well-coordinated TCIM self-care for advancing community-based and focused interventions to help contain health system expenditure for those living post-stroke.

Conclusion

Rehabilitation care is an identified priority of post-stroke treatment and research and although there is a lack of solid evidence regarding the efficacy of TCIM for the management of stroke, TCIM self-care programs are commonly used by stroke survivors and their carers. To strengthen this important field of post-stroke patient care, more TCIM self-care research projects are needed in order to ensure in-depth understanding of how those living post-stroke navigate all the broad and complex treatment options available to them. Insights from such work will be of significance to all involved in post-stroke care. Regardless of professional judgement or perspective regarding TCIM, it is essential that those providing rehabilitation care for stroke survivors engage with both practitioner-based and self-care TCIM practices in order to maintain and ensure safe, effective care delivery.

References

Adams, J., Prior, J., Sibbritt, D., Connon, I., Dunston, R., McIntyre, E., Lauche, R. (2018). The use of self-care practices and products by women with chronic illness: a case study of older women with osteoarthritis and osteoporosis. In Adams, J., Steel, A., Broom, A. and Frawley, J. (eds.), *Women's Health and Complementary and Integrative Medicine*, Routledge, New York, pp. 89–105.

Adams, J., Kroll, T., Broom, A. (2014). The significance of complementary and alternative medicine (CAM) as self-care: Examining 'hidden' health-seeking behaviour for chronic illness in later life. *Advances in Integrative Medicine*, *1*(3), 103–104.

American Stroke Assocation. (2016). Let's talk about stroke patient information sheets http://www.strokeassociation.org/STROKEORG/AboutStroke/Lets-Talk-About-Stroke-Patient-Information-Sheets_UCM_310731_Article.jsp#. Wz8j11UzaUm.

Australian Institute of Health and Welfare (2011). Trenmds in palliative care. AIHW, Canberra.

Australian Institute of Health and Welfare (2012). Older Australians at a glance. AIHW, Canberra.

Australian Stroke Foundation. (2017a). Clinical guidelines for stroke management 2017 https://informme.org.au/Guidelines/Clinical-Guidelines-for-Stroke-Management-2017.

Australian Stroke Foundation (2017b). Stroke risk factors. https://stroke foundation.org.au/About-Stroke/Preventing-stroke/Stroke-risk-factors.

Australian Stroke Foundation (2018). Stroke symptoms. https://strokefoundation. org.au/About-Stroke/Stroke-symptoms.

Banks, E., Redman, S., Jorm, L., Armstrong, B., Bauman, A., Beard, J., Lujic, S. (2008). Cohort profile: The 45 and up study. *International Journal of Epidemiology*, *37*(5), 941–947.

Caruana, E., Roman, M., Hernández-Sánchez, J., Solli, P. (2015). Longitudinal studies. *Journal of Thoracic Disease*, *7*(11), E537–E540.

Cerniauskaite, M., Quintas, R., Koutsogeorgou, E., Meucci, P., Sattin, D., Leonardi, M., Raggi, A. (2012). Quality-of-life and disability in patients with stroke. *American Journal of Physical Medicine & Rehabilitation*, *91*(13), S39–S47.

D'souza, E. (2016). Modified fatigue impact scale — 5-item version (MFIS-5). *Occupational Medicine*, *66*(3), 256–257.

Deloitte Access Economics. (2018). The economic impact of stroke in Australia. https://www2.deloitte.com/au/en/pages/economics/articles/economic-impact-stroke-australia.html.

Demaerschalk, B., Hwang, H., Leung, G. (2010). US cost burden of ischemic stroke: A systematic literature review. *American Journal of Managed Care*, *16*(7), 525–533.

Fang, J., Chen, L., Ma, R., Keeler, C. L., Shen, L., Bao, Y., Xu, S. (2016). Comprehensive rehabilitation with integrative medicine for subacute stroke: A multicenter randomized controlled trial. *Scientific Reports*, *6*, 25850.

Feigin, V. (2007). Herbal medicine in stroke: Does it have a future? *Journal of the American Heart Association*, *38*, 1734–1736.

Feigin, V., Forouzanfar, M., Krishnamurthi, R., Mensah, G., Connor, M., Bennett, D., Murray, C. (2014). Global and regional burden of stroke during 1990–2010: Findings from the Global Burden of Disease Study 2010. *Lancet*, *383*(9913), 245–254.

Frost, Y., Weingarden, H., Zeilig, G., Nota, A., Rand, D. (2015). Self-care self-efficacy correlates with independence in basic activities of daily living in individuals with chronic stroke. *Journal of Stroke and Cerebrovascular Diseases*, *24*(7), 1649–1655.

Guidetti, D., Spallazzi, M., Baldereschi, M., Di Carlo, A., Ferro, S., Rota, E. M. N., Inzitari, D. (2014). Post-stroke rehabilitation in Italy: Inconsistencies across regional strategies. *European Journal of Physical and Rehabilitation Medicine, 50*(3), 335–341.

Hankey, G. J. (2014). Secondary stroke prevention. *Lancet Neurology, 13*(2), 178–194.

Hart, J. (2010). Poststroke recovery: Emerging complementary therapies. *Alternative and Complementary Therapies, 16*(5), 277–280.

Hughes, G., Aboyade, O., Hill, J., Rasu, R. (2015). The role and importance of economic evaluation of traditional herbal medicine use for chronic non-communicable diseases. *Comparative Effectiveness Research, 2015*(5), 49–55.

Jan, S. (2012). Falling through the cracks. *Medical Journal of Australia, 196*, 29–31.

Jones, F. (2013). Self-management: Is it time for a new direction in rehabilitation and post stroke care? *Panminerva Medica, 55*(1), 79–86.

Jones, F., Riazi, A., Norris, M. (2013). Self-management after stroke: Time for some more questions? *Disability and Rehabilitation, 35*(3), 257–264.

Langhorne, P., Bernhardt, J., Kwakkel, G. (2011). Stroke rehabilitation. *Lancet, 377*(9778), 1693–1702.

Lennon, S., McKenna, S., Jones, F. (2013). Self-management programmes for people post stroke: A systematic review. *Clinical Rehabilitation, 27*(10), 867–878.

Miller, K., Liebowitz, R., Newby, L. (2004). Complementary and alternative medicine in cardiovascular disease: A review of biologically based approaches. *American Heart Journal, 147*(3), 401–411.

Mukherjee, D., Patil, C. (2011). Epidemiology and the global burden of stroke. *World Neurosurgery, 76*(6), S85–S90.

National Heart Lung and Blood Institute. (2015). *Stroke.* https://www.nhlbi.nih.gov/health-topics/stroke.

National Stroke Foundation. (2015). National Stroke Audit — Acute Services Report 2015. https://www.aihw.gov.au/getmedia/c420f6f1-0464-4f43-b55a-62f995a0f8f3/ah16-3-6-stroke.pdf.aspx.

O'Donnell, M., Chin, S., Rangarajan, S., Xavier, D., Liu, L., Zhang, H., Yusuf, S. (2016). Global and regional effects of potentially modifiable risk factors associated with acute stroke in 32 countries (INTERSTROKE): A case-control study. *Lancet, 388*(10046), 761–775.

Papanicolas, I., Woskie, L., Jha, A. (2018). Health care spending in the united states and other high-income countries. *Journal of the American Medical Association, 319*(10), 1024–1039.

Pierce, L., Gordon, M., Steiner, V. (2004). Families dealing with stroke desire information about self care needs. *Rehabilitation Nursing Journal, 29*(1), 14–17.

Pinedo, S., Erazo, P., Tejada, P., Lizarraga, N., Aycart, J., Miranda, M., Bilbao, A. (2014). Rehabilitation efficiency and destination on discharge after stroke. *European Journal of Physical and Rehabilitation Medicine, 50*(3), 323–333.

Riegel, B., Moser, D., Buck, H., Dickson, V., Dunbar, S., Lee, C., Webber, D. (2017). Self care for the prevention and management of cardiovascular disease and stroke: A scientific statement for healthcare professionals from the American Heart Association. *Journal of the American Heart Association, 6*(9), e006997.

Rouillard, S., De Weerdt, W., De Wit, L., Jelsma, J. (2012). Functioning at 6 months post stroke following discharge from inpatient rehabilitation. *South African Medical Journal, 102*(6), 545–548.

Savage, J. (2009). Models of carefor chronic disease. Background paper for the Models of Access and Clinical Service Delivery Project. Australasian Society for HIV Medicine: Sydney.

Sax Institute. (2009). 45 and Up Study. https://www.saxinstitute.org.au/our-work/45-up-study/.

Shah, S., Engelhardt, R., Ovbiagele, B. (2008). Patterns of complementary and alternative medicine use among United States stroke survivors. *Journal of the Neurological Sciences, 271*(1–2), 180–185.

Shaul, M. (2012). Transitions in chronic illness. *Rehabilitation Nursing, 22*, 199–205.

Straus, S., Majumdar, S., McAlister, F. (2002). New evidence for stroke prevention: scientific review. *Journal of the American Medical Association, 288*(11), 1388–1395.

Taylor-Piliae, R. E., Hoke, T. M., Hepworth, J. T., Latt, L. D., Najafi, B., Coull, B. M. (2014). Effect of Tai Chi on physical function, fall rates and quality of life among older stroke survivors. *Archives of Physical Medicine and Rehabilitation, 95*(5), 816–824.

Tse, T., Binte Yusoff, S. Z., Churilov, I., Ma, H., Davis, S., Donnan, G. A., START research team. (2017). Increased work and social engagement is associated with increased stroke specific quality of life in stroke survivors at 3 months and 12 months post-stroke: A longitudinal study of an Australian stroke cohort. *Topics in Stroke Rehabilitation, 24*(6), 405–414.

Walsh, M., Galvin, R., Macey, C., Mccormack, C., Horgan, F. (2015). Community re-integration and long-term need in the first five years after stroke: Results from a national survey. *Disability and Rehabilitation, 37*(20), 1834–1838.

Wardle, J., Adams, J. (2014). Indirect and non-health risks associated with complementary and alternative medicine use: An integrative review. *European Journal of Integrative Medicine*, 6(4), 409–422.

White, J. H., Bynon, B. L., Marquez, J., Sweetapple, A., Pollack, M. (2013). Masterstroke: Apilot group stroke prevention program for community dwelling stroke survivors. *Disability and Rehabilitation*, *35*(11), 931–938.

Willison, K., Lindsay, S., Taylor, M., Schroeder, H., Andrew, G. (2012). Complementary and integrative medicine, ageing and chronic illness: Towards an interprofessional approach in primary health care. In Adams, J., Magin, P. and Broom, A. (eds.), *Primary Health Care and Complementary and Integrative Medicine: Practice and Research*. Imperial College Press, London.

Wilson, J., Hareendran, A., Grant, M., Baird, T., Schulz, U., Muir, K., Bone, I. (2002). Improving the assessment of outcomes in stroke: Use of a structured interview to assign grades on the modified Rankin Scale. *Stroke*, *33*(9), 2243–2246.

Wu, H., Tang, J., Lin, X., Lau, J., Leung, P., Woo, J., Li, Y. (2008). Acupuncture for stroke rehabilitation. *Stroke*, *39*(2), 517–518.

Zhang, J., Wang, D., Liu, M. (2014). Overview of systematic reviews and meta-analyses of acupuncture for stroke. *Neuroepidemiology*, *42*(1), 50–58.

Chapter 11

Low Back Pain and Manual Therapies: Examining Care via Non-Conventional Approaches

Eric Roseen, Jon Adams and Bradley Leech

Introduction

Low back pain (LBP) has been described as a complex condition incorporating many psychological factors, biophysical factors, social factors, comorbidities and pain-processing mechanisms which contribute to both pain and disability (Hartvigsen *et al.*, 2018). Many modestly effective treatments for LBP exist, including a range of both conventional medical and non-pharmacological treatments. This chapter will focus on the role of manual practitioners (e.g. chiropractors, osteopaths, massage therapists) who provide a range of non-pharmacologic treatments for the management of LBP. Manual practitioners often sit outside of mainstream health care systems. The integration of manual practitioners alongside conventional medical providers and within the formal health care system remains, in most cases, highly contested and not without its challenges (Wardle *et al.*, 2012). Nevertheless, a better understanding of such a large readily available workforce for treating LBP and other common musculoskeletal conditions may hold much potential for ensuring safe, effective and coordinated patient care for this major chronic health issue.

This chapter includes an overview of what is currently known about manual practitioners in high-income countries, where these manual practitioners are most commonly trained, the locations in which these practitioners are widely available to the public and where most research relating to their practices for LBP has been performed. A highlight on research related to what is known about these providers, their approach to managing LBP and how they interact with conventional medical settings will be discussed. Additionally, gaps in the literature, including important health services research questions that remain unanswered are explored. Specifically, we consider patients with LBP, and factors that may hinder or facilitate their access to manual practitioners and manual therapy.

The Burden of Low Back Pain

LBP is an extremely common health problem affecting all age groups with disability highest among working-age individuals (Hartvigsen *et al.*, 2018). Most adults experience LBP at some point in their lives, (i.e. the lifetime prevalence of LBP has been estimated to be over 80%) (Hoy *et al.*, 2012; Balague *et al.*, 2012) and LBP is the cause of more years lived with disability than any other condition (GBD, 2015).

Back pain is often separated into acute (0–6 weeks), sub-acute (6 weeks to 6 months) and chronic (greater than 6 months) LBP. Very often, acute LBP will resolve within a few weeks. However, recurrences of LBP are common — roughly one-third of LBP experiences will reoccur within 1 year (Machado *et al.*, 2017). Additionally, for most adults with LBP it is not possible to identify a single pain generating structure responsible for their pain and, as such, it is almost always the case that multiple structures (e.g. intervertebral disc, facet joint, vertebral endplate, or soft tissues [ligament, muscle, fascia]) contribute to back pain (Hartvigsen *et al.*, 2018). Specific less common causes of LBP include: radicular pain/ radiculopathy from disk herniation or spinal stenosis. Serious, albeit very rare, causes of LBP include: fractures, tumours, infections, inflammatory diseases and cauda equina syndrome.

The cost associated with LBP, incorporating both health care and work disability expenses, varies between countries and is suggested to be determined by social factors, health care and legislation (Hartvigsen *et al.*, 2018). The direct costs associated with LBP in the US have been estimated to be between US$12 and 91 billion, (Luo *et al.*, 2004) while indirect costs, such as lost productivity, are thought to well exceed this estimate (Dagenais *et al.*, 2008). Costs associated with LBP are thought to be similar to other common costly conditions (e.g. cardiovascular disease, cancer) (Maniadakis and Gray, 2000). In Australia, women with back pain have been estimated to spend out-of-pocket in excess of 1.4 billion AUD per year on back pain care (Kirby *et al.*, 2013). However, the total costs including public expenditure and across both adult men and women is likely to be much greater. Given the significant burden of LBP related disability and costs, it is important to understand the cost-effectiveness of common and promising LBP treatments.

Due to high prevalence and the difficulties in targeting specific cause, LBP is challenging to manage. For adults with chronic or recurring LBP, long-term treatment to manage important fluctuations, or flairs, over the life course, may be necessary (Sibbritt and Adams, 2010; Sibbritt *et al.*, 2016; Broom 2012a) and the effective, safe and coordinated management of LBP symptoms, over time, constitutes a key public health and health services research issue.

Conventional Medical Care for LBP

Adults with LBP commonly seek medical care from general practitioners/ family doctors and speciality care physicians (Licciardone, 2008). Commonly used conventional medications include paracetamol and nonsteroidal anti-inflammatory drugs (NSAIDs) with many general practitioners prescribing medications, most of which are NSAIDs (Spijker-Huiges *et al.*, 2015). However, paracetamol, also known as acetaminophen, is not thought to be effective for managing LBP (Williams *et al.*, 2014) and is no longer recommended by clinical guidelines (National Institute for Health and Care Excellence) in England (Bernstein *et al.*, 2017) or the US (Qaseem *et al.*, 2017). NSAIDs are thought to be a modestly effective short-term treatment for LBP (Roelofs *et al.*, 2008). However, neither paracetamol nor NSAIDs should be used long-term given potential associated side-effects — liver failure and gastrointestinal bleeding, respectively (Moore *et al.*, 2015). Paracetamol and NSAIDs can be prescribed but are also readily available as over-the-counter medications — perhaps making it difficult to discourage use over the longer term of a patient's experience of and attempts to manage their LBP. Other conventional medications include tricyclic antidepressants, and muscle relaxers, which are recommended by some guidelines; both may cause drowsiness. Opioid medications, are recommended as a potential treatment for acute LBP in the United Kingdom (Bernstein *et al.*, 2017) but are discouraged in the US, where opioids are considered a treatment of last resort (Qaseem *et al.*, 2017). There is no support for the effectiveness of opioids for chronic LBP. Currently, potentially severe risks associated with opioid use, including addiction, overdose and death, are a major concern in many countries (Martins *et al.*, 2015). Less severe common side-effects from opioid use include constipation, dizziness and sedation (Turk *et al.*, 2011).

Alongside medication prescription, medical procedures (e.g. epidural injections) are also a mainstay of conventional medicine, particularly by specialists trained in these techniques. When back pain persists, or reoccurs, particularly following medication prescription, injection therapies are commonly recommended by conventional medical providers. Common injections include epidural steroid injections and injections of the facet and sacroiliac joints. While there has been an increase in epidural and facet injection use for LBP (Manchikanti *et al.*, 2010), there is limited evidence to support the effectiveness in LBP (Staal *et al.*, 2009). Similarly, while epidural injections may provide short-term effect for back pain that radiates down one or both legs (i.e. radiculopathy) there is no evidence supporting the use of epidural steroid injections for non-radiating LBP (Friedman and Dighe, 2013; Chou *et al.*, 2015). Potential side effects of injections include infection/meningitis (Benoist *et al.*, 2012).

Many patients with LBP consider surgery as a treatment option. However, non-specific LBP surgery does not appear any more effective than conservative non-pharmacologic approaches (Chou *et al.*, 2009). In the US, despite limited evidence, and guidelines that do not recommend surgery, the use of surgery for LBP has nevertheless increased. For example, over twice as many spinal fusion surgeries were performed in 2008, compared to 1998, (Rajaee *et al.*, 2012). Whereas in the Netherlands general practitioners referred only 9% of their patients presenting with LBP to undergo surgery (Spijker-Huiges *et al.*, 2015).

The Demand for Non-Pharmacological Approaches

While conventional medical treatments have to date been somewhat underwhelming in their effectiveness in the management of LBP, a number of non-pharmacological therapies are available and have grown in popularity. While a number of clinical guidelines from the US (Chou *et al.*, 2016; Qaseem *et al.*, 2017), Canada (Bussieres *et al.*, 2018), the United Kingdom (Bernstein *et al.*, 2017), and Denmark (Stochkendahl *et al.*, 2018), among other countries, have recommended the use of common manual therapies, such as spinal manipulation or massage, these treatments remain in most cases located outside of mainstream health care settings. This is due, in part, to the poor integration of those providers of non-pharmacological treatments, particularly manual practitioners, into conventional medical care approaches and settings. Furthermore, manual practitioners are often educated in separate private institutions, and manual practitioner students may have limited opportunities to interact with their conventional medicine colleagues, and vice versa, during their formative training experience.

Overview of Manual Practitioners

Common manual practitioners include chiropractors, osteopaths and massage therapists. Each of these providers is readily accessible in many high-income countries, usually in the community-based private practice setting. This section below provides a brief overview of the three main manual practitioner groups and their practice in high-income countries.

Chiropractors

Chiropractors are commonly consulted in high income countries. According to the American Chiropractic Association, chiropractors 'practice a hands-on, drug-free approach to health care that includes patient examination, diagnosis and treatment. Chiropractors have broad diagnostic skills and are also trained to recommend therapeutic and rehabilitative exercises, including spinal manipulation' (American Chiropractic Association, 2018). Chiropractors most commonly provide care for musculoskeletal conditions, particularly back and neck pain, worldwide (Adams *et al.*, 2017; Charity *et al.*, 2016).

Osteopaths

Osteopathy is commonly described as a distinctive modality that applies a hands-on approach, focusing on musculoskeletal disorders, improving physiologic function and promoting homeostasis (Seffinger *et al.*, 2010). In the US, osteopaths are trained similar to medical doctors (MDs) but receive training in osteopathic manipulation, a form of spinal manipulation. In other high-income countries, while training and scope of practice can vary, osteopaths are more likely to perform spinal manipulation as well as other manual therapies.

Massage therapists

Massage therapists commonly provide a range of massage therapy techniques and are trained in private colleges or other institutions across high-income countries. In general, massage therapists press, rub and otherwise manipulate the muscles and other soft tissues of the body.

Prevalence of Manual Therapy Use for Low Back Pain

Among high-income countries such as Australia, Canada, Germany and the US the use of manual therapy for the management of back pain is common (Murthy *et al.*, 2015). Back pain sufferers commonly consult complementary and alternative medicine practitioners with manual therapists being the most frequently consulted practitioner type. The estimated prevalence of manual therapy use for back pain is 16.1–74.0% (mean 38.1%) for chiropractic treatment, 14.0–62.7% (mean 30.1%) for massage therapy and 4.1–48.4% (mean 14.4%) for osteopathic care (Murthy *et al.*, 2015).

Integrative care is common for the management of LBP with back pain sufferers utilizing a combination of conventional and complementary care (Broom *et al.*, 2012b). However, women who seek conventional medical care are subsequently less likely to consult with a chiropractor (Murthy *et al.*, 2014). The prevalence of manual therapy for LBP varies between countries with many independent factors influencing patients' decisions around manual therapy use (Murthy *et al.*, 2015).

Health Service Challenges

In many high-income countries some manual therapies are considered first-line therapies (before over-the counter or prescribed medications) for the management of LBP (Qaseem *et al.*, 2017). Nevertheless, a number of important issues around education, inter-professional communication, cost and personalized care are all influential upon the use of manual therapy for LBP.

Lack of Inter-Professional Education

Inter-professional education is necessary to create collaborative relationships between medical providers and manual therapy providers. Primary health care doctors often have a very limited understanding of what manual therapists do (Allareddy *et al.*, 2007) and nurse practitioners and physicians assistants, who have increasing autonomy in primary health care settings, also require (and are open to receiving) more information regarding manual providers (Bowden and Ball, 2016). It is this lack of knowledge, or limited opportunities for inter-professional education, that can prevent or delay appropriate referrals to manual providers for patients with LBP.

Poor Communication Between Manual Providers, Medical Providers and Patients

Manual therapies are often not well coordinated with primary care or specialty care. A major political challenge is the response and approach of conventional medical providers toward manual therapists.

Previous experiences, knowledge and beliefs may prevent conventional medical doctors from referring to manual therapists (Dikkers *et al.*, 2016). However, in recent years patients appear to be increasingly communicating with their primary care physician about the use of manual therapy (Murthy *et al.*, 2015). It is interesting to note, back pain sufferers have been reported to perceive less benefit from manual therapy when such therapy is referred by a conventional medical practitioner (Kanodia *et al.*, 2010).

Increasingly, manual therapies are being incorporated into mainstream health care settings. In Norway, while most primary health care providers have initiated at least one referral to a chiropractor over 12 months, most primary health care providers report referring to chiropractors infrequently, and less than 10% of primary health care providers communicate regularly with chiropractors (Langworthy *et al.*, 2001). The use of a 'curbside' consult, which primary health care providers commonly use in patient care with other medical specialists, is less common with manual providers. For example, primary health care providers report not engaging in curbside consults with chiropractors due to having insufficient information about chiropractic care or training (Allareddy *et al.*, 2007). These barriers to communication, as well as geographic distance from medical settings to chiropractic clinics, have been identified as major barriers that prevent referrals from chiropractors to primary health care providers. Similar themes around difficulty developing collaboration and trust, which prevent referrals to manual therapies, have been identified in the Netherlands among primary health care providers, physical therapists and other manual therapists (Dikkers *et al.*, 2016).

Cost

From a societal perspective (i.e. considering costs of intervention, loss of productivity at work and other associated health care costs) manual therapies are cost-effective treatments (Tsertsvadze *et al.*, 2014). However, care from manual providers may not be covered by health insurers and patients may have to provide substantial out-of-pocket contributions. A lack of insurance coverage, or prohibitive cost sharing in the form of high co-payments, may render manual therapies financially inaccessible for some, and limit the overall use of these services (Whedon *et al.*, 2017). Furthermore, in the US the likelihood of services being reimbursed for a chiropractic consult has been found to be 71% lower than that for a primary care physician (Whedon *et al.*, 2017). Additionally, patients often require a series of treatments to successfully manage an episode of LBP, and costs for each visit can compound. These are major financial barriers, particularly for lower-income populations. Expanding coverage of manual therapy by insurers, and expanded access to manual practitioners, may reduce overall costs to patients and increase utilization of these service.

Limited Understanding of Life Course Care for Chronic or Recurrent Low Back Pain

While manual therapists may most often see patients for symptomatic relief in an episode or flair of LBP, it is also fairly common that manual providers and their patients have long-term relationships. There is little, if any, research on the long-term use of manual therapies for LBP that begins in adolescence and persists or recurs throughout the life course. Patients may also seek ongoing maintenance care for symptoms that persist or are hard to manage with self-care alone. Alternatively, patients may try multiple different therapies seeking a complete resolution of back symptoms, which can lead to an escalation of care, from more conservative treatments (manual therapies) to more invasive treatments (injections or surgery). It is also common for patients to use over-the-counter medications, such as Tylenol or NSAIDs, for chronic pain, which have potentially serious risks if used long-term. Indeed, little is understood about best practices in managing back pain longitudinally as clinical trials, for manual and other back pain treatments, almost always assess short-term outcomes. Emerging evidence suggests maintenance care with manual therapies is cost-effective compared to caring for symptomatic episodes over a 12 month period (Eklund *et al.*, 2014). However, the cost-effectiveness of manual therapies over many years remains unknown.

Individualized Care

There is currently little guidance available to identify patients likely to respond to a particular LBP treatment. However, promising approaches for subgrouping patients into meaningful clinical categories have not been widely disseminated. Identifying the right treatment for the right patient with LBP has been a major area of clinical research (i.e. clinical prediction rules, treatment-based classification, etc.) (Alrwaily *et al.*, 2016). Patient expectations or preferences may also be valuable in identifying likely manual therapy responders (George and Robinson, 2010).

New Models for Training Manual Providers and Conventional Medical Providers

Students of manual therapy and conventional medicine that train together are more likely to work together. In Denmark and Switzerland, fully integrated training programs have realized this goal (Myburgh and Mouton, 2008; Humphreys and Peterson, 2016). However, in the US and elsewhere well-established training programs for manual providers and conventional medicine providers have developed separately, and the merging of these institutions may not be feasible. Additional research is needed to understand the effectiveness of inter-professional education curricula. Opportunities for a wide range of health care students to co-manage patients across institutions may further bridge gaps of knowledge that prevent collaboration in real-world health care settings.

New Models for Integrated Care Delivery

Few opportunities exist for manual practitioners in conventional medical settings. In the US, the Veterans Health Administration has broadly implemented non-pharmacological approaches, including manual providers, for the management of musculoskeletal pain. This research has largely been a response to the opioid epidemic. However, while civilian populations throughout North America, Europe and Australia are similarly affected by opioid medications, there is limited integration of manual providers in conventional health care settings in the US (Salsbury *et al.*, 2018).

In Canada, chiropractors have been integrated successfully into a number of community health centres, increasing access to manual therapies for low income and racially diverse populations (Kopansky-Giles *et al.*, 2007; Garner *et al.*, 2008). Research can leverage this public health need, to design innovative multidisciplinary models that improve collaboration of manual and conventional medicine providers.

New Payment Models

Fee for service models, particularly when insurance does not cover manual therapy, or when there are high co-payments, limits the utilization of manual providers (Whedon *et al.*, 2017). At the same time, in a fee for service payment model, other more expensive treatments (injections, surgery) or imaging techniques (MRIs) are perceived as more affordable, because they are completely covered or require only a single co-payment. Health services researchers must explore alternative value-based payment models that would incentivize effective relatively low-cost treatments such as manual therapies. One such model is a capitated system, where a universal payment covers all health care costs and providers are incentivized to provide essential cost-effective care. A second model, bundled payments, is where reimbursement for a particular condition (e.g. low back pain) is always the same, and again, the care provided must be relatively low cost and effective for the health care system to make a profit.

Conclusions

Osteopaths, chiropractors and massage therapists are accessible and popular in most high-income countries. Clinical guidelines increasingly recommend spinal manipulation, massage and other manual therapies for the management of common musculoskeletal conditions, with low back pain being an excellent example. As this chapter illustrates, there remain a number of important challenges requiring attention in order to achieve a closer relationship or interface between manual therapies and mainstream health care systems in most high income countries. The benefits of improved coordination and integration of manual therapists within LBP care are potentially significant — helping possibly save substantial costs for the health system and highlighting a wider range of treatment options, that appear relatively safe and effective, for LBP patients.

References

Adams, J., Peng, W., Cramer, H., *et al.* (2017). The Prevalence, Patterns, and Predictors of Chiropractic Use Among US Adults: Results From the 2012 National Health Interview Survey. *Spine (Phila Pa 1976)*, *42*(23), 1810–1816.

Allareddy, V., Greene, B. R., Smith, M., Haas, M., Liao, J. (2007). Facilitators and barriers to improving interprofessional referral relationships between primary care physicians and chiropractors. *Journal of Ambulatory Care Management, 30*(4), 347–354.

Alrwaily, M., Timko, M., Schneider, M., Stevans, J., Bise, C., Hariharan, K., Delitto, A. (2016). Treatment-based classification system for low back pain: Revision and update. *Physical Therapy*, *96*(7), 1057–1066.

American Chiropractic Association (2018). What is a Doctor of Chiropractic. https://www.acatoday.org/Patients/Why-Choose-Chiropractic/What-is-Chiropractic Accessed on 14 August 2018.

Balague, F., Mannion, A.F., Pellise, F., Cedraschi, C. (2012). Non-specific low back pain. *Lancet, 379*(9814), 482–491.

Benoist, M., Boulu, P., Hayem, G. (2012). Epidural steroid injections in the management of low-back pain with radiculopathy: An update of their efficacy and safety. *European Spine Journal*, *21*(2), 204–213.

Bernstein, I. A., Malik, Q., Carville, S., Ward, S. (2017). Low back pain and sciatica: Summary of NICE guidance. *BMJ, 356*, i6748.

Bowden, B. S., Ball, L. (2016). Nurse practitioner and physician assistant students' knowledge, attitudes, and perspectives of chiropractic. *Journal of Chiropractic Education, 30*(2), 114–120.

Broom, A., Kirby, E., Sibbritt, D., Adams, J. Refshauge, K. (2012a). Back pain amongst mid-age Australian women: A longitudinal analysis of provider use and self-prescribed treatments. *Complementary Therapies in Medicine, 20*, 275–282.

Broom, A. F., Kirby, E. R., Sibbritt, D. W., Adams, J., Refshauge, K. M. (2012b). Use of complementary and alternative medicine by mid-age women with back pain: A national cross-sectional survey. *BMC Complementary and Alternative Medicine, 12*, 98.

Bussieres, A. E., Stewart, G., Al-Zoubi, F., Decina, P., Descarreaux, M., Haskett, D., Hincapie, C., Page, I., Passmore, S., Srbely, J., Stupar, M., Weidberg, J., Ornelas, J. (2018). Spinal manipulative therapy and other conservative treatments for low back pain: A guideline from the canadian chiropractic guideline initiative. *Journal of Manipulative and Physiological Therapeutics*, *41*(4), 265–293.

Charity, M. J., Britt, H. C., Walker, B. F., *et al.* (2016). Who consults chiropractors in Victoria, Australia? Reasons for attending, general health and lifestyle habits of chiropractic patients. *Chiropractic and Manual Therapies*, *24*(1), 28.

Chou, R., Baisden, J., Carragee, E. J. Resnick, D. K., Shaffer, W. O., Loeser, J. D. (2009). Surgery for low back pain: A review of the evidence for an American Pain Society Clinical Practice Guideline. *Spine (Phila Pa 1976)*, *34*(10), 1094–1109.

Chou, R., Hashimoto, R., Friedly, J., *et al.* (2015). Pain management injection therapies for low back pain. *Rockville Agency for Healthcare Research and Quality.*

Chou, R., Gordon, D. B., de Leon-Casasola, O. A., Rosenberg, J. M., Bickler, S., Brennan, T., Wu, C. L. (2016). Management of postoperative pain: A Clinical Practice Guideline From the American Pain Society, the American Society of Regional Anesthesia and Pain Medicine, and the American Society of Anesthesiologists' Committee on Regional Anesthesia, Executive Committee, and Administrative Council. *The Journal of Pain*, *17*(2), 131–157.

Dagenais, S., Caro, J., Haldeman, S. (2008). A systematic review of low back pain cost of illness studies in the United States and internationally. *The Spine Journal*, *8*, 8–20.

Dikkers, M. F., Westerman, M.J., Rubinstein, S.M., van Tulder, M.W., Anema, J.R. (2016). Why neck pain patients are not referred to manual therapy: A qualitative study among dutch primary care stakeholders. *PLoS One*. *11*(6), e0157465.

Eklund, A., Axen, I., Kongsted, A., Lohela-Karlsson, M., Leboeuf-Yde, C., Jensen, I. (2014). Prevention of low back pain: effect, cost-effectiveness, and cost-utility of maintenance care — study protocol for a randomized clinical trial. *Trials*, *15*, 102.

Friedman, J. H., Dighe, G. (2013). Systematic review of caudal epidural injections in the management of chronic back pain. *Rhode Island Medical Journal*, *96*(1), 12–16.

Furlan, A. D., Giraldo, M., Baskwill, A., Irvin, E., Imamura, M. (2015). Massage for low-back pain. *Cochrane Database of Systematic Reviews* (8)4: CV001929.

Garner, M. J., Birmingham, M., Aker, P., *et al.* (2008). Developing integrative primary healthcare delivery: Adding a chiropractor to the team. *EXPLORE: The Journal od Science and Healing, 4*(1), 18–24.

GBD (2015). Disease and Injury Incidence and Prevalence Collaborators. (2016). Global, regional, and national incidence, prevalence, and years lived with disability for 310 diseases and injuries, 1990–2015: A systematic analysis for the Global Burden of Disease Study 2015. *Lancet. 388*, 1545–1602.

George, S. Z., Robinson, M. E. (2010). Preference, expectation, and satisfaction in a clinical trial of behavioral interventions for acute and sub-acute low back pain. *Journal of Pain, 11*(11), 1074–1082.

Hartvigsen, J., Hancock, M. J., Kongsted, A., *et al.* (2018). What low back pain is and why we need to pay attention. *Lancet. 391*(10137), 2356–2367.

Hoy, D., Bain, C., Williams, G., *et al.* (2012). A systematic review of the global prevalence of low back pain. *Arthritis Rheumatology, 64*(6), 2028–2037.

Humphreys, B. K., Peterson, C. K. (2016). The Swiss master in chiropractic medicine curriculum: Preparing graduates to work together with medicine to improve patient care. *The Journal of Chiropractic Humanities, 23*(1), 53–60.

Kanodia, A. K., Legedza, A. T., Davis, R. B., Eisenberg, D. M., Phillips, R. S. (2010). Perceived benefit of Complementary and Alternative Medicine (CAM) for back pain: A national survey. *Journal of the American Board of Family Medicine, 23*(3), 354–362.

Kirby, E., Broom, A., Sibbritt, D., Refshauge, K., Adams, J. (2013). Health care utilization and out-of-pocket expenditure associated with back pain: A nationally representative survety of Australian women. *PloS One, 8*(12), e83559.

Kjaer, P., Kongstep, A., Hartvigsen, J., Isenberg-Jorgensen, A., Schiottz-Christensen, B., Soborg, B., Kroe, C., Moller, C. M., Halling, C. M. B., Lauridsen, H. H., Hansen, I. R., Norregaard, J., Jorgensen, K. J., Hansen, L. V., Jakobsen, M., Jensen, M. B., Melbye, M., Dvel, P., Christensen, S. W., Povlsen, T. M. (2018). National Clinical Guidelines for non-surgical treatment of patients with recent onset low back pain or lumbar radiculopathy. *European Spine Journal, 27*(1), 60–75.

Kopansky-Giles, D., Vernon, H., Steiman, I., *et al.* (2007). Collaborative community-based teaching clinics at the Canadian Memorial Chiropractic College: Addressing the needs of local poor communities. *Journal of Manipulative and Physiological Therapeutics. 30*(8), 558–565.

Langworthy, J. M., Birkelid, J. (2001). General practice and chiropractic in Norway: How well do they communicate and what do GPs want to know? *Journal of Manipulative and Physiological Therapeutics, 24*(9), 576–581.

Licciardone, J. C. (2008). The epidemiology and medical management of low back pain during ambulatory medical care visits in the United States. *Osteopathic Medicine and Primary Care, 2*, 11.

Lisi, A. J., Salsbury, S. A., Twist, E. J., Goertz, C. M. (2018). Chiropractic Integration into Private Sector Medical Facilities: A Multisite Qualitative Case Study. *The Journal of Alternative and Complementary Medicine, 24*(8), 792–800.

Luo, X. Pietrobon, R., Sun, S. X., Liu, G. G., Hey, L. (2004). Estimates and patterns of direct health care expenditures among individuals with back pain in the United States. *Spine, 29*, 79–86.

Machado, G. C., Maher, C. G., Ferreira, P. H., Latimer, J., Koes, B. W., Steffens, D., Ferreira, M. L. (2017). Can recurrence after an acute episode of low back pain be predicted? *Physical Therapy*, *97*(9), 889–895.

Manchikanti, L., Pampati, V., Boswell, M.V., Smith, H. S., Hirsch, J. A.. (2010). Analysis of the growth of epidural injections and costs in the Medicare population: A comparative evaluation of *1997*, 2002, and 2006 data. *Pain Physician*, *13*(3), 199–212.

Maniadakis, N., Gray, A. (2000). The economic burden of back pain in the UK. *Pain, 84*(1), 95–103.

Martin, B. I., Deyo, R. A., Mirza, S. K., Turner, J. A., Comstock, B. A., Hollingworth, W., Sullivan, S. D. (2008). Expenditures and health status among adults with back and neck problems. *The Journal of Alternative and Complementary Medicine, 299*, 656–664.

Martins, S. S., Sampson, L., Cerda, M., Galea, S. (2015). Worldwide prevalence and trends in unintentional drug overdose: A systematic review of the literature. *American Journal of Public Health*, *105*(11), e29–e49.

Moore, N., Pollack, C., Butkerait, P. (2015). Adverse drug reactions and drug-drug interactions with over-the-counter NSAIDs. *Therapeutics and Clinical Risk Management*, *11*, 1061–1075.

Murthy, V., Sibbritt, D., Adams, J., Broom, A., Kirby, E., Refshauge, K. M. (2014). Consultations with complementary and alternative medicine practitioners amongst wider care options for back pain: A study of a nationally representative sample of 1,310 Australian women aged 60–65 years. *Clinical Rheumatology, 33*(2), 253–262.

Murthy, V., Sibbritt, D. W., Adams, J. (2015). An integrative review of complementary and alternative medicine use for back pain: A focus on prevalence, reasons for use, influential factors, self-perceived effectiveness, and communication. *Spine Journal, 15*(8), 1870–1883.

Myburgh, C., Mouton, J. (2008). The development of contemporary chiropractic education in Denmark: An exploratory study. *Journal of Manipulative and Physiological Therapeutics. 31*(8), 583–592.

Qaseem, A., Wilt, T. J., McLean, R. M., Forciea, M. A. (2017). Noninvasive treatments for acute, subacute, and chronic low back pain: A clinical practice guideline from the american college of physicians. *Annals of Internal Medicine, 166*(7), 514–530.

Rajaee, S. S., Bae, H. W, Kanim, L. E, Delamarter, R. B. (2012). Spinal fusion in the United States: Analysis of trends from 1998 to 2008. *Spine (Phila Pa 1976), 37*(1), 67–76.

Roelofs P. D. D. M., Deyo R. A., Koes B. W., Scholten R. J. P. M., van Tulder M. W. (2008). Non-steroidal anti-inflammatory drugs for low back pain. *Cochrane Database of Systematic Reviews.* (1).

Salsbury, S. A., Goertz, C. M., Twist, E. J., & Lisi, A. J. (2018). Integration of Doctors of Chiropractic Into Private Sector Health Care Facilities in the United States: A Descriptive Survey. *Journal of Manipulative and Physiological Therapeutics, 41*(2), 149–155.

Seffinger, M. A., Buser, B. R., Licciardone, J. C., Lipton, J. A., Lynch, J. K., Patterson, M. M., Snow, R., Trovtman, M. E. (2010). American Osteopathic Association guidelines for osteopathic manipulative treatment (OMT) for patients with low back pain. *Journal of the American Osteopathic Association, 110*(11), 653–666.

Sibbritt, D., Adams, J. (2010). Back pain amongst 8,910 young Australian women: A longitudinal analysis of the use of conventional providers, complementary and alternative medicine (CAM) practitioners and self-prescribed CAM. *Clinical Rheumatology, 29,* 25–32.

Sibbritt, D., Lauche, R., Sundberg, T., Peng, W., Moore, C., Broom, A., Kirby, E., Adams, J. (2016). Severity of back pain may influence choice and order of practitioner consultations across conventional, allied and complementary health care: A cross-sectional study of 1851 mid-age Australian women. *BMC Musculoskeletal Disorders, 17,* 393.

Spijker-Huiges, A., Groenhof, F., Winters, J. C., van Wijhe, M., Groenier, K. H., van der Meer, K. (2015). Radiating low back pain in general practice: Incidence, prevalence, diagnosis, and long-term clinical course of illness. *Scandinavian Journal of Primary Health Care, 33*(1), 27–32.

Staal, J. B., de Bie, R. A., de Vet, H. C., Hildebrandt, J., Nelemans, P. (2009). Injection therapy for subacute and chronic low back pain: An updated Cochrane review. *Spine (Phila Pa 1976), 34*(1), 49–59.

Tsertsvadze, A., Clar, C., Court, R., Clarke, A., Mistry, H., Sutcliffe, P. (2014). Cost-effectiveness of manual therapy for the management of musculoskeletal conditions: A systematic review and narrative synthesis of evidence from randomized controlled trials. *Journal of Manipulative and Physiological Therapeutics, 37*(6), 343–362.

Turk, D. C., Wilson, H. D., Cahana, A. (2011). Treatment of chronic non-cancer pain. *Lancet. 377*(9784), 2226–2235.

Wardle, J., Steel, A., Adams, J. (2012). A review of the tensions and risks in naturopathic education and training in Australia: A need for regulation. *The Journal of Alternative and Complementary Medicine, 18*(4), 363–370.

Whedon, J., Tosteson, T. D., Kizhakkeveettil, A., Kimura, M. N. (2017). Insurance reimbursement for complementary healthcare services. *The Journal of Alternative and Complementary Medicine, 23*(4), 264–267.

Williams, C. M., Maher, C. G., Latimer, J., *et al.* (2014). Efficacy of paracetamol for acute low-back pain: A double-blind, randomised controlled trial. *Lancet, 384*(9954), 1586–1596.

Chapter 12

Traditional, Complementary and Integrative Medicine in the Brazilian Public Health Service: Opportunities and Limitations

Islândia Maria Carvalho de Sousa, Adriana Falangola Benjamin Bezerra, Maria Beatriz Guimarães, Iracema de Almeida Benevides and Charles Dalcanale Tesser

Introduction

This chapter presents an overview of the current status of the integration and development of Complementary and Integrative Medicine (TCIM) — known locally as Integrative and Complementary Practices in health care (*Práticas Integrativas e Complementares em Saúde* — [PICS]) — in the Brazilian Unified Health System (*Sistema Único de Saúde;* SUS). The limitations of such integration will also be discussed.

In Brazil, PICS refers to a wide set of integrative and complementary health approaches whose origins are in other countries and culture but which have been exported and assimilated by local Brazilian culture. Complex whole medical systems such as Ayurveda, traditional Chinese medicine, homeopathy and anthroposophic medicine are also include under the rubric of PICS. PICS can be organized according to the treatment method: phytotherapy and medicinal plants; manual care (acupuncture, chiropractic, osteopathy, massage therapy), mind–body therapies (tai chi chuan, yoga, lian gong, meditation, bioenergetics) or support group therapy — a Brazilian approach known as Community Integrative Therapy (Brazil, 2008). A caveat should be made about the term PICS in Brazil, for it does not include indigenous or traditional medicine. Indeed, indigenous public health care has its own specific model in Brazil providing primary care for indigenous populations through multidisciplinary health teams and organized in conjunction with local indigenous authorities as a sub-system of care and provision (Brasil, 2016; Cardoso, 2014).

In this chapter we briefly introduce SUS and Brazilian Primary Health Care (PHC) provision — both essential for understanding key aspects of the situation of PICS in the wider Brazilian health care system. Other aspects such as relevant milestones, the role of different levels of government in health care provision and the organization of PICS services in the SUS are also detailed in order to explain the characteristics of the different health services, types of practices delivered, geographic distribution, the status of all professionals involved in PICS training and related workplace distribution. This information will help in highlighting some reflections on the limits and possibilities of the integration of PICS into the Primary Health Care level within the SUS. It is important to highlight that the Health System in Brazil is based upon a private health sub-system covering 25% of the population (Vieira and Martins, 2015) and offering PICS (via health insurance companies and independent self-employed practitioners), Unfortunately, access to information regarding this private health sub-system is extremely limited and as a result will not be a focus of this chapter.

The Unified Health System and the Primary Health Care Strategy in Brazil

The SUS system was established within the Brazilian Federal Constitution in 1988, to provide universal health care offering comprehensive, preventive and curative care as a duty of the state and as a right for all citizens. The management of SUS is decentralised, and operates at the three levels of government (union, states and municipalities), with each level of government holding specific responsibilities for the planning and execution of different health services. Community participation is defined at all levels (Paim *et al.*, 2011). The SUS is financed by the three government levels via citizen taxes (Gurgel *et al.*, 2017). Overall, despite a number of limitations that can be expected in all health systems, SUS has achieved good coverage and positive results in some areas and topics at different levels of the Brazilian system: primary health care as well as hospital and specialized care.

The Family Health Program (now called the Family Health Strategy, or FHS) was introduced at the close of the 1990s and has since evolved into a robust approach to provide primary care for defined populations by deploying interdisciplinary health care teams. The nucleus of each Family Health (FH) team includes a physician, a nurse, a nurse assistant, and four to six full-time community health agents. FH teams are organized geographically, covering up to 1000 households each (Macinko and Harris, 2015). Currently, there are more than 30,000 FH teams responsible for about 50% of all primary care coverage across Brazil.

Implementation and TCIM Service Organization in SUS

The implementation of PICS into SUS was enhanced in the 1980s, based on the recommendations of the 1978 Alma Ata Conference (WHO, 1978). The SUS final report contained a series of recommendations based on guiding principles, one of which advocated the introduction of 'alternative' practices within health services, allowing citizens the right to choose preferred therapy (Brasil, 1987: 10). This report was key in introducing homeopathy and acupuncture in the SUS in 1989, making it possible to collect data on these practices via relevant health information systems.

In 2006, after 3 years of consultations and mediations with specific professional groups, a range of PICS were institutionalized through the National Policy on Integrative and Complementary Practices (Política Nacional de Práticas Integrativas e Complementares, PNPIC) (Brazil, 2008) as issued by the Brazilian Ministry of Health. However, at this time (2006), it was already known that several PICS practices had already been implemented by municipalities in their jurisdictions — a survey undertaken by the Ministry of Health in 2004 revealed PICS in 232 municipalities across Brazil (Brazil,2008). In most cases, such a development had been to address the needs of the local population/community, and were almost always established through grassroot initiatives involving PHC professionals, in some cases on a voluntary basis (Santos *et al.*, 2011; Nagai and Queiroz, 2011; Salles and Schraiber, 2009). By 2008, the Ministry of Health reported that more than 800 municipalities in Brazil were providing some form of PICS practices (Brazil, 2010).

When PNPIC was established in the SUS in 2006, one of its priorities was the introduction and strengthening of PICS practices at the primary level of care, focusing in five modalities and different medical systems: homeopathy; traditional Chinese medicine; anthroposophic medicine; termalism/crenotherapy; and medicinal plants and phytotherapy (Brazil, 2008).

In 2017, 10 years after its implementation, the PNPIC was expanded, broadening the scope of PICS. The Brazilian Ministry of Health defined new rules incorporating 14 new practices (art therapy, Ayurveda, biodance, circular dance, meditation, music therapy, naturopathy, osteopathy, chiropractic, reflexology, shantala, integrative community therapy and yoga) to be considered in the guidelines for training, implementation and research within the SUS (Brasil, 2017a).

In March 2018 the Ministry of Health promoted a wide international conference in Rio de Janeiro (First International Congress of Complementary and Integrative Medicine in Public Health) with around 70 acknowledged international keynote speakers together with other 200 national speakers, counting on the support of the Brazillian Parliament (a Parlamentary Alliance in favor of PICS), World Health Organization (WHO) and the Pan American Health Organization (PAHO). During the event, the Minister of Health communicated the recognition and incorporation of a new range of therapies in PNPIC, reaching a total of 29 modalities (Brasil, 2017b).

Another meaningful step towards strengthening PNPIC at the federal level followed the new ordinance, issued on March 2018, was the creation of the national coordination for PICS inside the official schedule/calendar of the Minister of Health (Brasil, 2017b). The role of states in this legislation is focused on planning and supporting municipalities in all health actions. As such, in the case of the PNPIC, technical support can be provided to the process of training professionals, structuring of services and the evaluation of services. In Brazil, seven states (Bahia, Rio Grande do Norte, Rio Grande do Sul, Espírito Santo, Minas Gerais, Goias, São Paulo) have laws in addition to the Federal District and Amapá that offer policies regarding PICS.

Municipalities have the autonomy to implement the PICS modalities considered more appropriate to their context and territory, whether these are officially integrated with the PNPIC or not. PICS management and coordination activities are organized according to the specific context — some municipalities have a specific coordination for PICS services and provision while others add and direct such PICS coordination policy to the requirements and duties of those professionals responsible for the primary health care or general health service coordination (Brazil, 2008).

Provision and Distribution of PICS Across Brazil

Drawing upon data collected from a number of sources (the current Brazilian government public health database, newsletters and reports of the Ministry of Health and a national phone and online survey of municipal managers of Brazilian municipalities (Sousa *et al.*, 2016)) this section overviews the distribution of PICS across Brazil.

Tabnet Datasus — the Brazilian health information system — contains data on the physical structure of health services, on health professionals as well as equipment and operations relating to SUS at the federal, state and municipal levels (Brasil, 2018). This database was accessed between December 3rd and 27th, 2017, and January 10th, 2018 (http://tabnet.datasus.gov.br/cgi/deftohtm.exe?cnes/cnv/servc2br.def). For clarity and convenience we restricted our analysis of this database to the following years (2008–2017) which contained the most comprehensive data.

Most of the PICS provided in Brazil's public health system is available in health services that offer conventional health care. Currently, the practice and provision of PICS are recorded in the information system even when it refers to only one professional performing a specific modality of PICS (e.g. one practitioner offering two PICS modalities is recorded as offering two modalities). As such, it is possible to verify different types and modalities of PICS in the same health facility.

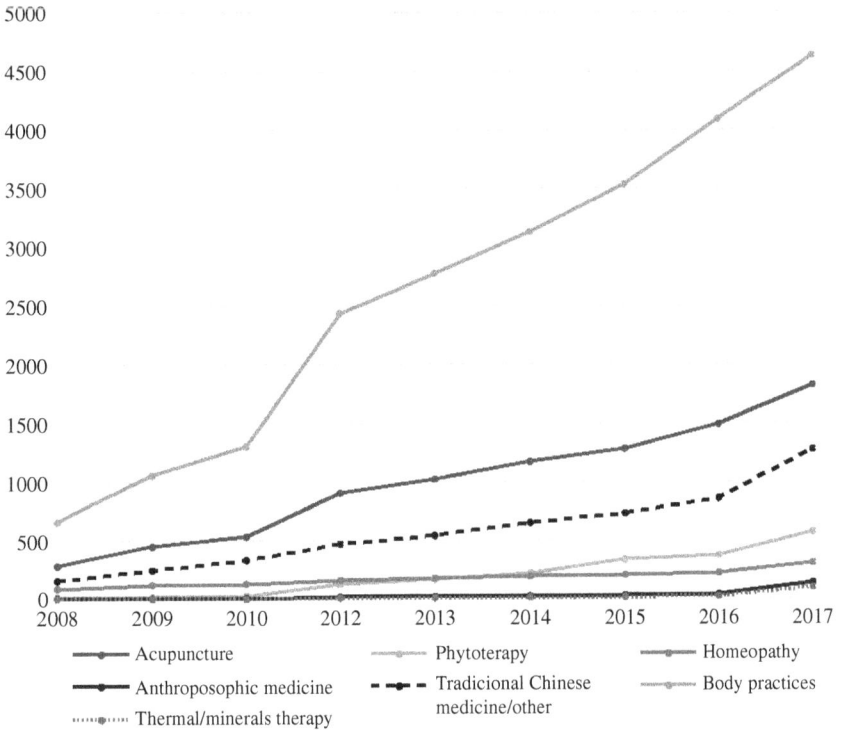

Figure 1.   TCIM provision in unified health system Brazil, 2008–2017.

Note: There were not available data for 2011; It was selected the data of December of each year, except for 2010 which the last available month was May.
Source: TABNET Datasus (17).

Figure 1 shows the types of services registered in the information system and their growth in recent years.

The modalities registered as 'services' in the information system are those recognized by the Ministry of Health and available in the PNPIC. Between 2008 and 2017, official data shows a growth in all these PICS services. However, some service offerings expanded more than others, such as phytotherapy, which increased 33% (17 services in 2008 to 566 in 2017), followed by mind-body practices, which grew 7% (657 services in 2008 to 4629 in 2017) (Figure 1). Our analysis shows PICS approaches provided only by physicians, such as medical consultation in homeopathy

Table 1.   Provision by type of health facility and modalities of PICS (number e percentual per 100.000 inhabitants[a]), Brazil 2008–2017.

Description	2008			2017		
	n	%	100.000h	n	%	100.000h
Health fitness center	0	—	—	424	4.9	0.21
Family Health Support Center	1	0.2	—	167	1.9	0.08
Psicossocial Center	13	2.3	0.01	222	2.6	0.11
Health Center/Family Health Team[b]	322	56.4	0.16	5547	64.7	2.69
Specialized Clinic	76	13.3	0.04	1105	12.9	0.54
Private practice	27	4.7	0.01	337	3.9	0.16
Hospitals[c]	50	8.8	0.02	294	3.4	0.14
Polyclinics	71	12.4	0.03	325	3.8	0.16
Others	11	1.9	0.01	154	1.8	0.07
Total	571	100	0.28	8575	100	4.16
Modalities of TCIM offered	**n**	**%**	**100.000h**	**n**	**%**	**100.000h**
Traditional Chinese medicine/ acupuncture	283	23.1	0.14	1753	20.4	0.85
Phytoterapy	17	1.4	0.01	547	6.4	0.27
Homeopathy	92	7.5	0.04	300	3.5	0.15
Anthroposophic Medicine	10	0.8	—	129	1.5	0.06
Traditional Chinese medicine/other[d]	161	13.1	0.08	1213	14.1	0.59
Body practices[e]	657	53.6	0.32	4539	52.9	2.20
Thermal/minerals therapy	6	0.5	—	94	1.1	0.05
Total	1226	100		8575	100	—

Sources: All date are from the same source TABNET Datasus (tabnet.datasus.gov.br) LEGEND: (a) population estimates in 2016 (206.114.067 million of inhabitants); (b) Strategy expansion of PHC in Brazil; (c) General and specialized Hospitals; (d) includes auriculotherapy and other chinese practices; (e) include yoga, tai chi chuan, liang gong and other body practices.

and anthroposophic medicine, have recently experienced a slower growth in their PNPIC service provision.

Analysis of data since 2008 indicates that there has been a gradual increase in the deployment of PICS in primary care services, that already account for more than 50% of all PICS care in 2017 (Table 1).

The provision of PICS located in specialized care environments includes public and private settings. However, private health care settings that offer PICS services account for less than 10% of all registered health care settings.

In recent years, the Ministry of Health implemented a quality assessment and an improvement program aimed at the FH Strategy and Primary Health Care teams in SUS called Improvement of Quality and Access Program (Programa de Melhoria do Acesso e da Qualidade — PMAQ) (Macinko *et al.*, 2017). One of the self-assessment modules (questionnaire) was designed to collect information on the presence and modalities of PICS in the Family Health Strategy (FHS) or PHC team as they are considered resources that can expand both access and quality of care. The assessment cycles have been frequent and show that the care is spread and presents a rather diversified and heterogeneous pattern around the country. During 2016 and 2017 it was observed that 5,600 FHS/PHC teams out of more than a total of 30,000 were performing PICS in SUS. The most commonly offered modalities could be organized in four main groups: mind-body therapies, phytotherapy, acupuncture and integrative community therapy — the latter being a psychological group meeting that using singing and music (Brasil, 2017a).

PICS provision in Brazil has also been investigated via a national telephone interview study (Sousa *et al.*, 2016). Out of 1,617 municipal health authority managers interviewed, 432 (26.7%) reported offering some type of PICS in SUS in their municipality, with 84.0% of such provision (corresponding to 365 municipalities) offered in PHC settings via the Family Health Strategy (Sousa *et al.*, 2016)). A comparison of the Ministry of Health data (Brasil, 2017a) with this interview survey data (Sousa *et al.*, 2016), it is noticeable that a major component of the PICS provision registered in PHC appears to be the product of spontaneous, uncoordinated action on behalf of individual health professionals working in the FHS strategy rather than planned and organized activities put together by health authorities at that level. While such initiatives have undoubtedly made the expansion of PICS in SUS possible and visible, such actions do not seem sustainable due to their informality. This could signalize concerns for long-term survival and

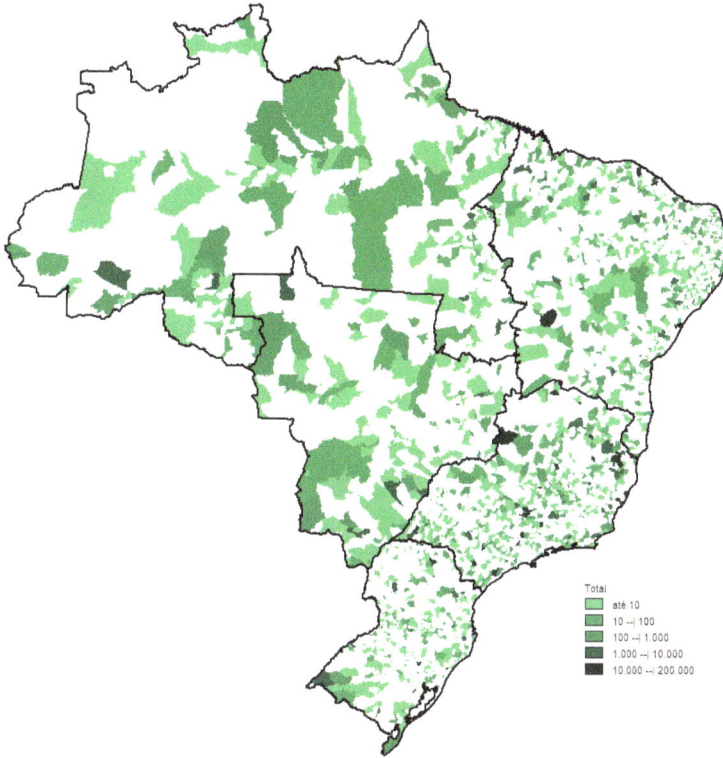

Figure 2.   Interventions of TCIM in care in PHC in SUS Brazil, 2017.

Source: Ministry of *Health/PNPIC Report* November 2016.

growth of PICS provision in the Brazilian public health care system over coming years.

Figure 2 shows the geographic distribution of PICS in PHC in Brazil. It shows that integrative care is being offered in the majority of Brazilian municipalities across the country. However, when compared to coverage data (Figure 3), large inequalities exist which render access to PICS a challenge in many locations/regions across Brazil. There is a major concentration of PICS services in the metropolitan regions, such as São Paulo and Rio de Janeiro. Data demonstrate the provision of PICS across the three levels of care in 3,097 (56%) municipalities (Figure 2).

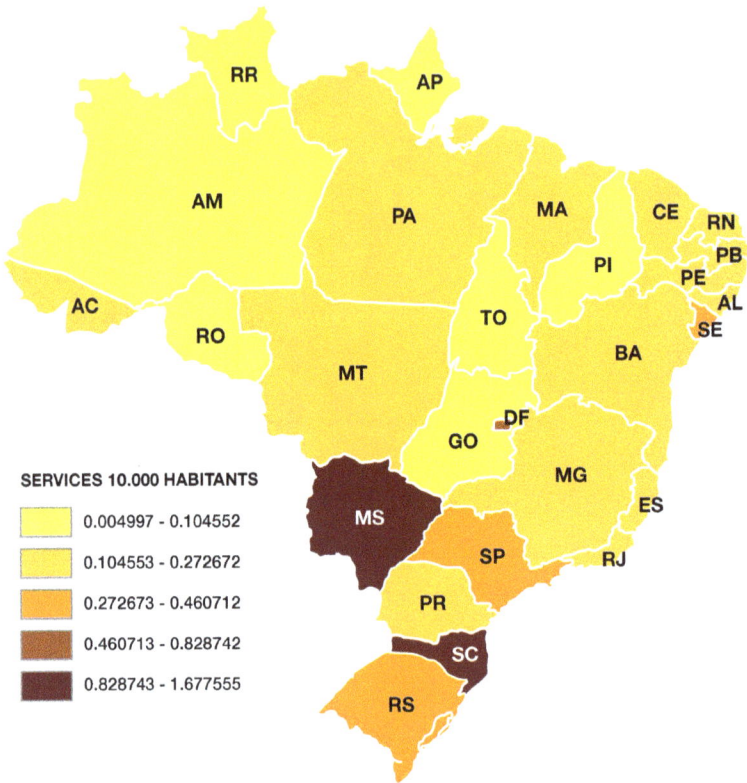

Figure 3.   Health services and TCIM coverage in SUS Brazil, 2017.
Sources: Fortunato, (2015) and Sousa *et al.* (2016).

Sousa and Tesser (2017) analyzed and deepened the discussion about the possibilities and limitations of the implementation of PICS in primary care in five large Brazilian cities. These authors recommend that PICS can be successfully implemented and practiced in PHC when the FHS/PHC teams are working in an integrated way, in a coordinated PHC care model (*matriciamento*[1]) (Oliveira and Campos, 2015) in which specialized PICS teams or practitioners provide practices — this could be considered as the best and more sustainable strategy for expanding PICS in public services in Brazil.

---

[1] *matriciamento*, this is a Brazilian term referring to Family Health Strategy.

PICS Task-force and Professional Regulations

As previously mentioned, PICS provision in PHC setting in Brazil can be compared to a patchwork formed by a complex mix of modalities and multiprofessional network of health practitioners, not completely clear and visible in the database. Only a small fraction of this practitioner population are hired exclusively to work with PICS (Sousa and Tesser, 2017), here titled 'PICS specialists'. In contrast, the major PICS task-force in SUS is hired as conventional health practitioners who later promote the necessary conditions to introduce PICS in their care setting. However, the data collected usually does not record such nuance. Barros (2000) has referred to these practitioners as 'hybrid professionals' — conventional health professionals who have a dual competence and training in both conventional medical and PICS practice. This leads to an under-reporting of PICS health practitioners in the official database and a more in-depth study is required to help ensure that such double competence can be registered and made visible (as connected to each professional). Such information is not only relevant to help identify the full range of services offered within the SUS but also to inform practice evaluations and, ultimately, improvements in patient care.

The Brazilian Ministry of Health established the practice of PICS in SUS through the PNPIC in a multiprofessional base (Brazil, 2008). It is important to point out that in Brazil, the Ministry of Health's participation in the regulation of health professionals is significantly indirect in comparison to neighbouring countries such as Argentina, where the Ministry of Health is directly responsible for registering and supervising health professionals. In Brazil, a joint commission formed by representatives of Minister of Health and Minister of Labor defines which professionals can work in the SUS and their field of action in this system. Nevertheless, the institution of a profession is made by specific law, through the Legislative power and afterwards, it is regulated by the specific professional council. In the case of doctors, nurses, physiotherapists and dentists, for example, the respective professional council regulates if or which PICS they are allowed to practice.

On the other hand, the Ministry of Labor, through the Brazilian Classification of Occupations (CBO) defines the fields of occupations and has established approximately 40 occupations in the field of health (Brazil, 2010). Most of these occupations are well-established professions, such as doctors, physiotherapists, nurses, psychologists, just to name a few. They have their own formal, self-regulating institutions and Boards of professional practice standards. Through specific laws, such professions ensure exclusive fields of practice. The CBO is used by the Minister of Health to identify the professional in the information system and also to attribute specific competencies in the policies.

For example, in Brazil acupuncture is considered a medical specialty by the Federal Council of Medicine, which advocates the exclusivity of its practice by doctors (Kornin, 2016). However, other health professional councils (for physiotherapists, nurses, psychologists) also recognize acupuncture as a specialty (Rocha *et al.*, 2015). As a result, acupuncture is practiced by a wide range of professionals in Brazil, including acupuncturists trained abroad, some practitioners trained in acupuncture via free courses in Brazil, acupuncture technicians (practitioners that have not completed formal graduation programs in the health field), and acupuncture specialists (conventionally graduated health practitioners that completed a post-graduation program). Such a landscape of care with acupuncture has resulted in major ethical–legal dilemmas and legal conflicts regarding the right to practice acupuncture across Brazil (Rocha *et al.*, 2015; Câmara dos Deputados, 2016).

In the context of PNPIC and therefore in SUS, acupuncture can be practiced by various professionals (physicians, physiotherapists, pharmacists, conventional medical practitioners, speech therapists and psychologists) throughout the country, provided they have a post-grad degree in acupuncture and can be recognized as specialists by their own professional council (Brazil, 2008). There is a substantial number of professional acupuncturists in Brazil ($n = 2,586$) (Sousa *et al.*, 2012), but there is also a strong political and legal dispute over the right to practice acupuncture, in which the greatest controversy lies between the competency to practice across physicians and non-physicians who provide acupuncture services.

Indeed, according to Nascimento (1998), during the process of expansion of acupuncture in Brazil, factions were formed within the corporations. The Brazilian Association of Acupuncture, founded in the 1970s, gathered medical and non-medical professionals among its associates. In the 1980s, a movement was initiated to defend the practice of acupuncture as restricted to physicians, resulting in the founding of the Brazilian Medical Society of Acupuncture (SMBA) and the Paulista Medical Association of Acupuncture, currently named Associação Médica Brasileira de Acupuntura (AMBA). Similarly, the Medical College of Acupuncture considers acupuncture a line of treatment to be performed exclusively by a qualified medical professional. According to the Federal Council of Medicine (2012), acupuncture treats diseases and, in Brazil, 'to diagnose and treat diseases are activities exclusively for doctors' (Conselho Federal de Medicina, 2012). The contest between physician versus non-physician acupuncturists, their relative merits and right to practice still remains, even with the acceptance and extension of acupuncture provision among the ranks of other health professional groups.

The case of homeopathy also raises relevant points for consideration. Homeopathy has been recognized as a medical specialty in Brazil since 1980 (Galhardi and Barros, 2008) and it was officially included as a practice within the Brazilian Health System in 1999 (Santos *et al.*, 2009). Currently, Homeopathy it is also recognized as a specialty for other health professionals (Conselho Federal de Farmácia, 2018) In 2007, ordinance number 3.237 of the Ministry of Health included the homeopathic medicines of the Brazilian Homeopathic Pharmacopoeia (about 450 medicines) to be made available to SUS users, in accordance with the PNPIC. The tensions around rights to practice as outlined earlier with regard to acupuncture have also been experienced in relation to homeopathy. The Brazilian Homeopathic Medical Association (Associação Médica Homeopática Brasileira, AMHB) claims that homeopathy should only be available to patients through a medically trained doctor (Galhardi and Barros, 2008). The prescription of drugs by non-medical professionals is prominent and a strong point of tension in the debate between physicians and non-physicians practicing homeopaths in Brazil.

In the case of anthroposophic medicine, the coverage is still considered low, although some increase has been observed in SUS lately. Interesting to observe that this complex system that has its roots in Europe at the beginning of the 1920s proposes a multiprofessional team (anthroposophic physician, nurse, art therapist, rhythmic massage therapist, etc.) practicing under the same referential with specific competencies for each profession. In the specific case of the anthroposophic physician, this constitutes a development of medical practice along with the necessary background in conventional medicine (double competence) (Kienle *et al.*, 2013; Benevides, 2014).

One of the features that differentiates PICS in the context of the Brazilian health system is the existence of an extensive PHC network. Over more recent decades, PHC has been the main setting for PICS expansion across the country. One of the factors influencing this scenario is the behaviour of PHC professionals, who independently seek training in PICS and often introduced PICS practice in PHC health services even prior to the necessary regulation of such practices was introduced by the Ministry of Health in 2006 (Santos *et al.*, 2011). However, more recently the Brazilian Ministry of Health has begun to invest in PICS training through distance education.

Several sources of information point to the existence of a large network of professionals working in PICS in the SUS, predominantly in PHC, representing different modalities and with different types of insertion, levels of training and stages of integration with the health service. This can be considered as a favorable scenario for the development of collaborative experiences for the research and production of knowledge in a shared way as in the Australian experience of TCIM Problem Based Research Network initiatives (Adams *et al.*, 2015, 2016, 2017).

Final Remarks

Since the Unified Health System was established in Brazil in the 1980s, there has been positive consideration and demand for PICS. The benchmarks for PICS practice were defined in 2006 with the PNPIC, and expanded in 2017 to include 14 new modalities of TCIM, including other medical rationalities — achieving a total of 19 TCIM modalities whose practices are now benchmarked. In 2018 there was a new revision and the set of TCIM in PNPIC reached 29 modalities. However, federal funding of these TCIM practices has been severely limited (with TCIM provision costs the responsibility almost entirely of the municipalities). Moreover, while there has been a more recent concentrated effort to facilitate and fund PICS training courses, federal investment in vocational training in PICS and regulation / standardization of these practices has been scarce until very recently. As a result, almost all the affiliated institutions and training courses in PICS are now privately run, without regulation and with neither official nor academic accreditation (Galhardi and Barros, 2008). In addition, despite the federal level government wide effort to introduce PICS into the curricula of the various health professions in public universities, this has been negligible for the largest, most important and most respected universities across Brazil. Indeed, it was only in early 2018 that, as far as is acknowledged, the first public tender specifically focused on the topic of PICS and aimed at higher education teachers at a Brazilian public university was floated.

There has been little investment in health professional development, in research, and an evaluation in order to strengthen evidence about their contribution to the health care offered to users of the SUS. Nevertheless, regardless of a lack of wider coordinated financial support or policy, Brazilian municipalities continue to provide these services over the last decade, with some investing their own funds to support such service offerings and a significant proportion of such services being implemented by grassroots health professionals working as volunteers (Sousa *et al.*, 2011).

Despite the existence of a national policy for PICS, federal government investments remain restricted to small incentives in training and the payment of some activities. Such underwhelming investments in PICS infrastructure and development are also mirrored in the research space in Brazil. Only a single one-off call for PICS-research focused grant submissions has been initiated in 2013 by the National Council for Scientific and Technological Development. It is widely acknowledged that the growth and rigor of health professions and modalities and their standards of professional practice are well aided by the growth of a relevant research base (Conselho Nacional de Pesquisa, 2017) and without adequate research investment it is unlikely that the full opportunity and challenges of PICS practice and provision can be realized or addressed within the Brazilian health care system.

However, data indicate a consistent and progressive institutional presence of these PICS practices in Brazilian PHC. Among a range of factors that have been influential in the expansion of PICS in Brazilian PHC are: the increased recognition and authorization of PICS - almost symbolic – by federal regulators including the PNPIC; the expansion of primary health care over the last two decades; individually-led PICS initiatives headed by municipal managers; and the broader growing consumer and cultural interest in 'natural' approaches to health and wellbeing. This emerging presence and strengthening of PICS in PHC seems to be feasible in a peculiar way in Brazil, mainly through the practice of PICS by conventional medical professionals who gain PICS training largely via their own motivation or, in a few cases, through in-service training provided by the local health municipality (Santos and Tesser, 2012).

The few and insufficient regulations regarding PICS in Brazil have generated a number of legal conflicts, but these do not seem to have prevented or obstructed the growth of PICS in PHC. Indeed, despite some fragility in regulation, inconsistency and lack of sustainability of PICS provision in Brazilian PHC, the continental dimension of SUS and its PHC (although this only serves approximately 65% of the Brazilian population) make the Brazilian experience with PICS a *sui generis* case. The social and cultural context, permeated by broad-based multiculturalism, which characterizes the Brazilian population (Cardoso, 2014), has favoured the construction of a plurality of care within PHC services. A plurality in which TCIM practices are slowly but progressively incorporated and offered in a blended and integrated manner with relative success through the grassroots initiatives of hybrid professionals sometimes supported by municipal managers.

Overall, despite a number of contemporary challenges threatening to dismantle and destroy the construction of SUS as a universal public system which values the integral care of all citizens, the growth of PICS in SUS and PHC appears to have remained steady. The integration of PICS in the Brazilian health care system is desirable both to widen choice and access to health services across the population and to help improve the overall quality, safety and efficiency of health service provision (including both PICS and conventional medicine) across the Brazilian health care system.

References

Adams, J., Steel, A., Chang, S., Sibbritt, D. (2015). Helping address the national research and research capacity needs of Australian chiropractic: Introducing the Australian Chiropractic Research Network (ACORN) project. *Chiropractic & Manual Therapies, 23*, 12.

Adams, J., Steel, A., Moore, C., Amorin-Woods, L., Sibbritt, D. (2016). Establishing the ACORN national practitioner database: Strategies to recruit practitioners to a national practice-based research network. *Journal of Manipulative Physiological Therapeutics. 39*(8), 594–602.

Adams, J., Lauche, R., Peng, W., Steel, A., Moore, C., Lyndon G. Amorin-Woods, Sibbritt, D. (2017). A workforce survey of Australian chiropractic: The profile and practice features of a nationally representative sample of 2,005 chiropractors. *BMC Complementary and Alternative Medicine, 17*, 14.

Barros, N. F. (2000). Medicina Complemetar: Uma reflexao sobre o outra lado da practica medica. Sao Paulo: Annablume/Fapesp.

Benevides, I. (2014). Resultado do estudo de campo: A medicina e o médico antroposófico nas vozes de quatro gerações brasileiras distintas. In Luz, M. T. and Afonso, V. W. *Organizadores. Medicina Antroposófica como Racionalidade Médica e prática integral de cuidado à saúde.* Juiz de Fora: UFJF, 195.

Brasil (1987). Ministério da Saúde. Ministério da Previdência e Assistencial Social. Relatório da 8a Conferência Nacional de Saúde. Brasília, 1987, p. 29. http://bvsms.saude.gov.br/bvs/publicacoes/8_conferencia_nacional_saude_relatorio_final.pdf.

Brasil (2016). Secretaria Especial de Saúde Indígena — SESAI. Brasília, DF, 2018. http://portalms.saude.gov.br/saude-indigena.

Brasil (2017a). Departamento de Atenção Básica. Coordenação de Práticas Integrativas e Complementares. PNPIC (2017) — Informe Maio 2017. Departamento de Atenção Básica, MS–DAB/MS, 2017. http://189.28.128.100/dab/docs/portaldab/documentos/informe_pics_maio2017.pdf. Accessed on 3 December 2017.

Brasil (2017b). Portal do Ministério da Saúde. Ministério da Saúde inclui 10 novas práticas integrativas no SUS. http://portalms.saude.gov.br/noticias/agencia-saude/42737-ministerio-da-saude-inclui-10-novas-praticas-integra-tivas-no-sus. Accessed on 9 April 2018.

Brasil (2018). Cadastro Nacional de Estabelecimentos de Saúde (CNES). http://datasus.saude.gov.br/sistemas-e-aplicativos/cadastros-nacionais/cnes. Accessed on 27 November 2017.

Brazil (2008). Ministry of Health of Brazil. Secretary of Health Care. Department of Primary Care. PNPIC: National Policy on Integrative and Complementary Practices of the SUS: access expansion initiative / Ministry of Health of Brazil, Secretary of Health Care, Department of Primary Care. — Brasília: Ministry of Health of Brazil, 2008. http://189.28.128.100/dab/docs/publicacoes/geral/pnpic_ingles.pdf.

Brazil (2010). 3._Departamento de Atenção Básica, Secretaria de Atenção à Saúde, Ministério da Saúde. Relatório do 1° Seminário Internacional de Práticas Integrativas e Complementares em Saúde. http://dab.saude.gov.br/semi_praticas_integrativas.php. Accessed on 20 January 2010.

Câmara dos Deputados (2016). Portal Câmara dos Deputados. http://www2.camara.leg.br/camaranoticias/noticias/SAUDE/542073-ASSOCIACOES-DIVERGEM-SOBRE-PROPOSTA-QUE-REGULAMENTA-A-PRATICA-DA-ACUPUNTURA.html.

Cardoso, M. D. (2014). Saúde e povos indígenas no Brasil: notas sobre alguns temas equívocos na política atual. *Cadernos de Saúde Pública* [online], *30*(4), 860–866. https://doi.org/10.1590/0102-311X00027814>. ISSN 1678-4464. https://doi.org/10.1590/0102-311X00027814. Accessed on 10 July 2018.

Conselho Federal de Medicina (2012). Publicado acórdão do TRF que restringe exercício da acupuntura somente a médicos. Conselho Federal de Medicina. 2012. [documento da internet]. http://portal.cfm.org.br/index.php?option=com_content&view=article&id=22788:publicado-acordao-do-trf-que-restringe-exercicio-da-acupuntura-somente-a-medicos&catid=3. Accessed on 13 January 2013.

Conselho Nacional de Pesquisa (2017). Diretório Nacional dos grupos de pesquisa no Brasil. http://lattes.cnpq.br/web/dgp.

Conselho Federal de Farmácia (2018). Portal do Conselho Federal da Farmácia. http://www.cff.org.br/noticia.php?id=653.

Galhardi, W. M. P., Barros, N. F. (2008). The teaching of homeopathy and practices within Brazilian public health system (SUS). *Interface — Comunicação, Saúde, Educação*, *12*(25), 247–266. https://dx.doi.org/10.1590/S1414-32832008000200003.

Gurgel Jr., G. D., Sousa, Jr., I. M. C., Oliveira, S. R. A., De Assis, F. S., Direrichsen, F. (2017). The national health services of Brazil and Northern Europe: Universality, equity, and integrality-time has come for the latter. *International Journal of Health Services*, *47*, 002073141773254.

Kienle, G. S., Albonico, H.-U., Baars, E., Hamre, H. J., Zimmermann, P., Kiene, H. (2013). Anthroposophic medicine: An integrative medical system originating in Europe. *Global Advances in Health and Medicine*, *2*(6), 20–31.

Kornin, A. (2016). O processo de regulamentação da acupuntura no Brasil: um mapeamento dos discursos de atores e entidades protagonistas. Dissertação (mestrado) — Universidade Federal de Santa Catarina, Centro de Ciências da Saúde, Programa de Pós-Graduação em Saúde Coletiva, Florianópolis. https://core.ac.uk/download/pdf/78554608.pdf.

Macinko, J., Harris, M. J. (2015). Brazil's family health strategy — delivering community-based primary care in a universal health system. *New England Journal of Medicine*, *372*(23), 2177–2181.

Macinko, J., Harris, M. J., Rocha, M. G. (2017). Brazil's national program for improving Primary Care Access and Quality (PMAQ): Fulfilling the potential of the world's largest payment for performance system in primary care. *The Journal of Ambulatory Care Management*, *40*(2 Suppl), S4–S11. http://doi.org/10.1097/JAC.0000000000000189.

Nagai, S. C., Queiroz, M. S. (2011). Alternative and complementary medicine in the basic health system network in Brazil: A qualitative approach. *Ciência & Saúde Coletiva*, *16*(3), 1793–1800. https://dx.doi.org/10.1590/S1413-81232011000300015.

Nascimento, M. C. (1998). De panacéia mística a especialidade médica: A acupuntura na visão da imprensa. *História, Ciências e Saúde*, *1*, 99–113.

Oliveira, M. M., Campos, G. W. S. (2015). Matrix support and institutional support: analyzing their construction. *Ciência & Saúde Coletiva*, *20*(1), 229–238. https://dx.doi.org/10.1590/1413-81232014201.21152013.

Paim, J., Travassos, C., Almeida, C. Bahia, L., Macinko. J. (2011). The Brazilian health system: History, advances, and challenges. *Lancet*. DOI: https://doi.org/10.1016/S0140-6736(11)60054-8.

Rocha, S. P., Benedetto, M. A. C., Fernandez, F. H. B, Gallian, D. M. C. (2015). The trajectory of the introduction and regulation of acupuncture in Brazil: recollections of the challenges and struggles.Ciênc. saúde coletiva [online]. *20*(1), 155–164. ISSN 1413-8123. http://dx.doi.org/10.1590/1413-81232014201.18902013.

Salles, S. A. C., Schraiber, L. B. (2009). Support for and resistance to Homeopathy among managers of the unified national health system. Cad. Saúde Pública [online]. *25*(1), 195–202. ISSN 0102-311X. http://dx.doi.org/10.1590/S0102-311X2009000100021.

Santos, M. C., Tesser, C. D. (2012). Um método para a implantação e promoção de acesso às Práticas Integrativas e Complementares na Atenção Primária à Saúde. *Ciênc. saúde coletiva*, *17*(11), 3011–3024.

Santos, FAS, Gouveia, GC, Martelli, PJL, & Vasconcelos, EMR. (2009). Acupuncture in the Brazilian National Health System (SUS) and the inclusion of non-medical professionals. *Brazilian Journal of Physical Therapy*, *13*(4), 330–334. Epub 28 August 2009. https://dx.doi.org/10.1590/S1413-35552009005000043.

Santos, F. A. S., Sousa, I. M. C., Gurgel, I. G. D., Bezerra, A. F. B., Barros, N. F. (2011). Integrative practice policy in Recife, Northeastern Brazil: An analysis of stakeholder involvement. *Revista de Saúde Pública*, *45*(6), 1154–1159. https://dx.doi.org/10.1590/S0034-89102011000600018.

Sousa, I. M. C., Bodstein, R. C. A., Tesser, C. D., Santos, F. A. S., Hortale, V. A. (2012). Integrative and complementary health practices: The supply and production of care in the Unified National Health System and in selected municipalities in Brazil. *Cadernos de Saúde Pública*, *28*(11), 2143–2154. https://dx.doi.org/10.1590/S0102-311X2012001100014.

Sousa, I. M. C., *et al.* (2016). Relatório de Pesquisa do CNPq- Avaliação dos Serviços em Práticas Integrativas e Complementares no SUS em todo o Brasil e a efetividade dos serviços de plantas medicinais e Medicina Tradicional Chinesa/práticas corporais para doenças crônicas em estudos de caso no Nordeste. http://cnpq.br/relatorios-de-pesquisa?p_p_id=relatoriopes quisabuscaportlet_WAR_relatoriopesquisabuscaportlet&p_p_lifecycle= 0&p_p_state=normal&p_p_mode=view&p_p_col_id=column-2&p_p_col_ pos=1&p_p_col_count=2&modoBusca=textual.

Sousa, I. M. C., Tesser, C. D. (2017). Medicina Tradicional e Complementar no Brasil: inserção no Sistema Único de Saúde e integração com a atenção primária. Cadernos de Saúde Pública, *33*(1), e00150215. Epub January 23, 2017.

Vieira Jr., W. M., Martins, M. (2015). The elderly and healthcare plans in Brazil: analysis of the complaints received by the National Regulatory Agency for Private Health Insurance and Plans. *Ciência & Saúde Coletiva*, *20*(12), 3817–3826. https://dx.doi.org/10.1590/1413-812320152012.11082014.

World Health International Organization (1978). *International Conference on Primary Health Care*. Report of the International Conference on Primary Health Care jointly sponsored by the Word Health Organization and the united Nations Organization and United Nations Children's Fund, [Geneva], Alma Ata, URSS), p. 61. http://www.who.int/publications/almaata_declaration_ en.pdf.

Chapter 13

Traditional Medicine and Relational Ecological Public Health: Challenges and Opportunities

Erica McIntyre, Jason Prior and Jon Adams

Introduction

The recent emergence of relational ecological public health — also referred to as planetary health — has highlighted how far-reaching changes to the Earth's natural systems represent a growing threat to human health (Horton, 2016). These changes to the environment, ranging from climatic change, ocean acidification, land degradation through to water scarcity and biodiversity loss, pose serious challenges to the global health gains of the past several decades and are likely to become increasingly dominant during the second half of the 21ˢᵗ Century and beyond (Whitmee *et al.*, 2015).

Planetary health calls for a transdisciplinary approach to understanding human health outcomes as emerging from complex interactions between natural and social systems (Whitmee *et al.*, 2015). Despite planetary health's calls for more integrated understandings of the link between environment and health it has been remarkably silent on its relationship to traditional medicine (TM). This is surprising given that TM is often strongly grounded in both natural and social systems. Within this chapter we address this silence, by highlighting the opportunities that might arise from contemplating planetary health through the lense of TM, and conversely the challenges that may face these medicine systems as a result of the anticipated environmental challenges that are the focus of planetary health. Before outlining these challenges and opportunities we provide the reader with an understanding of planetary health and conclude the chapter by outlining a research agenda at the intersection of planetary health and TM.

Planetary Health

In 2015, a Rockefeller Foundation–Lancet Commission introduced a new field reflecting relational ecological public health called 'planetary health'. Planetary health is defined as 'the health of human civilization and the state of the natural systems on which it depends' (Whitmee *et al.*, 2015). Planetary health presents an opportunity to adopt a transdisciplinary approach to developing strategies with a view to reducing and preventing risks to human health and natural systems (Butler *et al.*, 2015). The opportunity to improve and sustain human health through enhancing the stewardship of natural systems and reducing the exploitative use of resources linked to unsustainable consumption and production patterns is a surprisingly new concept for global health and health care practice — both of which have until now been dominated by the biomedical approach to health (Horton *et al.*, 2014).

The definition of health in late modern societies has been focused on the individual. For example, the World Health Organization's simplistic definition of health states that 'health is a state of complete physical, mental and social wellbeing and not merely the absence of disease', has not been updated since it was first enacted in 1948 (WHO, 1946). In contrast, planetary health has redefined the concept of health to incorporate all its complexities and acknowledges the natural systems on which it depends. The Lancet Commission on Planetary Health defined health as, 'the achievement of the highest attainable standard of health, wellbeing, and equity worldwide through judicious attention to the human systems — political, economic and social — that shape the future of humanity and the

Earth's natural systems that define the safe environmental limits within which humanity can flourish' (Whitmee *et al.*, 2015, p. 15). This new definition represents a more holistic view, aligned with the philosophies and approaches of TM systems and fundamentally moves beyond the reductionist biomedical approach to health.

Natural systems are deteriorating at an alarming rate as a result of human exploitation of the environment for resources (Whitmee *et al.*, 2015). Despite the deterioration of the Earth's ecosystems, human health outcomes have continued to improve; for example, the average life expectancy is now 69 years compared to just 47 in the 1950s (Whitmee *et al.*, 2015). Possible explanations for this paradox include: increased productivity (e.g. higher crop yields) in food systems (Bereuter and Glickman, 2015); increased efficiency of technology and infrastructure that allow separation from natural environments (e.g. allowing food production to be independent of ecosystems); and the proposed time delay between ecosystem deterioration and effects on human wellbeing where we have yet to see the effects on younger generations (Whitmee *et al.*, 2015).

It is clear that the current rate of ecosystem deterioration is unsustainable. Increasing pressure on the global environment from human activity has led to environmental change resulting in a range of unprecedented public health challenges that include: direct health effects (e.g. pollution exposure, heatwaves, natural disasters); ecosystem-mediated health effects (e.g. infectious disease, mental health, reduced food yields); and indirect or deferred health effects (e.g. loss of livelihood, displacement of populations, conflict) (Whitmee *et al.*, 2015). In order to mitigate these health effects it is critical that the health of ecosystems is conserved and placed central to our ongoing attempts to investigate, understand and improve health outcomes for all.

Traditional Medicine and Planetary Health

There are a number of challenges and opportunities for TM related to a rapidly changing environment. The health effects of deteriorating ecosystems and environmental change will impact on TM in various ways presenting both challenges and opportunities. This section will discuss two significant challenges to TM and two potential opportunities with consideration of ethnopharmacology and socioecological systems in the context of planetary health. Addressing these challenges and opportunities will require a transdisciplinary approach to ensure optimal human health and environmental health across cultures.

The Impact of Environmental Change on Traditional Medicine

It is quite clear that TM is not immune to the environmental crisis facing our planet. Significant changes in ecosystems and vegetation types have impacted on the procurement, preparation and cost of plant medicines (Barata *et al.*, 2016; Biswas *et al.*, 2017). Loss of plant medicines from over-harvesting, habitat loss and global change is a significant concern for TM and conventional medicine (Schippmann *et al.*, 2002). Anthropogenic change is causing an estimated global loss of plant species at between 100 and 1000 times greater than natural extinction rates, with approximately 15,000 endangered medicinal plant species (Chen *et al.*, 2016). This section focuses on the challenges that climatic change, land degradation, water scarcity, pollution and biodiversity loss, may pose to the production and consumption of TM and complementary medicine (CM) products. The challenges discussed here are important given that improving the health of the world's 370 million indigenous people remains heavily dependent among other factors upon the access to and use of TM (Adams *et al.*, 2015; Gall *et al.*, 2018).

Loss of natural resources and sustainability

Ecosystem destruction and biodiversity loss is occurring at an alarming rate. Indigenous TM and CM (primarily sold as commercial products) rely heavily on natural resources for production. Healthy ecosystems with biological diversity are essential for ensuring plant foods and medicines are available in their natural (wild) growing environments and agricultural systems (cultivated) (Heywood, 2013). Biodiversity is also essential for ensuring optimal macro- and micronutrient status of foods and phytochemicals in plant medicines (Heywood, 2011). Consequently, ecosystem conservation and sustainable agriculture represent core strategy in helping prevent the loss of plant species and ensure access to quality food and medicine (Heywood, 2013).

Guaranteeing the sustainability of plant foods and medicines is critical for the ongoing future of TM. This is particularly challenging as there are many interacting sociocultural, political and environmental factors involved; for example, the high demand for plant foods and medicines, will continue to increase with population growth (Cordell, 2017). Population growth is increasing urban development, and increasing the populations reliance on large scale agriculture to produce plant foods and medicines (Whitmee *et al.*, 2015). Over one-tenth of all plant species globally are used to produce pharmaceutical and CM products (Chen *et al.*, 2016). There is also a lack of medical plant diversity globally with only two countries, China and India, using the largest number of medicinal plants (Chen *et al.*, 2016). While research for the efficacy of TM is essential, as the evidence-base grows for the efficacy of specific herbs so does the global demand for these medicines increasing the strain on ecosystems (Cordell, 2015).

Rhodiola rosea is an example of a plant medicine that has been impacted as a result of increased commercial production to meet global demand. *Rhodiola* has traditionally been used for a range of medical purposes throughout Europe, Asia and Russia for thousands of years (Camfield *et al.*, 2017). Due to the evidence for *Rhodiola's* efficacy in treating anxiety, as a cognition enhancer and an adaptogen (Camfield *et al.*, 2017) the use of this herbal medicine has increased rapidly throughout the world resulting in a reduction of the species in natural habitats due to unsustainable wildcrafting (Booker *et al.*, 2016). This unsustainable use has caused *Rhodiola* to become endangered (Booker *et al.*, 2016).

The safety of herbal medicines is also affected by environmental change. For example, there have been many cases of adulteration in which one plant species is replaced for another, and contamination with pollutants such as heavy metals (Posadzki *et al.*, 2013). Adulteration can occur when a particular plant species is in short supply, or the medicine is in high demand or expensive (Booker *et al.*, 2016). The herb *Rhodiola* has often been replaced with other species that do not confer the same medicinal properties or contain potentially harmful constituents (Booker *et al.*, 2016).

Contamination has frequently occurred in products manufactured in China and India (Posadzki *et al.*, 2013). For example, Ayurvedic medicines have been found to contain lead, arsenic and mercury (Saper *et al.*, 2008). Heavy metal contamination is likely to become an increasing problem for herbal medicine production as the majority of countries growing and producing these medicines (e.g. China, India) have significant problems with water and soil contamination (Kulhari *et al.*, 2013; Song *et al.*, 2018).

Reduction of micronutrients in soil is another concern related to a changing environment and loss of biodiversity that will have implications for TM, CM and human health more generally. Vitamin and mineral deficiency is already a major public health concern, especially in low income countries. For example, vitamin A deficiency is noted as one of the world's biggest undernutrition crisis (Heywood, 2011). The primary approach to addressing this deficiency has been to provide medicinal doses of vitamin A to children in order to meet the international developmental goal of reducing child mortality (Heywood, 2011). The importance of this goal is not in dispute. However, high dose supplementation in this context (i.e. a symptom of social and economic disadvantage) is not a long-term solution and is not a response that aligns with a planetary health perspective or TM approaches to health. High dose supplementation is also frequently used in complementary and integrative medicine to address nutritional deficiencies (Litchy, 2011). However, the same health benefits are not inferred from taking supplements as ingesting nutrients from a diversity of whole foods when consumed within traditional food systems (Heywood, 2011). In addition, vitamin and mineral supplementation increases the use of a broad range of natural recourses placing further strain on ecosystems (Cordell, 2015). Socio-ecological systems approaches should be used to preserve biological diverse ecosystems and food security (Wittman *et al.*, 2016) to develop sustainable food systems that aim to prevent macro- and micronutrient shortage and address social, economic and geographical disadvantage (Heywood, 2011).

It is also argued that a large amount of the CM products being consumed may be of little or no health benefit to consumers or pose health risks (Wardle and Adams, 2014). For example, CM products are primarily self-prescribed by consumers, and studies have found that these medicines are not necessarily taken for their evidence-based indications (McIntyre *et al.*, 2015). Considering the global supplement industry is estimated to turn over US$120 billion by 2020 (World Health Organization, 2014), this is extremely concerning from a planetary health perspective. There are issues related to profit motives in health care, equity, the unnecessary use of natural resources and questionable treatment decision-making in health care. Self-care is a critical component of health care that has benefits for individuals and health care systems. However, effective decision-making related to self-care relies on adequate health literacy and access to reliable information about TM and CM (Wardle and Adams, 2014).

Ensuring sociocultural equity while addressing the challenges that result from environmental change is a critical consideration for TM. This is particularly important for indigenous peoples as they are likely most affected by climate change and environmental disasters and rely on TM as primary health care (Adams *et al.*, 2012; Suswardany *et al.*, 2015). The over-harvesting of some foods and medicines has resulted in a loss of access to traditional foods and medicines for indigenous people. Local traditional foods and medicines that are not resilient to climate change may disappear (Heywood, 2011), contamination from technological and natural disasters may prevent access to traditional sources of foods and medicines (Chen *et al.*, 2016) and displacement and migration of indigenous people into urban environments may result in the loss of access to their TM and difficulties with accessing conventional health care (Alves and Rosa, 2007).

Traditional medicine is strongly dependent on local agriculture

Traditional medicine systems are complex socio-ecological systems that are primarily dependent on indigenous small-scale agriculture systems for foods and plant (herbal) medicines (Heywood, 2011). Many of these foods and medicines have been used for thousands of years, and the concept of food as medicine is embodied within traditional knowledge (Heywood, 2011). A changing climate is already presenting significant challenges to longstanding cultural practices resulting from loss of farming land, water insecurity, contamination, natural disasters and climate change (Ford, 2012). These environmental changes will require indigenous communities to adapt and be resilient to change (Ford, 2012). It may no longer be possible to grow some traditional medicines and foods because of these environmental changes. Loss of access to TM demands local communities consider other non-traditional medicines or identify traditional plant medicines that are more robust in adapting to changing climactic conditions (e.g. draught resistant, nutrient dense). This is a challenging situation as TM knowledge is accumulated over long periods of time — in some cases thousands of years (Barata *et al.*, 2016).

The loss of access to traditional foods and medicines will present unique challenges related to cultural sensitivity and sociocultural equity. The capacity of indigenous communities to adapt to a changing environment is compromised as they face unique vulneraries such as economic poverty, a lack of technological capacity (e.g. access to health care), social-political inequality, reduced institutional capacity (e.g. human and financial resources) and information deficits (e.g. lack of understand about climate change health risks) (Ford *et al.*, 2010). These vulnerabilities will need to be addressed by governments to reduce poverty and inequality and build capacity in order to adapt to a changing environment and ensure their health care needs can be met (Ford *et al.*, 2010). Health professionals outside TM systems will have a critical role in helping indigenous communities adapt and address the changing health needs of communities (Adams *et al.*, 2015). However, indigenous cultures, belief systems and interpretations of the meaning of health and wellbeing must be respected and applied in the context of person-centred care with open communication and shared decision-making (Gall *et al.*, 2018). Other supportive strategies may include the provision of plant medicine education from other indigenous and non-indigenous communities related to medicines from outside the local area that may be more robust to the changing environmental conditions.

Despite this challenge to TM there are important initiatives underway to address the conservation of ecosystems and social systems. For example, indigenous communities in the Eastern Kimberly in Australia use traditional ecological knowledge to inform how natural resources are managed and help plan for various environmental changes (Leonard *et al.*, 2013).

This traditional ecological knowledge is helping scientists to further understand ecosystems.

The Ability of Traditional Medicine to Adapt to Changing Health Issues Resulting from Environmental Change

This section focuses on the ability of TM to adapt to environmental change by finding new ways to address transforming health issues (e.g. increased vector born disease) brought about by climatic change, ocean acidification, land degradation, water scarcity and biodiversity loss among others. This raises concerns about the impact environmental change may have on the management of health care through TM.

Conventional biomedicine needs to urgently consider greater collaboration and integration with TM in order to adapt to and mitigate challenges posed to human health with a changing environment. As recommended by the WHO, an important priority should be to achieve integrative health care in which TM and CM are incorporated into national health care systems (2014). This is particularly important given that modern health care systems are resource-intense and are significant contributors to climate change (Whitmee *et al.*, 2015). It is also important because conventional health care will need to respectfully support traditional indigenous communities who face health-related challenges caused by loss of access to TM, increasing vector-borne disease and climate-related health risk (Whitmee *et al.*, 2015). An integrative health care system that draws from the strengths of both TM and biomedicine could provide the best of each medical paradigm. For example, increased access to the medical technologies developed by biomedicine would benefit traditional indigenous communities (e.g. vaccination), and engagement with traditional indigenous knowledge could benefit modern health care systems.

The current displacement of populations (Whitmee *et al.*, 2015) will also impact upon the access to TM among different populations. As communities and peoples are increasingly driven to relocate to urban environments, they may no longer have access to TM employed for their primary health care needs in their native area (Heywood, 2011). In addition, pharmaceutical medicines and conventional health care may be unaffordable for displaced people reducing their access to health care. Consequently, health care systems will need to adapt and be resilient to population changes and consider sociocultural needs of displaced people to ensure equitable culturally appropriate access to health care. Incorporating traditional healers from displaced communities into these health care systems may assist in managing such challenges. In addition, the use of TM where possible in conventional health care systems may be more culturally appropriate (Gall *et al.*, 2018) and help displaced indigenous people adapt to an unfamiliar environment.

TM systems may also face challenges within their communities related to new health risks emerging as a consequence of changing environments. These challenges may relate to food security (e.g. undernutrition), environmental contamination (e.g. chemical exposure), climate change (e.g. heat stress and infectious disease) and natural disasters (e.g. displacement) (Whitmee *et al.*, 2015). These increased health risks will be a significant challenge for traditional indigenous communities and require new ways of treating illness with unfamiliar medicines and potentially more intervention from conventional biomedicine (Whitmee *et al.*, 2015). For example, sub-Saharan Africa is considered one of the most vulnerable regions to climate change (Berrang-Ford *et al.*, 2012). Uganda is a country in this region that has limited economic and health care resources making it difficult to adapt to a changing environment (Berrang-Ford *et al.*, 2012). The Batwa are indigenous peoples of Uganda who have been displaced as a consequence of conservation strategies; consequently, they have lost access to the forests that were their traditional lands that contained their traditional foods, medicines and livelihoods. The Batwa now experience a higher burden of disease as they are exposed to new infectious diseases (e.g. HIV, malaria), water and food insecurity, extreme weather events and access less health services compared to the general population of Uganda (Berrang-Ford *et al.*, 2012).

In this section we focused on just two examples of the complex challenges faced by TM with a rapidly changing environment: the impact of environmental change on TM, and the ability of TM to adapt to a changing environment. While these examples have significant implications for human health, TM may also help to address planetary health challenges. For example, we can learn from TM systems and integrate approaches that have co-benefits for environmental and human health, such as focusing on preventive health and wellness (Adams *et al.*, 2013). This approach has the potential to prevent future health challenges and ease the burden on resource intense health care systems. A discussion of the opportunities for TM related to planetary health follows.

Advancing Planetary Health Through Traditional Medicine Ideas of Environment and Human Relationships

In this section we focus on the philosophies underpinning medicine systems, in particular the difference between the philosophies underpinning planetary health and the dominant biomedical approach. We also explore the opportunity for informing and strengthening the more integrated philosophies underpinning planetary health — including the human relationship with the natural environment — through a consideration of philosophies underpinning TM (e.g. 'vitalism' and 'holism') (Coulter, 2004). Attention should be given to the lessons that TM offer for planetary health and the development of a truly integrated health care system.

The philosophies of TM systems have historically been aligned with the natural environment and align with the concept of planetary health. These medicine systems recognize that the health of the environment is critical for human health and primarily rely on the use of natural medicines (Alves and Rosa, 2007). Unlike conventional biomedicine, traditional and complementary medicine perspectives consider the concepts of food, medicine and health as interrelated and dependent on the health of the environment (Alves and Rosa, 2007). This is a philosophy that has been originally learnt from indigenous traditional knowledge and is imbedded in indigenous cultural beliefs and ways of being (Heywood, 2011). Indigenous traditional knowledges also include the concept of people being custodians of the land; acknowledging the important responsibly humans have to respect and care for the Earth (Leonard *et al.*, 2013).

Unlike biomedicine, TM systems adopt a philosophy of holism that aligns with planetary health, as they consider all interrelated aspects of a person's health (Litchy, 2011). These healing philosophies require TM health practitioners to ensure the health of the planet. For example, naturopathic philosophy adheres to a therapeutic order that begins with establishing conditions for health by assisting patients with self-care practices. The next stage is referred to as 'vis medicatrix naturae', which is focused on stimulating body systems through the understanding that healing forces in the natural environment (e.g. water, air, light) are needed for the body to heal itself (Litchy, 2011).

The philosophies of TM and CM have been described as being diametrically opposed with conventional biomedicine. For example, traditional and complementary medicine is considered to be holistic, empowering, inductive and intuitive; compared to conventional biomedicine being reductionist, controlling, deductive and scientific (Barrett *et al.*, 2003). This lack of alignment between the two paradigms presents challenges to integrative health care that would benefit planetary health (Whitmee *et al.*, 2015). In contrast, CM is focused on individual health with little consideration of public health (Barrett *et al.*, 2003).

It is important to note that as CM attempts to become legitimised in modern health care systems (and similarly, TM may attempt to become legitimised in low to middle income countries) there is a risk of alignment with a number of late capitalist [neoliberal] ideals and goals primarily focused on the health of individuals (as opposed to wider collectives or human kind) and ensuring a profit from health care (as opposed to focusing upon other less limiting and short-term non-economic outcomes). These neoliberal ideals contradict the philosophies of planetary health as they value materialism, over-consumption and economic wealth over social equality and environmental sustainability (Prescott and Logan, 2018). The profit motive can already be seen in the highly lucrative CM supplement industry as described previously in this chapter. Integrating TM and CM into conventional health systems would help reduce profit motives, as it would provide more equitable access to TM and CM in countries where there is universal health care (WHO, 2014).

Advancing Planetary Health Through Traditional Medicine as a Preventative and Educational Approach

In this section we discuss how the underlying philosophies and practice of TM more broadly align with the planetary health approach, and how TM might contribute to ensuring planetary health. It is now well recognized that healthy dietary and lifestyle behaviours are critical for the health of humans and the planet (Whitmee *et al.*, 2015) and some CM practitioners, such as naturopaths and Western herbalists, have adopted knowledges of food and medicine from a range of different TM systems across the globe. The concept of health prevention and education (although described differently) originated from TM systems that are thousands of years old and continue to be practiced toady (Pal *et al.*, 2015). Traditional indigenous cultures incorporate their food and medicine growing and gathering into their way of life. As such, they are intimately connected to their environment. These traditional agricultural and wild plant gathering practices are taught from within each community, often by community elders or healers (Heywood, 2011). This passing down of traditional knowledge means that cultural ecological values and practices endure over time (Heywood, 2011). This has been demonstrated in ethnobotanical research, which has found that indigenous traditional agricultural systems (home gardens in particular) result in increased access to foods that are high in energy, and macro- and micronutrients (Heywood, 2011).

Wild edible foods have been found to provide higher amounts of micronutrients, and are usually consumed by traditional communities to supplement locally cultivated foods (Bodeker and Kronenberg, 2002). These traditional agricultural systems are considered to be agriculturally and ecologically diverse and suited to local climactic conditions (Heywood, 2011). Home gardens also mitigate food security risk and provide opportunities for additional income (Heywood, 2011). Local indigenous food production coupled with gathering of wild foods is considered a sustainable approach to ensuring food security and a preventative health strategy that enhances human-ecological wellbeing consistent with planetary health (Heywood, 2011).

In contrast to TM, CM is primarily practised in high income countries, and the way it is used can differ across cultures and the various health professions (Herman *et al.*, 2012). For example, CM can be used within more biomedically oriented paradigms. General practitioners may adopt CM and use them without consideration of TM philosophies (Coulter, 2004). Conversely, some CM practitioners, such as Western herbalists, continue to follow TM principles embodied in traditional ways of knowing, such as food as medicine (Niemeyer *et al.*, 2013). As some CM practitioners (e.g. naturopaths, Western herbalists) focus on prevention of disease and enhancing wellbeing (Litchy, 2011; Niemeyer *et al.*, 2013) they are well positioned to draw on preventative health strategies by educating and empowering their patients (and their communities) to adopt similar approaches to food growing and consumption used by those in traditional communities.

In this context CM practitioners are an underutilized resource that if integrated into modern health care systems could make a significant contribution to advancing planetary health. This is particularly important in urban environments in high income countries in which there is high reliance on CM products that are resource intensive (Cordell, 2011), food is primarily produced from large scale agriculture (also resource intense) and often lower in essential nutrients (Heywood, 2011), and there is high consumption of un-healthy diets (Whitmee *et al.*, 2015).

Across various cultures and regions there is a strong emphasis on the role of TM and CM practitioners as teachers and guides who assist people to eliminate obstacles to health, achieve good health outcomes and maintain wellness (Williams-Piehota *et al.*, 2011). Within their educational role TM and CM practitioners have an important role to play in adaptation and mitigation of environmental change, by supporting people to engage in health promoting behaviours. A primary role of both TM and CM practitioners is to educate patients about healthy eating and using food to prevent and treat illness (Williams-Piehota *et al.*, 2011). Given their role in health prevention and education TM and CM practitioners also have an important role to play in increasing planetary health literacy. This can be achieved in dialogue with patients about health promoting behaviours and self-care. For example, research has demonstrated that adopting a health promoting diet can reduce greenhouse gas emissions

(Macdiarmid *et al.*, 2012). These conversations with patients could also be used as educational opportunities to increase knowledge about the use of plant medicines and supplements to help consumers make sustainable treatment choices.

Encouraging the adoption of self-care practices and health promoting behaviours is an important focus of TM. The holistic approach adopted by CM practitioners requires them to address potential causes of disease with the aim of preventing future illness and promoting wellness. An emphasis on healthy eating with a diet based on whole foods and active lifestyles will help reduce acute and chronic illness, which consequently will reduce burden on health care systems helping to mitigate climate change (Whitmee *et al.*, 2015). People who consult CM practitioners have been found to engage in more health promoting behaviours, such as healthy eating and physical activity, compared to non-users in a number of Western countries where there is a high prevalence of chronic illness (Williams-Piehota *et al.*, 2011).

Research has also found that those who consult with CM practitioners develop self-awareness and an understanding of their health needs that led to changes in their health behaviours (Williams-Piehota *et al.*, 2011). Possible explanations for increased uptake in health promoting behaviours may be related to the strategies used by some CM practitioners to facilitate behaviour change. These include informational strategies, such as increasing knowledge of risk factors for disease, and acting as role models by engaging in healthy behaviours themselves (Steg and Vlek, 2009).

Mind–body therapies, such as yoga and meditation, are complementary therapies originating from ancient traditional knowledges, and continue to be used in TM systems. These therapies have been more recently been adopted and adapted in various forms (e.g. mindfulness-based cognitive therapy) in more conventional approaches to health care, and have an increasing empirical evidence-base for their efficacy in a range of health problems (Cramer *et al.*, 2017; Goyal *et al.*, 2014; Piet and Hougaard, 2011). These therapies are often used as self-care practices to enhance health and wellbeing (Cramer *et al.*, 2016a, 2016b, Sibbritt *et al.*, 2011). Yoga practice incorporates elements of mindfulness (a form of meditation), and mindfulness has been found to increase self-awareness, compassion and influence behaviour change (Cook-Cottone and Guyker, 2017). Mindfulness is a particularly important TM practice for planetary health, as mindfulness-based interventions have been shown to increase pro-environmental behaviours (Barbaro and Pickett, 2016; Barrett *et al.*, 2016).

Health behaviour change is challenging at an individual level; consequently, for timely and significant change to occur at a larger population level there needs to be a shift in social norms (Keyes and Galea, 2016). Given that people who use CM are more likely to engage in more health promoting behaviours, integrating TM and CM into mainstream health care may be one solution to increasing the rate of change in social norms related to healthy living that aligns with planetary health.

Concluding Discussion and Research Agenda

This chapter has discussed some challenges and opportunities for TM within the context of planetary health. Considering the primary drivers of biodiversity loss (i.e. habitat loss, global change, invasive species, overexploitation of resources, pollution) are directly related to access to and production of foods and medicines essential for health, it is clear that TM has an important role to play in reducing biodiversity loss and conserving ecosystems. In this section, we highlight some research and policy priorities that will have co-benefits for human and environmental health.

As recognized by the Convention on Biological Diversity, agricultural biodiversity is a critical consideration for mitigating biological and ecosystem diversity while conserving social benefits for communities (Heywood, 2011). There are a number of research priorities related to ensuring the ecological diversity needed to maintain access to plant foods and medicines. These include identification of underutilized species and nutrient dense micronutrient efficient species, and conservation of the genetic diversity of plants to ensure their chemical features are retained so they maintain their medicinal and nutritional properties (Heywood, 2011). Identification of climate resilient plant species is also important, as traditional foods and medicines provide a source of community resilience to food insecurity, conserves local food biodiversity and helps to sustain local economies and cultures (Heywood, 2011).

Improved and consistent regulation of TM and CM across all countries is a goal of the WHO (2014) that aligns with planetary health. As there is variable regulation of herbal medicine product manufacturing across the globe, there needs to be consistency of good manufacturing practice across regions to ensure access to effective, safe, affordable, culturally appropriate and sustainable access to plant medicines (2014). As proposed by Cordell (2017), the CM product industry urgently needs to adopt the concept of 'sustainable medicines'. This requires working with indigenous peoples to preserve traditional medicine knowledge, and future planning with consideration of the role of traditional and complementary medicines with changing global health needs (Cordell, 2017). This will also require consideration of the role of TM and CM within health care systems.

Governments and policymakers need to create more equitable health care systems, and integrate TM into these systems (WHO, 2014). This will assist with improving the delivery of TM (Heywood, 2011). This integration will require researchers and policymakers to prioritise the development of strategies to create sustainable integrative health care systems that are culturally sensitive and informed by traditional indigenous knowledges.

References

Adams, J., Andrews, G., Barnes, J., Broom, A., Magin, P. (eds.), (2012). *Traditional, Complementary and Integrative Medicine: An International Reader*: Macmillan International Higher Education.

Adams, J., Sommers, E., Robinson, N. (2013). Public health and health services research in integrative medicine: An emerging, essential focus. *European Journal of Integrative Medicine*, 5(1), 1–3. doi:10.1016/j.eujim.2012.11.004.

Adams, J., Valery, P. C., Sibbritt, D., Bernardes, C. M., Broom, A., Garvey, G. (2015). Use of traditional indigenous medicine and complementary medicine among indigenous cancer patients in Queensland, Australia. *Integrative Cancer Therapies*, 14(4), 359–365. doi:10.1177/1534735415583555.

Alves, R. R., Rosa, I. M. (2007). Biodiversity, traditional medicine and public health: Where do they meet? *Journal of Ethnobiology and Ethnomedicine*, 3, 14. doi:10.1186/1746-4269-3-14.

Barata, A. M., Rocha, F., Lopes, V., Carvalho, A. M. (2016). Conservation and sustainable uses of medicinal and aromatic plants genetic resources on the worldwide for human welfare. *Industrial Crops and Products*, *88*, 8–11. doi:10.1016/j.indcrop.2016.02.035.

Barbaro, N., Pickett, S. M. (2016). Mindfully green: Examining the effect of connectedness to nature on the relationship between mindfulness and engagement in pro-environmental behavior. *Personality and Individual Differences*, *93*, 137–142. doi:10.1016/j.paid.2015.05.026.

Barrett, B., Grabow, M., Middlecamp, C., Mooney, M., Checovich, M. M., Converse, A. K., Yates, J. (2016). Mindful climate action: Health and environmental co-benefits from mindfulness-based behavioral training. *Sustainability*, *8*(10). doi:10.3390/su8101040.

Barrett, B., Marchand, L., Scheder, J., Plane, M. B., Maberry, R., Appelbaum, D., Rakel, D., Rabago, D. (2003). Themes of holism, empowerment, access, and legitimacy define complementary, alternative, and integrative medicine in relation to conventional biomedicine. *The Journal of Alternative and Complementary Medicine*, *9*(6), 937–947.

Bereuter, D., Glickman, D. (2015). *Healthy Food for a Healthy World: Leveraging Agriculture and Food to Improve Global Nutrition*. http://www.thechicago-council.org/sites/default/files/GlobalAg-HealthyFood_FINAL.pdf.

Berrang-Ford, L., Dingle, K., Ford, J. D., Lee, C., Lwasa, S., Namanya, D. B., Henderson, J., Llanos, A., Carcamo, C., Edge, V. (2012). Vulnerability of indigenous health to climate change: A case study of Uganda's Batwa Pygmies. *Social Science and Medicine*, *75*(6), 1067–1077. doi:10.1016/j.socscimed.2012.04.016.

Biswas, S., Rawat, M. S., Tantray, F. A., Sharma, S. (2017). Medicinal plants conservation and development areas (MPCDAs) — An initiative towards conservation of medicinal plants. *Medicinal Plants*, *9*(3), 143–149. doi:10.5958/0975-6892.2017.00013.

Bodeker, G., Kronenberg, F. (2002). A public health agenda for traditional, complementary, and alternative medicine. *Public Health Matters*, *92*, 1582–1591.

Booker, A., Zhai, L., Gkouva, C., Li, S., Heinrich, M. (2016). From traditional resource to global commodities: A comparison of rhodiola species using NMR spectroscopy-metabolomics and HPTLC. *Front Pharmacol*, *7*, 254. doi:10.3389/fphar.2016.00254.

Butler, C., Dixon, J., Capon, A. (eds.), (2015). *Health of People, Places and Planet. Reflections based on Tony McMichael's Four Decades of Contribution to Epidemiological Understanding*. ANU Press, ACT, Australia.

Camfield, D., McIntyre, E., Sarris, J. (eds.), (2017). *Evidence-Based Herbal and Nutritional Treatment for Anxiety in Psychiatric Disorders.* Springer International Publishing, Switzerland.

Chen, S. L., Yu, H., Luo, H. M., Wu, Q., Li, C. F., Steinmetz, A. (2016). Conservation and sustainable use of medicinal plants: Problems, progress, and prospects. *Chinese Medical Journal, 11,* 37. doi:10.1186/s13020-016-0108-7.

Cook-Cottone, C. P., Guyker, W. M. (2017). The Development and Validation of the Mindful Self-Care Scale (MSCS): An Assessment of practices that support positive embodiment. *Mindfulness, 9*(1), 161–175. doi:10.1007/s12671-017-0759-1.

Cordell, G. A. (2011). Sustainable medicines and global health care. *Planta Medica, 77*(11), 1129–1138. doi:10.1055/s-0030-1270731.

Cordell, G. A. (2015). Ecopharmacognosy and the responsibilities of natural product research to sustainability. *Phytochemistry Letters, 11,* 332–346. doi:10.1016/j.phytol.2014.09.003.

Cordell, G. A. (2017). Cognate and cognitive ecopharmacognosy — in an anthropogenic era. *Phytochemistry Letters, 20,* 540–549. doi:10.1016/j.phytol.2016.10.009.

Coulter, I. (2004). Integration and paradigm clash: The practical difficulties of integrative medicine. In Tovey, P, G., Easthope and Adams, J. (eds.), *Mainstreaming Complementary and Alternative Medicine,* London: Routledge, London, pp. 103–122.

Cramer, H., Anheyer, D., Lauche, R., Dobos, G. (2017). A systematic review of yoga for major depressive disorder. *Journal of Affective Disorders, 213,* 70–77. doi:10.1016/j.jad.2017.02.006.

Cramer, H., Hall, H., Leach, M., Frawley, J., Zhang, Y., Leung, B., Adams, J., Lauche, R. (2016a). Prevalence, patterns, and predictors of meditation use among US adults: A nationally representative survey. *Scientific Reports, 6,* 36760. doi:10.1038/srep36760.

Cramer, H., Ward, L., Steel, A., Lauche, R., Dobos, G., Zhang, Y. (2016b). Prevalence, patterns, and predictors of yoga use: Results of a U.S. nationally representative survey. *American Journal of Preventive Medicine, 50*(2), 230–235. doi:10.1016/j.amepre.2015.07.037.

Ford, J. D. (2012). Indigenous health and climate change. *American Journal of Public Health, 102*(7), 1260–1266.

Ford, J. D., Berrang-Ford, L., King, M., Furgal, C. (2010). Vulnerability of aboriginal health systems in Canada to climate change. *Global Environmental Change, 20*(4), 668–680. doi:10.1016/j.gloenvcha.2010.05.003.

Gall, A., Leske, S., Adams, J., Matthews, V., Anderson, K., Lawler, S., Garvey, G. (2018). Traditional and complementary medicine use among indigenous cancer patients in Australia, Canada, New Zealand, and the United States: A systematic review. *Integrative Cancer Therapies*, 1–14. doi: //10.1177/1/ 1534735418775821.

Goyal, M., Singh, S., Sibinga, E. M., Gould, N. F., Rowland-Seymour, A., Sharma, R., Beuger, Z., Sleicher, D., Maron, D. D., Shihab, H. M., Ranasinghe, P. D., Linn, S., Saha, S., Bass, E. B., Haythornthwaite, J. A. (2014). Meditation programs for psychological stress and well-being: A systematic review and meta-analysis. *JAMA Internal Medicine*, *174*(3), 357–368. doi:10.1001/jamainternmed.2013.13018.

Herman, P. M., Poindexter, B. L., Witt, C. M., Eisenberg, D. M. (2012). Are complementary therapies and integrative care cost-effective? A systematic review of economic evaluations. *BMJ Open*, *2*(5). doi:10.1136/bmjopen-2012-001046.

Heywood, V. H. (2011). Ethnopharmacology, food production, nutrition and bio-diversity conservation: Towards a sustainable future for indigenous peoples. *J Ethnopharmacology*, *137*(1), 1–15. doi:10.1016/j.jep.2011.05.027.

Heywood, V. H. (2013). Overview of agricultural biodiversity and its contribution to nutrition and health. In Fanzo, J., Hunter, D., Borelli, T., Mattei, F. (eds.), *Diversifying Food and Diets*. Routledge, London.

Horton, R. (2016). Offline: Planetary health — where next? *The Lancet*, *387*(10028), 1602. doi:http://dx.doi.org/10.1016/S0140-6736(16)30196-9.

Horton, R., Beaglehole, R., Bonita, R., Raeburn, J., McKee, M., Wall, S. (2014). From public to planetary health: a manifesto. *The Lancet*, *383*(9920), 847. doi:http://dx.doi.org/10.1016/S0140-6736(14)60409-8.

Keyes, K. M., Galea, S. (2016). *Population Health Science*. Oxford University Press, London.

Kulhari, A., Sheorayan, A., Bajar, S., Sarkar, S., Chaudhury, A., Kalia, R. K. (2013). Investigation of heavy metals in frequently utilized medicinal plants collected from environmentally diverse locations of north western India. *SpringerPlus*, *2*, 676.

Leonard, S., Parsons, M., Olawsky, K., Kofod, F. (2013). The role of culture and traditional knowledge in climate change adaptation: Insights from East Kimberley, Australia. *Global Environmental Change*, *23*(3), 623–632. doi:10.1016/j.gloenvcha.2013.02.012.

Litchy, A. P. (2011). Naturopathic physicians: Holistic primary care and integrative medicine specialists. *Journal of Dietary Supplements*, *8*(4), 369–377. doi:10.3109/19390211.2011.623148.

Macdiarmid, J. I., Kyle, J., Horgan, G. W., Loe, J., Fyfe, C., Johnstone, A., McNeill, G. (2012). Sustainable diets for the future: Can we contribute to reducing greenhouse gas emissions by eating a healthy diet? *American Journal of Clinical Nutrition*, *96*(3), 632–639. doi:10.3945/ajcn.112.038729.

McIntyre, E., Saliba, A. J., Wiener, K. K. K., Sarris, J. (2015). Prevalence and predictors of herbal medicine use in adults experiencing anxiety: A critical review of the literature. *Advances in Integrative Medicine*, *2*(1), 38–48. doi:10.1016/j.aimed.2015.04.002.

Niemeyer, K., Bell, I. R., Koithan, M. (2013). Traditional Knowledge of Western Herbal Medicine and Complex Systems Science. *Journal of Herbal Medicine*, *3*(3), 112–119. doi:10.1016/j.hermed.2013.03.001.

Pal, R., Mohanta, P. K., Sarker, G., Rustagi, N., Ghosh, A. (2015). Traditional Healers and Evidence-Based Medicine. *American Journal of Public Health Research*. doi:10.12691/ajphr-3-5A-41.

Piet, J., Hougaard, E. (2011). The effect of mindfulness-based cognitive therapy for prevention of relapse in recurrent major depressive disorder: A systematic review and meta-analysis. *Clinical Psychology Review*, *31*(6), 1032–1040. doi:10.1016/j.cpr.2011.05.002.

Posadzki, P., Watson, L., Ernst, E. (2013). Contamination and adulteration of herbal medicinal products (HMPs): An overview of systematic reviews. *European Journal of Clinical Pharmacology*, *69*(3), 295–307. doi:10.1007/s00228-012-1353-z.

Prescott, S., Logan, A. (2018). Larger than life: injecting hope into the planetary health paradigm. *Challenges*, *9*(1). doi:10.3390/challe9010013.

Saper, R. B., Phillips, R. S., Sehgal, A., Khouri, N., Davis, R. B., Paquin, J., Thuppil, V., Kales, S. N. (2008). Lead, mercury, and arsenic in US- and Indian-manufactured Ayurvedic medicines sold via the Internet. *JAMA*, *300*(8), 915–923.

Schippmann, U., Leaman, D. J., Cunningham, A. B. (2002). *Impact of Cultivation and Gathering of Medicinal Plants on Biodiversity: Global Trends and Issues*. Paper presented at the Biodiversity and the Ecosystem Approach in Agriculture, Forestry and Fisheries. Satellite event on the occasion of the Ninth Regular Session of the Commission on Genetic Resources for Food and Agriculture, Rome.

Sibbritt, D., Adams, J., van der Riet, P. (2011). The prevalence and characteristics of young and mid-age women who use yoga and meditation: Results of a nationally representative survey of 19,209 Australian women. *Complementary Therapies of Medicine*, *19*(2), 71–77. doi:10.1016/j.ctim.2010.12.009.

Song, Y., Hou, D., Zhang, J., O'Connor, D., Li, G., Gu, Q., Liu, P. (2018). Environmental and socio-economic sustainability appraisal of contaminated land remediation strategies: A case study at a mega-site in China. *Science of the Total Environment*, 610–611, 391–401. doi:10.1016/j.scitotenv.2017. 08.016.

Steg, L., Vlek, C. (2009). Encouraging pro-environmental behaviour: An integrative review and research agenda. *Journal of Environmental Psychology, 29*(3), 309–317. doi:10.1016/j.jenvp.2008.10.004.

Suswardany, D. L., Sibbritt, D. W., Supardi, S., Chang, S., Adams, J. (2015). A critical review of traditional medicine and traditional healer use for malaria and among people in malaria-endemic areas: contemporary research in low to middle-income Asia-Pacific countries. *Malaria Journal, 14*(1), 98.

Wardle, J. L., Adams, J. (2014). Indirect and non-health risks associated with complementary and alternative medicine use: An integrative review. *European Journal of Integrative Medicine*, *6*, 409–422. doi:10.1016/j. eujim.2014.01.001.

Whitmee, S., Haines, A., Beyrer, C., Boltz, F., Capon, A. G., de Souza Dias, B. F., Yach, D. (2015). Safeguarding human health in the Anthropocene epoch: Report of The Rockefeller Foundation–Lancet Commission on planetary health. *The Lancet, 386*(10007), 1973–2028. doi:10.1016/s0140-6736(15)60901-1.

Williams-Piehota, P. A., Sirois, F. M., Bann, C. M., Isenberg, K. B., Walsh, E. G. (2011). Agents of change: How do complementary and alternative medicine Providers play a role in health behavior change? *Alternative Therapies, 17*(1), 22–30.

Wittman, H., Chappell, M. J., Abson, D. J., Kerr, R. B., Blesh, J., Hanspach, J., Fischer, J. (2016). A social–ecological perspective on harmonizing food security and biodiversity conservation. *Regional Environmental Change, 17*(5), 1291–1301. doi:10.1007/s10113-016-1045-9.

World Health Organization. (1946). *Official Records of WHO*. Preamble to the Constitution of WHO as adopted by the International Health Conference. Geneva: World Health Organization.

World Health Organization. (2014). *WHO Traditional Medicine Strategy* 2014–2023. Geneva: World Health Organization.

Chapter 14

The Need for Research on the Use of Traditional, Complementary and Integrative Medicine in Emerging and Re-Emerging Infectious Disease Outbreaks: Ebola as a Case Study

Peter Bai James, Jon Wardle, Amie Steel and Jon Adams

Introduction

Infectious diseases are considered a global health threat to human progress and survival especially those caused by emerging and re-emerging pathogens (Jones *et al.*, 2008; Morens *et al.*, 2004). Emerging infections are 'infections that have either not previously affected human or have already appeared in small human population and isolated regions but are rapidly increasing in incidence or geographic range (e.g. Ebola virus, Zika virus and Severe Acute Respiratory Synticial (SARS) virus)' whereas re-emerging infectious diseases are 'ones that were previously a significant local or global public health problem, and then declined dramatically, but are again becoming health problems for a significant proportion of the population (malaria and tuberculosis are examples)' (Heymann and Lee, 2009).

Over the past few decades, the world has witnessed an increased incidence in both emerging and re-emerging infectious diseases all due to biological, ecological, political and socioeconomic factors (Jones *et al.*, 2008; Morse, 2004). Ease of international travel as well as global trade and commerce have amplified the global spread of emerging and re-emerging infectious diseases (Hsu and Shih, 2010; Scotto, 2011; Tatem *et al.*, 2006). The World Health Organization (WHO) estimates that 52% of all deaths in low income countries are due to emerging and re-emerging infectious disease (WHO, 2017b). Women and children in low to middle income countries usually bear the greater burden of both morbidity and mortality for these diseases (Mathers, 2008) and higher incidence of these types of infectious diseases often occurred in places where health systems are under-resourced or over-burdened and where therapeutic pluralism — the use of a range of (sometimes competing) modalities and knowledge systems to treat illness and maintain health — is common. Recent reports of antimicrobial resistance among emerging and re-emerging pathogens as well as concerns over the safety of antimicrobials (McCormick, 1998) have helped rekindle the interest in traditional, complementary and integrative medicine (TCIM), in part based on a perception that TCIM is natural and is therefore safe and effective (WHO, 2013).

In recent times, the worldwide interest in and the utilization of TCIM, has grown rapidly (WHO, 2013) with TCIM use available as both self-administered practices or via consultation with a TCIM practitioner. In recognition of the role of TCIM in the health and wellbeing of individuals across the globe, the WHO has put forward strategies that promote the appropriate integration of TCIM into primary health care systems and its rational use by consumers (WHO, 2013). In middle to low income countries, where the highest prevalence of infectious diseases such malaria, tuberculosis and HIV/AIDS have been recorded (Mathers and Loncar, 2005), current evidence also suggests TCIM is being used to manage and treat these diseases (Nguta *et al.*, 2015; Peltzer *et al.*, 2011; Ranasinghe *et al.*, 2015; Suswardany *et al.*, 2017). The concomitant use of TCIM with conventional therapies have been reported in certain emerging infectious disease outbreaks such as SARS (Hsu *et al.*, 2008; Lau *et al.*, 2005), pandemic influenza (Hsu *et al.*, 2006; Wang *et al.*, 2014) and Zika virus infection (Deng *et al.*, 2016). Alongside this growing evidence of use, the antiviral activity of TCIM products against dengue (Kasture *et al.*, 2016) and chinkunkuya disease (Murali *et al.*, 2015) fever has also been reported. Emerging evidence from preclinical reports or phase one clinical trials suggest some TCIM such as Chinese herbs and other herbal remedies (*Houttuynia cordata* and *Glycyrrhiza* spp. (liquorice)) may be effective in treating these viral infections (Liu *et al.*, 2006, 2012; Yarnell, 2016). While there is a growing body of evidence of TCIM use with regard to some of these recent emerging infectious diseases, the role of TCIM in terms of scale and impact among Ebola patients and survivors has received no research attention since the discovery of the disease. In response, this chapter highlights what is currently known on this topic and identifies the current research gaps that require focus and resource. Our aim is to help draw attention to the need for the inclusion of TCIM regarding the contemporary Ebola research agenda. We will first present an overview of the origins of the Ebola virus disease, mode of spread, prevalence, reactions to the disease as well as prevention and control policies and strategies. This is then followed by a discussion of the role of TCIM during previous and recent Ebola virus disease (EVD) outbreaks and the current picture of TCIM and post-Ebola survivors' syndrome as well as the need for further research.

Ebola Virus Disease: Origin, Mode of Spread, Prevention and Control Strategies

Ebola virus disease is a fatal zoonotic disease transmitted through close human contact with an infected animal or human (dead or alive). Most recently, sexual transmission among EVD survivors has been proposed but more surveillance and clinical research data is required to confirm whether the virus can be transmitted through sexual means (Thorson *et al.*, 2016). Common symptoms and signs include fever, nausea and vomiting, diarrhoea, red eyes, body ache and pain and bleeding. Signs and symptoms take 2–21 days to manifest after contracting the EVD virus (Chertow *et al.*, 2014).

EVD was first discovered in 1976 as a result of two simultaneous outbreaks in east and central Africa (Sudan and Democratic Republic of Congo) (Pourrut *et al.*, 2005). Since the discovery of the disease, thirty-five outbreaks have occurred worldwide but predominantly in Africa, with an average case fatality of 50% (25–90%) (WHO, 2018). The recent 2014–2016 EVD outbreak in West Africa is considered the largest and most complex outbreak to date on the history of the disease. Morbidity and mortality rates were higher compared to all previous outbreaks combined and across all of the three most affected countries (Guinea, Sierra Leone and Liberia), urban in addition to rural settlements were heavily affected. The unprecedented scale, severity, and complexity of the 2014–2016 EVD outbreak in West Africa was further enhanced due to existing poverty, weak health systems and social customs and traditions that makes it difficult to reduce or eliminate the spread of human transmission (Shoman *et al.*, 2017; WHO, 2015b).

There is currently no proven treatment for EVD although several experimental therapies are under evaluation (Martínez *et al.*, 2015). Treatment is purely symptomatic with rehydration with oral and intravenous fluids. A recent EVD vaccine (rVSV-ZEBOV) has shown promising signs of effectiveness in a clinical trial conducted in Guinea (Henao-Restrepo *et al.*, 2017). A package of prevention and control interventions have proven effective and these include active case management, surveillance and contact tracing, a good laboratory service, safe burials, social mobilization and community engagement (Lokuge *et al.*, 2016; WHO, 2015a). Raising awareness on the risk of infection transmission and the use of protective measures (vaccination) through social mobilization and community engagement is crucial in the control and prevention of EVD (Kirsch *et al.*, 2017; Marais *et al.*, 2015).

The Role of TCIM During Ebola Virus Disease Outbreak

The recent 2014–2016 outbreak of the Ebola virus disease (EVD) in West Africa has been described by WHO as the most devastating public health emergency the world has witnessed since the discovery of the virus 40 years ago in the Democratic Republic of the Congo (CDC, 2015; WHO, 1978, 2018). As of May 11, 2016,current statistics put the number of EVD cases (confirmed, probable and suspected) as 28,616 with 11,310 reported deaths (confirmed, probable and suspected) and over 10,000 survivors (WHO, 2015c, 2016). Evidence of the use of TCIM during Ebola outbreaks in East-central and West Africa is minimal and primarily serves to draw attention to the potential significance of the issue without affording insight to the scale or impact. For instance, in a study by De Roo and colleagues in the Democratic Republic of the Congo, nine (26%) of the 34 survivors of the 1995 outbreak self-medicated with traditional medicines after experiencing symptoms suggestive of Ebola (De Roo *et al.*. 1998). In the most recent outbreak in Sierra Leone, the death of a traditional healer from the Ebola virus who is believed to have been infected when treating Ebola patients was the original locus of spread nationally (WHO, 2017a). Also, given that there is no cure for EVD, there are widespread yet unconfirmed claims that TCIM practices administered by traditional healers have effectively prevented or treated the disease (Hewlett and Amola, 2003; Manguvo and Mafuvadze, 2015; Dixon, 2014; Umeora *et al.*, 2014). A case in point was the recommendation by traditional healers to bath with warm salt water to prevent against EVD (Umeora *et al.*, 2014). In the 2000–2001 EVD outbreak in Uganda, drinking bleach was believed to cure the disease (Kinsman, 2012) while communities in the Democratic Republic of the Congo believed the assertions of traditional healers that cursed hunters were the cause of the EVD outbreak (Nkoghe *et al.*, 2011). In the most recent 2018 EVD outbreak in the Democratic Republic of Congo (Rimmer, 2018), three EVD patients were removed from an Ebola treatment centre and taken to church for prayers by their relatives (BBC, 2018). In instances where health care services were inaccessible, EVD patients self-medicated with traditional medicines and relatives used TCIM to treat their infected family members at home (Schwerdtle *et al.*, 2017). Given the lack of knowledge about the Ebola virus disease among traditional healers (Aminu, 2017) and the potential of these healers to spread false information as well as non-adherence to prevention and control measures such as the use of proper protective equipment, it appears traditional healers spread false messages about EVD as well as being prone to infection and being sources of the spread of EVD to others (WHO, 2017a).

The absence of a proven cure for EVD can potentially increase the potential of patients who are suspected of being EVD positive to seek TCIM health care during the EVD outbreak in West Africa. The treatment

of EVD is purely supportive and symptomatic although potential therapeutics such drugs, immune therapies and blood products are still under
investigation (WHO, 2018). Although recent interim results of an EVD
vaccine study show promising signs of being effective and safe, more data
on the efficacy of the vaccine is required to ensure its widespread use
(Henao-Restrepo *et al.*, 2017). In addition, during the West African EVD
outbreak, health facilities were perceived by communities to be highly
infectious and a place of high-risk for mortality further promoting non-
adherence to early care seeking among those infected with Ebola virus
(WHO, 2015b).

The recent prevention and control response to the Ebola outbreak in
West Africa highlighted that the use of biomedical intervention without
incorporating other socio-cultural factors unique to the local setting is
insufficient to prevent and control the disease. For example, community
resistance to biomedical approaches to halt the spread of the Ebola virus
have been observed during the outbreak in West Africa. This was due to
community perception that biomedicine was in conflict with their local
religious, cultural and traditional beliefs and practices (Fairhead, 2016).
Notwithstanding the effects of traditional medicine practices in promoting
the spread of the disease, clear insights into the ethno-social dynamics are
valuable in understanding how traditional practices can be leveraged to
help control infectious disease like Ebola (Adams *et al.*, 2013).

The claims by traditional healers of a cure for Ebola and the utilization of TCIM by those suspected of carrying the Ebola virus during the
outbreak (Hewlett and Amola, 2003; Manguvo and Mafuvadze, 2015) call
for inclusion rather than exclusion of traditional medicine practitioners
into every aspect of future Ebola outbreak response. While traditional
healers are highly revered and easily accessible and provide affordable
health care service to their local communities, their knowledge of Ebola
has been identified as inadequate (Mueller, 2014; Aminu, 2017). As such,
training for traditional medicine practitioners raising their EVD awareness
regarding the disease's cause, pathogenesis, disease symptoms and prevention and control measures is crucial. With such knowledge, traditional
medicine practitioners can be better placed and equipped to discern
potential symptoms of Ebola in the many patients who consult them. In
doing so, they can act as a source of referral to Ebola treatment centres.

Also, with such knowledge, traditional medicine practitioners can serve as a valuable resource with which to dispel myths and false rumours about Ebola in their communities and help promote effective Ebola prevention and control practices. However, it is important to note that training of traditional healers should be followed by monitoring and supervision to ensure that they convey the correct information to their patients and the public over time and back in the community. Going forward, it is important that well-designed studies seek to determine the role of TCIM in the social and cultural life of Ebola-affected communities. Findings from such research will help provide a clear insight as to how TCIM can be leveraged in EVD control and prevention interventions. Such information will not only provide valuable insights for the current and any future EVD outbreaks but can also possibly illustrate how TCIM and traditional health care practitioners may be useful in the ongoing attempts to prevent and control other infectious diseases affecting low to middle income countries.

TCIM and Post-Ebola Survivors' Syndrome: The Need for Further Research

The unprecedented scale of the 2013–2016 Ebola outbreak in West Africa has led to the highest number of survivors in the history of the disease. Currently, there are over 10,000 survivors in all of the three most affected countries. (WHO, 2016) It is apparent that in addition to the psychological trauma experienced during admission most survivors are presenting with physical and psychosocial complications immediately post-discharge and over the long-term, some of which are severe. The commonly reported post-Ebola sequalae include musculoskeletal, ocular, abdominal, auditory, skin, neurological, mental and sexual health disorders (Clark *et al.*, 2015; Qureshi *et al.*, 2015). Despite the high number of people who use TCAM in West Africa (Busia and Kasilo, 2010), and the interest among the scientific community in understanding post-Ebola sequelae among survivors (WHO, 2016), the role of TCIM in addressing the health needs of survivors has received little or no attention. Preliminary data suggest that Ebola survivors are seeking the services of traditional healers (Yoon-Cho, 2016), however, more robust and large scale studies are required to determine the extent to which this early finding can be corroborated and applicable to the wider population of Ebola survivors. Bearing that in mind, we identify areas in the following paragraphs that need for further exploration.

While there is research evidence that demonstrates the use of TCIM therapies among survivors of similar emerging infectious diseases such as SARS (Siu, 2016; WHO, 2004), Ebola survivors' use of TCIM remains largely unexamined. It is imperative that well-designed population-based studies explore the health-seeking behaviour of Ebola survivors battling with post-Ebola complications. Findings describing whether EVD survivors self-medicate, visit traditional healers or seek care in conventional health care facilities and the factors that influence their choice of health care will provide valuable insights that will inform how best health care delivery interventions should be structured to better respond to the health needs of EVD survivors. With regards to TCIM use, it will be necessary to explore the pattern of use such as the proportion TCIM users and non-users, frequency of use, type of TCIM product and practitioners being utilized and for which type of sequelae are TCIM products being used. In addition to understanding the TCIM prevalence and pattern of use, an examination of any push and pull factors (Gyasi *et al.*, 2016a) that influence TCIM utilization among Ebola survivors is also needed. In the context of TCIM use, push factors are issues related to the nature and process of conventional medical care delivery (ineffectiveness and safety of allopathic drugs, attitude of health care personnel, etc.) that may encourage people to seek an alternative health care whereas pull factors are issues related to the nature of TCIM therapies (holism, perceived safety and effectiveness, emotional support, low cost, accessibility etc.) that attract people into using them (Gyasi *et al.*, 2016b). Potentially, the inadequacy of the biomedical care being provided to EVD survivors as a result of the poorly understood nature and pathogenesis of post-Ebola sequelae may be considered a push factor. Also, health care providers hesitance, discrimination due to fear of being infected is a potential push factor to seeking TCIM. In addition, the inaptness to respond to the health needs of EVD survivors as a result of the absence of the competency required for health workers to adequately respond to the health challenges faced by Ebola survivors can potentially serve as a 'push' motivator to seeking TCIM. Pull factors such as societal stigma, isolation, exclusion and economic hardship due to loss of possessions, and means of livelihood as well as EVD survivor's perception and attitude towards TCIM can serve as strong drivers to seeking non-conventional forms of health care. Further, an insight into how TCIM use is influenced by factors such the severity, type and duration of post-Ebola sequelae, as well as survivor's sociodemographic factors (age sex, educational status, income level, etc.) need to be investigated. Such information is important as it helps decision makers and clinicians to identify who are potential users and non-users of TCIM and what motivates or limit survivor's use of TCIM which can help to better inform the current interim clinical care guidelines for EVD survivors (WHO, 2016).

The lived experiences of Ebola survivors as they utilised TCIM or conventional care is an area that requires research attention. Ebola survivor's experience with regard to the efficacy and safety of the TCIM being used needs to be explored. For EVD survivors that seek care from traditional healers, an insight into the perception of the nature of care received will help provide an in-depth understanding of the interplay of underlining factors that either promotes or limit the use of TCIM. The need to understand the perspectives of conventional health care and traditional complementary medicine practitioners providing care to EVD survivors about the use of TCIM is also essential to investigate. With regards to conventional practitioners, areas worth exploring include their perception of TCIM in general and as it relates to Ebola survivors as well as the nature and extent of communication with EVD survivors about TCIM. An understanding of this provider–patient interaction is crucial as it helps inform how best clinical care can be provided to maximize EVD survivor's health outcomes.

Conclusion

It is clear that medical pluralism is common among affected communities during and after an infectious disease outbreak like Ebola despite the dearth of research evidence. It is also known that TCIM practices are deeply rooted in traditional norms and the culture of their host society (Gyasi *et al.*, 2016a; Johnson, 2013), and that socio-cultural factors play an important role in the control and prevention of infectious disease outbreaks (Adongo *et al.*, 2016). As such, it is imperative that TCIM practices are explored, either as the stand-alone central focus of enquiry or as a major consideration in wider investigation, to help understand how relevant elements can be harnessed to maximize prevention and control efforts during and after emerging infectious disease outbreaks. With regards to EVD specifically, it is certainly clear that while there is huge research focus in understanding Ebola virus disease and its sequelae, research on the role of TCIM as a widely used form of health care on a global scale, during and after EVD outbreaks, has not received the research attention it deserves. It is essential that this overlooked area is included in the ongoing Ebola research agenda, as it will provide valuable insights for survivors, health care providers and policymakers.

References

Adams, J., Magin, P., Broom, A. (eds.), (2013). *Primary Health Care and Complementary and Integrative Medicine: Practice and Research*. World Scientific, London, UK.

Adongo, P. B., Tabong, P.T.-N., Asampong, E., Ansong, J., Robalo, M., Adanu, R. M. (2016). preparing towards preventing and containing an Ebola virus disease outbreak: What socio-cultural practices may affect containment efforts in Ghana? *PLoS Neglected Tropical Diseases*, *10*(7), e0004852.

Aminu, K. J. A. (2017). Traditional healers' knowledge of Ebola virus disease. *Annals of Public Health and Research*, *4*(1), 1054.

BBC (2018). *Ebola outbreak in DR Congo: Patients 'taken to church'*. British Broadcasting Corporation. https://www.bbc.com/news/world-africa-44229346. Accessed on 17 July 2018,

Busia, K., Kasilo, O. M. (2010). Overview of traditional medicine in ECOWAS member states. *African Health Monitor WHO/AFRO*, *13*, 16–24.

CDC (2015). *Outbreaks Chronology: Ebola Virus Disease*, Center for Disease Control and Prevention, Atlanta: CDC. https://www.cs.rutgers.edu/~mcgrew/Byrne2016/library/biologicalnightmare/Outbreaks%20Chronology:%20Ebola%20Virus%20Disease%20%7C%20Ebola%20Hemorrhagic%20Fever%20%7C%20CDC.pdf. Accessed on 17 July 2018.

Chertow, D. S., Kleine, C., Edwards, J. K., Scaini, R., Giuliani, R., Sprecher, A. (2014). Ebola virus disease in West Africa — clinical manifestations and management. *New England Journal of Medicine*, *371*(22), 2054–2057.

Clark, D. V., Kibuuka, H., Millard, M., Wakabi, S., Lukwago, L., Taylor, A., Eller, M. A., Eller, L. A., Michael, N. L., Honko, A. N., Jr, Olinger, G. G., Schoepp, R. J., Hepburn, M. J., Hensley, L. E. and Robb, M. L. (2015). Long-term sequelae after Ebola virus disease in Bundibugyo, Uganda: A retrospective cohort study. *Lancet Infectious Diseases, 15*(8), 905–912.

De Roo, A., Ado, B., Rose, B., Guimard, Y., Fonck, K., Colebunders, R. (1998). Survey among survivors of the 1995 Ebola epidemic in Kikwit, Democratic Republic of Congo: Their feelings and experiences. *Tropical Medicine & International Health, 3*(11), 883–885.

Deng, Y., Zeng, L., Bao, W., Xu, P., Zhong, G. (2016). Experience of integrated traditional Chinese and Western medicine in first case of imported Zika virus disease in China. *Zhonghua wei zhong bing ji jiu yi xue, 28*(2), 106–109.

Dixon, R. (2014). *Ebola Hits Home for a Liberian Faith Healer.* http://www.latimes.com/world/la-fg-c1-ebola-faith-healer-20141023-story.html#page=1.

Fairhead, J. (2016). Understanding social resistance to the Ebola response in the forest region of the Republic of Guinea: An anthropological perspective. *African Studies Review, 59*(3), 7–31.

Gyasi, R. M., Asante, F., Abass, K., Yeboah, J. Y., Adu-Gyamfi, S., Amoah, P. A. (2016a). Do health beliefs explain traditional medical therapies utilisation? Evidence from Ghana. *Cogent Social Sciences, 2*(1), 1–14.

Gyasi, R. M., Asante, F., Yeboah, J. Y., Abass, K., Mensah, C. M., Siaw, L. P. (2016b). Pulled in or pushed out? Understanding the complexities of motivation for alternative therapies use in Ghana. *International Journal of Qualitative Studies on Health and Well-being,* 11, doi: 10.3402/qhw.v11.29667.

Henao-Restrepo, A. M., Camacho, A., Longini, I. M., Watson, C. H., Edmunds, W. J., Egger, M., Carroll, M. W., Dean, N. E., Diatta, I., Doumbia, M., Draguez, B., Duraffour, S., Enwere, G., Grais, R., Gunther, S., Gsell, P.-S., Hossmann, S., Watle, S. V., Kondé, M. K., Kéïta, S., Kone, S., Kuisma, E., Levine, M. M., Mandal, S., Mauget, T., Norheim, G., Riveros, X., Soumah, A., Trelle, S., Vicari, A. S., Røttingen, J.-A., Kieny, M.-P. (2017). Efficacy and effectiveness of an rVSV-vectored vaccine in preventing Ebola virus disease: Final results from the Guinea ring vaccination, open-label, cluster-randomised trial (Ebola Ça Suffit!)'. *The Lancet, 389*(10068), 505–518.

Hewlett, B. S., Amola, R. P. (2003). Cultural contexts of Ebola in northern Uganda. *Emerging Infectious Diseases Journal,* 9, 1242–1248.

Heymann, D. L., Lee, V. (2009). Emerging and re-emerging infections, *Oxford Textbook of Public Health.* Oxford University Press, *Oxford,* pp. 1264–1276.

Hsu, C.-H., Hwang, K.-C., Chao, C.-L., Chang, S.G., Ho, M.-S. Chou, P. (2006). Can herbal medicine assist against avian flu? Learning from the experience of using supplementary treatment with Chinese medicine on SARS or SARS-like infectious disease in 2003'. *Journal of Alternative & Complementary Medicine*, *12*(6), 505–506.

Hsu, C.-H., Hwang, K.-C., Chao, C.-L., Chang, S. G., Ho, M.-S., Lin, J.-G., Chang, H.-H., Kao, S.-T., Chen, Y.-M., Chou, P. (2008). An evaluation of the additive effect of natural herbal medicine on SARS or SARS-like infectious diseases in 2003: A randomized, double-blind, and controlled pilot study. *Evidence-Based Complementary and Alternative Medicine*, *5*(3), 355–362.

Hsu, C. I., Shih, H. H. (2010). Transmission and control of an emerging influenza pandemic in a small-world airline network. *Accident Analysis and Prevention*, *42*(1), 93–100.

Johnson, P. (2013). Global use of complementary and alternative medicine and treatments, *Global Healthcare: Issues and Policies*. Jones & Bartlett Learning LLC, pp. 1–25.

Jones, K. E., Patel, N. G., Levy, M. A., Storeygard, A., Balk, D., Gittleman, J. L. Daszak, P. (2008). Global trends in emerging infectious diseases. *Nature*, *451*(7181), 990–993.

Kasture, P. N., Nagabhushan, K. H., Kumar, A. (2016). A multi-centric, double-blind, placebo-controlled, randomized, prospective study to evaluate the efficacy and safety of Carica papaya leaf extract, as empirical therapy for thrombocytopenia associated with dengue fever. *Journal of the Association of the Physicians of India*, *64*(6), 15–20.

Kinsman, J. (2012). "A time of fear": Local, national, and international responses to a large Ebola outbreak in Uganda. *Global Health*, *8*, 15.

Kirsch, T. D., Moseson, H., Massaquoi, M., Nyenswah, T. G., Goodermote, R., Rodriguez-Barraquer, I., Lessler, J., Cumings, D. A. T., Peters, D. H. (2017). Impact of interventions and the incidence of Ebola virus disease in Liberia — implications for future epidemics. *Health Policy and Planning*, *32*(2), 205–214.

Lau, J. T., Leung, P., Wong, E., Fong, C., Cheng, K., Zhang, S., Lam, C., Wong, V., Choy, K. Ko, W. (2005). The use of an herbal formula by hospital care workers during the severe acute respiratory syndrome epidemic in Hong Kong to prevent severe acute respiratory syndrome transmission, relieve influenza-related symptoms, and improve quality of life: a prospective cohort study. *Journal of Alternative & Complementary Medicine*, *11*, (1), 49–55.

Liu, X., Zhang, M., He, L., Li, Y. (2012). Chinese herbs combined with Western medicine for severe acute respiratory syndrome (SARS). *Cochrane Database of Systematic Reviews*, *10*, Cd004882.

Liu, X., Zhang, M., He, L., Li, Y. P., Kang, Y. K. (2006). Chinese herbs combined with Western medicine for severe acute respiratory syndrome (SARS). *Cochrane Database of Systematic Reviews*, *1*, Cd004882.

Lokuge, K., Caleo, G., Greig, J., Duncombe, J., McWilliam, N., Squire, J., Lamin, M., Veltus, E., Wolz, A., Kobinger, G., de la Vega, M.-A., Gbabai, O., Nabieu, S., Lamin, M., Kremer, R., Danis, K., Banks, E., Glass, K. (2016). Successful control of Ebola virus disease: Analysis of service based data from rural Sierra Leone. *PLoS Neglected Tropical Diseases*, *10*(3), e0004498.

Manguvo, A., Mafuvadze, B. (2015). The impact of traditional and religious practices on the spread of Ebola in West Africa: Time for a strategic shift. *The Pan African Medical Journal*, *22*(Suppl 1), 9.

Marais, F., Minkler, M., Gibson, N., Mwau, B., Mehtar, S., Ogunsola, F., Banya, S.S., Corburn, J. (2015). A community-engaged infection prevention and control approach to Ebola. *Health Promotion International*, *31*(2), 440–449.

Martínez, M. J., Salim, A. M., Hurtado, J. C., Kilgore, P. E. (2015). Ebola virus infection: overview and update on prevention and treatment. *Infectious Diseases and Therapy*, *4*(4), 365–390.

Mathers, C. (2008). *The global burden of disease: 2004 update*, World Health Organization.

Mathers, C. D., Loncar, D. (2005). Updated projections of global mortality and burden of disease, 2002–2030: Data sources, methods and results. *Geneva: World Health Organization*.

McCormick, J. B. (1998). Epidemiology of emerging/re-emerging antimicrobial-resistant bacterial pathogens. *Current Opinion in Microbiology*, *1*(1), 125–129.

Morens, D. M., Folkers, G. K., Fauci, A. S. (2004). The challenge of emerging and re-emerging infectious diseases. *Nature*, *430*(6996), 242–249.

Morse, S. S. (2004). Factors and determinants of disease emergence. *Scientific and Technical Review*, *23*(2), 443–451.

Mueller, K. (2014). *Turning to Traditional Healers to Help Stop the Ebola Outbreak in Sierra Leone*, International Federation of Rerd Cross and Red Crescent Societies., http://www.ifrc.org/en/news-and-media/news-stories/africa/sierra-leone/turning-to-traditional-healers-to-help-stop-the-ebola-outbreak-in-sierra-leone-66529/. Accessed on 1 November 2017.

Murali, K. S., Sivasubramanian, S., Vincent, S., Murugan, S. B., Giridaran, B., Dinesh, S., Gunasekaran, P., Krishnasamy, K., Sathishkumar, R. (2015). Anti—chikungunya activity of luteolin and apigenin rich fraction from Cynodon dactylon. *Asian Pacific Journal of Tropical Medicine, 8*(5), 352–358.

Nguta, J. M., Appiah-Opong, R., Nyarko, A. K., Yeboah-Manu, D., Addo, P. G. A. (2015). Medicinal plants used to treat TB in Ghana. *International Journal of Mycobacteriology, 4*(2), 116–123.

Nkoghe, D., Kone, M. L., Yada, A., Leroy, E. (2011). A limited outbreak of Ebola haemorrhagic fever in Etoumbi, Republic of Congo, 2005. *Transactions of the Royal Society of Tropical Medicine and Hygiene, 105*(8), 466–472.

Peltzer, K., Preez, N. F., Ramlagan, S., Fomundam, H., Anderson, J., Chanetsa, L. (2011). Antiretrovirals and the use of traditional, complementary and alternative medicine by HIV patients in a longitudinal study. *African Journal of Traditional Complementary Alternative Medicines, 8*(4), 337–345.

Pourrut, X., Kumulungui, B., Wittmann, T., Moussavou, G., Délicat, A., Yaba, P., Nkoghe, D., Gonzalez, J.-P., Leroy, E. M. (2005). The natural history of Ebola virus in Africa. *Microbes and Infection, 7*(7), 1005–1014.

Qureshi, A. I., Chughtai, M., Loua, T. O., Kolie, J. P., Camara, H. F. S., Ishfaq, M. F., N'Dour, C. T., Beavogui, K. (2015). Study of Ebola virus disease survivors in Guinea. *Clinical Infectious Diseases, 61*(7), 1035–1042.

Ranasinghe, S., Ansumana, R., Lamin, J. M., Bockarie, A. S., Bangura, U., Buanie, J. A., Stenger, D. A., Jacobsen, K. H. (2015). Herbs and herbal combinations used to treat suspected malaria in Bo, Sierra Leone. *Journal of Ethnopharmacology, 166*, 200–204.

Rimmer, A. (2018). New Ebola outbreak declared in Democratic Republic of the Congo. *BMJ, 361*, k2074.

Schwerdtle, P. M., De Clerck, V., Plummer, V. (2017). Experiences of Ebola Survivors: Causes of Distress and Sources of Resilience. *Prehospital and Disaster Medicine, 32*(3), 234–239.

Scotto, G. (2011). Globalization and infectious diseases: The past and future. *Infez Med, 19*(1), 56–61.

Shoman, H., Karafillakis, E., Rawaf, S. (2017). The link between the West African Ebola outbreak and health systems in Guinea, Liberia and Sierra Leone: A systematic review, *Globalization and Health, 13*(1), 1.

Siu, J.Y.m. (2016). 'Coping with future epidemics: Tai chi practice as an overcoming strategy used by survivors of severe acute respiratory syndrome (SARS) in post-SARS Hong Kong. *Health Expectations : An International Journal of Public Participation in Health Care and Health Policy, 19*(3), 762–772.

Suswardany, D. L., Sibbritt, D. W., Supardi, S., Pardosi, J. F., Chang, S., Adams, J. (2017). A cross-sectional analysis of traditional medicine use for malaria alongside free antimalarial drugs treatment amongst adults in high-risk malaria endemic provinces of Indonesia. *PLoS One*, *12*(3), e0173522.

Tatem, A. J., Rogers, D. J., Hay, S. I. (2006). Global transport networks and infectious disease spread. *Advances in Parasitology*, *62*, 293–343.

Thorson, A., Formenty, P., Lofthouse, C., Broutet, N. (2016). Systematic review of the literature on viral persistence and sexual transmission from recovered Ebola survivors: Evidence and recommendations. *BMJ Open*, *6*(1), e008859.

Umeora, O., Emma-Echiegu, N., Umeora, M., Ajayi, N. (2014). Ebola viral disease in Nigeria: The panic and cultural threat. *African Journal of Medical and Health Sciences*, *13*(1), 1–5.

Wang, C., Wang, H., Liu, X., Xu, D., Tang, Y., Luo, P. (2014). Traditional Chinese Medicine for the treatment of influenza: A systematic review and Meta-analysis of randomized controlled trials. *Journal of Traditional Chinese Medicine*, *34*(5), 527–531.

WHO (1978). Ebola haemorrhagic fever in Zaire, 1976. *Bull World Health Organ*, *56*(2), 271–293.

WHO (2004). *SARS: Clinical Trials on Treatmento Using a Combination of Traditional Chinese Medicine And Western Medicine.* World Health Organization, Geneva.

WHO (2013). *WHO Traditional Medicine Strategy 2014–2023.* World Health Organization, Geneva.

WHO (2015a). *2015 WHO Strategic Response Plan: West Africa Ebola outbreak.* World Health Organization, Geneva. http://apps.who.int/iris/bitstream/handle/10665/163360/9789241508698_eng.pdf;jsessionid=6A39AF7C681322E34C3EBABE57C543A6?sequence=1.

WHO (2015b). *Factors that contributed to undetected spread of the Ebola virus and impeded rapid containment*, World Health Organization, Geneva Switzerland http://www.who.int/csr/disease/ebola/one-year-report/factors/en/. Accessed on 1 November 2017.

WHO (2015c). *Ebola Data and Statistics.* http://apps.who.int/gho/data/view.cbola-sitrep.ebola-summary-20160511?lang=en. Accessed on 19 January 2017.

WHO (2016). *Clinical Care for Survivors of Ebola Virus Disease. Interim Guidance.* 2016 http://apps.who.int/iris/bitstream/10665/204235/1/WHO_EVD_OHE_PED_16.1_eng.pdf?ua=1.

WHO (2017a). *Sierra Leone: A Traditional Healer and a Funeral.* http://www.who.int/csr/disease/ebola/ebola-6-months/sierra-leone/en/'.

WHO (2017b) *The Top 10 Causes of Death. Leading Causes of Death by Economy Income Group*, World health Organization, Geneva, Switzerland. http://www.who.int/mediacentre/factsheets/fs310/en/index1.html. Accessed on 31 October 2017.

WHO (2018). *Ebola Virus Disease Key Facts.* World Health Organization Geneva, Switzerland, http://www.who.int/news-room/fact-sheets/detail/ebola-virus-disease. Accessed on 1 June 2017.

Yarnell, E. (2016). Herbs for emerging viral infectious diseases. *Alternative and Complementary Therapies*, 22(4), 164–274.

Yoon-Cho (2016). Experiences of Ebola survivors on healthcare access in Bombali District, Sierra Leone, University of Sheffield.

Chapter 15

Health Disparities and Traditional, Complementary and Integrative Medicine Use: Reflections and Recommendations from a Social Justice Perspective

Elizabeth Sommers and Jon Adams

'Health inequalities and social determinants of health are not footnotes to the determination of health. They are the main issues'.

Michael Marmot (Marmot, interview, 2011)

Introduction

Health inequities arc universal, ubiquitous and brutal. As a form of social injustice, health inequities know no borders. They are evident in every sphere and level of infrastructure of health care systems, whether we examine high income or low to middle income countries, urban or rural localities within countries, or across postal codes or districts within neighbourhoods or cities. This chapter will examine traditional, complementary and integrative medicine (TCIM) as part of a social justice agenda in the context of human and civil rights. The chapter will also provide a global perspective and examine health inequities in low to middle to high income country settings and health care systems.

The World Health Organization (WHO) has characterized health inequities as follows: 'Health inequities are the unjust differences in health between persons of different social groups, and can be linked to forms of disadvantage such as poverty, discrimination and lack of access to services or goods' (Hosseinpoor, 2013; World Health Organization, 2015). The right of access to health care as elucidated by the WHO Constitution has been further characterized by Margaret Chan, Director-General of WHO, in her remarks at the International Forum on Traditional Medicine in China:

> Modern medicine and traditional medicine make unique contributions to health, but both also have their limits and shortcomings. Countries, especially in the developing world, are wise to use the best of these two approaches in a carefully integrated and regulated way…For many millions of people, often living in rural areas of developing countries, herbal medicines, traditional treatments and traditional practitioners are the main, sometimes the only, source of health care (Chan, 2015).

Background

The underpinnings of determinants of health inequities include macro-environmental factors associated with every level of social structure (Braveman and Gottlieb, 2014). These social, political and individual factors interact in complex ways to affect all aspects of health. Since TCIM practitioners and researchers can appreciate the complexity of health and the body from a holistic perspective, this understanding may better equip us to consider, strategize and design plans to effectively address health inequities.

A matrix of social inequities that influences health and wellbeing has been described by Arcaya and colleagues; these factors include: income/poverty (individual and social); education; physical and mental health;

race/ethnicity; gender; age; physical ability/disability; sexual orientation and migrant worker status. Members of global society who are at highest risk of poor health outcomes include immigrants, asylum seekers, indigenous people, homeless individuals and travelers (Arcaya *et al.*, 2015).

Kawachi and colleagues distinguish between health inequalities and health inequities. The term *health inequality* is presented as a generic way of describing differences in the health of individuals or groups. It broadly includes measurable characteristics of health that may differ among individuals and populations. There is no inherent moral judgment associated with the term and no inference is made regarding fairness or justice. The term *health inequity,* however, is associated with health disparities or inequalities resulting from systemic bias or unjust appropriation of resources. Thus, there is a moral component to viewing health inequities as issues inherently connected to human rights and social justice (Kawachi *et al.*, 2002).

Health inequities are evident universally because all countries face shortages of resources and/or unequal resource allocation (Crombie *et al.*, 2005). The lack of economic resources or disparities in resource allotment may be apparent in a variety of ways in the health sphere. Services may not exist or may not be available to all citizens. Individuals or populations may not have timely and appropriate access to care. Language barriers may prevent individuals from receiving vital care. Resulting disparities in health may manifest in a variety of ways including reduced life expectancy, increased burden of illness, obstacles to maternal and child health and impaired psychosocial wellbeing (Crombie *et al.*, 2005).

Although there is evidence of broadening health inequities are broadening in the 21st century, adopting a public health perspective offers some affirmative strategies for addressing and bridging these circumstances (Elgar *et al.*, 2015; Olshansky *et al.*, 2012). This chapter will discuss some of the innovative and successful approaches, as well as best practices, that have been incorporated to address improving the health outcomes for vulnerable and underserved populations. These strategies encompass a variety of TCIM perspectives and have been implemented in low to middle income countries (in Latin America, South Africa and the Philippines) as well as in high income countries (such as Germany, Australia, Canada and the US).

To commemorate the 40th anniversary of the Declaration of Alma-Ata, the Pan American Health Organization (PAHO) and the WHO held a symposium in May, 2018 to further build upon the concepts raised four decades earlier (Pan American Health Organization, 2018). Representatives from PAHO's Universal Health Strategy group and the WHO Traditional Medicine Strategy 2014–2023 group met to examine the role of TCIM in primary health care. Presenters from Brazil, Belgium and the US described experiences in each of their respective countries. Brazil was represented byxDaniel Miele Amado, National Coordinator of Integrative and Complementary Practice in Health from the Brazilian Ministry of Health. Goals of national policy on TCIM in Brazil were summarized as follows, to: (1) incorporate and implement TCIM in national public health system; (2) increase citizens' access to TCIM; (3) continue to increase efficiency of the nation's health system; (4) promote best practices; (5) expand context of TCIM to include prevention, promotion and rehabilitation and (6) strengthen community participation (Pan American Health Organization, 2018).

From 2016 to 2017, Brazil expanded its state-sanctioned TCIM offerings from approaches such as anthroposophical medicine, Traditional Chinese medicine, homeopathy and herbal medicine to include Ayurveda, naturopathy, osteopathy, chiropractic, Reiki and yoga (Pan American Health Organization, 2018).

Vivian Camacho also addressed the joint gathering and offered her perspectives as an Indigenous activist and member of the PAHO High Level Commission for the 40th Anniversary of Alta-Ata. She urged conference participants to recognize and value the connections between Indigenous practices and the contemporary models of TCIM. She stressed the importance of developing public policy that addresses the fundamental role that TCIM plays in advancing universal health (Pan American Health Organization, 2018).

Examining Health Inequities from a TCIM Perspective

Our current global system of nation states hinges on interdependence, immigration, migration and social media connecting people in unprecedented ways. Reflecting our times and cultures, TCIM blends traditional, complementary and biomedical practices in new, evolving and pluralistic ways.

Through the lens of legislation

Stuttaford and her colleagues conducted surveys and examined related literature from England, South Africa, Kenya and Jordan to better understand themes related to the basic human right to health care and protection of citizens from harmful practices. Their findings highlight the evolving nature as well as gaps in international law related to the right to health (Stuttaford *et al.*, 2014). Dating as far back as 1966, the United Nations (UN) addressed implementing the right to health in its International Covenant on Social, Economic and Cultural rights (United Nations, 1966). Article 12 of this document specifies the right of all individuals to enjoy the highest attainable standard of physical and mental health. In 2000, the UN expanded on this concept by elaborating on the need for states to enact legislation and to devote administrative, economic and public health resources to actualize the right to health (United Nations, 2000). This UN document also addresses health rights for indigenous people, describing their right to health access and care:

> These health services should be culturally appropriate, taking into account traditional preventive care, health practices, and medicines. States therefore should provide resources for indigenous people to design, deliver, and control such services… in indigenous communities, the health of the individual is often linked to the health of the society as a whole and has a collective dimension (United Nations, 2000).

Illustrating key findings of Stuttaford *et al.*'s survey, South Africa and England have both enacted legal regulations related to biomedicine and some forms of TCIM, South Africa has developed legal requirements regulating traditional healing and Kenya has focused its regulatory powers on biomedicine (as of 2013). In Jordan Chinese medicine, acupuncture and reflexology are utilized by patients in private clinics while Indigenous populations and Muslims favour the use of herbs, prayers and reading the Quran and there is a lack of overarching regulation (Stuttaford *et al.*, 2014).

Stuttaford and her colleagues underscore associated rights and the need for legal implementation and oversight in the adoption of TCIM by countries (Stuttaford *et al.*, 2014). The issue of 'right to health in all its forms' is based on public health-related underpinnings such as accessibility, acceptability to populations (from both ethical and pragmatic perspectives), health promotion, right to information and the primary tenet of 'first do no harm'. The rights to equity and non-discrimination in health care that includes TCIM have also been addressed by other commentators (Nissen *et al.*, 2013; Yarney *et al.*, 2013). Although sentiment for the right to health in its many forms may be almost universally shared, implementing, monitoring and legislating this right vary considerably throughout the world. Understanding these gaps may assist in addressing disparities in TCIM availability, safety, efficacy and utilization.

TCIM: Substitute or complement?

Depending on the multilayered matrix of economic factors (such as individual, local or country-wide resources), TCIM may be a primary, secondary or non-option regarding health seeking. International literature provides us with a full spectrum of ways in which health integration has been effectively implemented in low to middle and high income countries. Due to the lack of access to conventional medical services in some cases and locales, TCIM may be the only type of healing or health care that is available; thus, it becomes essential to human health and healing (Hollenberg *et al.*, 2009).

In India, biomedical care for individuals diagnosed with cancer is expensive and thus unaffordable for most people (Broom *et al.*, 2009). Women with cancer tend to use TCIM approaches as a substitute for biomedical care. Likewise, in Kenya, users of TCIM tend to have fewer economic resources (Lambert *et al.*, 2011). Paradoxically, in high income countries such as Denmark, the choice of using TCIM is often made by individuals with higher economic status (Pederson *et al.*, 2009).

Mongolia suffered tremendous economic loss after the collapse of the Soviet Union in 1991 (Anderson, 2016). Despite a profound lack of health care resources, the Mongolian government rallied itself to restore and promote both conventional medicine as well as TCIM (World Health

Organization and Mongolian Ministry of Health, 2012). Although traditional health practices had been repressed for several decades, access to TCIM care has been increased and research institutes on traditional medicine and natural remedies have been established by Mongolia's government. Since much of the population lives outside the range of hospitals, traditional medicine is often the first approach to be utilized. Family medicine kits are available to citizens who live great distances from cities — these kits contain twelve types of traditional Mongolian medicine and are available at no cost (World Health Organization and Mongolian Ministry of Health, 2012).

Xu and Farrell used data from the Medical Expenditure Panel Surveys from 1996 and 1998 to examine TCIM utilization among racial and ethnic groups in the US. These surveys use a subset of data from the National Health Interview Survey (NHIS) which is administered by the US Federal Agency for Healthcare Research and Quality (Xu and Farrell, 2006). The NHIS collected data from 46,673 respondents. Although an earlier investigation by Druss and Rosenbeck determined that TCIM services complemented rather than substituted for conventional medical services, Xu and Farrell found that both substitution and complementarity could be observed across conventional and complementary medicine use and varied considerably for different racial and ethnic populations (Druss and Rosenbeck, 1999). Among non-Hispanic White respondents who were users of TCIM, chiropractic, acupuncture and nutritional counseling were complements to conventional medicine use. Prayer and spiritual healing were substitutes for conventional medicine utilization in some situations. Among Hispanic respondents, homeopathy and spiritual healing were found to be substitutes for conventional medical care. For African-American users of TCIM, acupuncture and massage were reported to be complements to conventional medical use while biofeedback and traditional practices were substitutes to use of conventional medicine. Asian-Americans reported frequent TCIM use as a substitute for conventional medical treatments. In particular, however, massage, herbal medicine, traditional medicine and spiritual healing were often used in conjunction with conventional medical care (Xu and Farrell, 2006).

No uniform patterns of substitution versus complementarity appear to be evident from US data or beyond at the international level.

Economic factors exert a profound influence regarding decisions about TCIM utilization. If countries or states cover costs of conventional medical treatment, while TCIM costs must be met via personal out-of-pocket expenditure, conventional medical care and services will often be the approach of choice (Lewando *et al.*, 2004).

The Stigma of TCIM

In a study conducted in Jordan assessing use of TCIM by individuals with mental health problems, it was noted that TCIM was often the first approach to be accessed (Gearing *et al.*, 2012). Underlying reasons for this choice included gender, cost and lack of stigma. Study respondents reported that traditional healing was easier to access and not stigmatized because it was embedded in their culture.

All types of TCIM have been subject to discussion and scrutiny in terms of efficacy, access, risks and costs. Some factors that may stigmatize TCIM approaches may include the fact that TCIM practitioners: may lack skills and training to diagnose or treat disease; do not work with conventional medical providers; do not have access to techniques or equipment needed for providing care; and may be unregulated (Anzat and Abdullah, 2008). In addition, stigmatization may also be due to the fact that TCIM techniques may be unproven; lack standardization; and may be associated with adverse effects or other risks to health. TCIM researchers and providers worldwide are attempting to address these deficiencies in order to remove or ameliorate the perceived stigma of TCIM (Anzat and Abdullah, 2008).

In the area of Traditional Chinese Medicine (TCM), efforts are underway to standardize terminology. Throughout 2018 the WHO will be working on developing a 'standard terminology in TCM' (Personal correspondence Daniel Gallego-Perez) and the WHO Traditional, Complementary and Integrative Medicine Department of Service Delivery and Safety are coordinating efforts to recruit experts in TCM from China as well as the US, Canada and Latin America to create a reference document for future relevant WHO material in the area of traditional, complementary and integrative medicine. Espinosa describes these efforts as 'in response to the increasing need for standardized TCM terminology in support of WHO technical documents in the area of TCM, such as the various benchmarks for practice and training. Such a standardized approach is also used for the list of diagnoses of 'traditional medicine of ancient Chinese origin' integrated as a chapter in the 11th revision of the International Classification of Diseases (ICD-11)'.

Evidence-based Practices for Addressing Health Inequities

A central tenet of our exegesis is that the international landscape consists of highly disparate segments in terms of economics, culture, values and infrastructure. Although all may share the fundamental desire to ensure health access for all citizens, economic and political realities may make this difficult to achieve. Since the determinants of health disparities are complex and often synergistic, multiple approaches to address inequities are needed. The adoption of TCIM practices may confer potential benefit as part of a comprehensive strategy to reduce health inequities (Struthers and Nichols, 2011).

To identify and examine evidence-based practices we propose using the following public health-related indicators listed in Table 1:

Table 1. Public health parameters.

Accessibility

Acceptability — individual and cultural

Cost — individual and societal

Evidence of clinical efficacy

Capacity to promote health — individual knowledge and empowerment

Evidence concerning lack of harm

Collaboration with biomedical partners

Training and monitoring of TCIM personnel

Regulatory oversight

Source: Adapted from Yamin (2016).

A Case Study: TCIM Use Among Individuals Diagnosed with HIV in South Africa, Uganda and the United States

The HIV/AIDS pandemic, which was first noted in the early 1980s, offers an example of a global health challenge through which we can evaluate the response and practice of TCIM communities. Although HIV/AIDS can be transmitted to anyone, the pandemic has disproportionately affected vulnerable populations who are socioeconomically disadvantaged and/or are at risk because of inadequate access to medical care (Sengupta *et al.*, 2010). Vulnerable individuals may lack resources for primary prevention — namely, health education and health promotion resources that are minimal or absent. Access to antiretroviral medication necessary to minimize the impact of the disease after it has been transmitted may also be sub-optimal (Johnson *et al.*, 2015).

The stigma of HIV/AIDS, which persists even after almost four decades of the pandemic, continues to isolate those affected by the virus, in particular, intravenous drug users and members of sexual minorities such as homosexual men, transsexual individuals and bisexuals. Women throughout the world also bear a disproportionate burden in terms of HIV-prevalence (Sommers, 2014).

The cost of antiretroviral treatment remained prohibitive until the advent of generic medicines made available through Brazil and India (Pinheiro Edos *et al.*, 2008). Until effective antiretroviral (conventional) treatment became available in the 1990s TCIM approaches were in some cases the exclusive options available to many individuals for symptom management or palliative care (Ludwig and Chittenden, 2008). Although no cure has yet been developed for HIV/AIDS, TCIM can be beneficial in managing certain symptoms (e.g. digestive side effects or pain); promoting antiretroviral medication adherence; reducing anxiety and depression; and promoting sobriety maintenance related to drug or alcohol use (Abou-Rizk *et al.*, 2016; Nlooto and Naidoo, 2016; Lorenc and Robinson, 2013).

South Africa, Uganda and the US present infrastructures that reflect varying stages of economic and resource development. Even within each country, multiple levels of economic status co-exist accompanied by

Table 2.   Economic health indicators — Uganda, South Africa, United States.

Country	Life expectancy (years) Females/Males	% GDP* spent on health	Per capita expenditure on health (US $ equivalent)
Uganda[a]	65/60	7.2	$144
South Africa[b]	67/60	8.8	$1148
United States[c]	81/76	17.1	$9403

Notes: *Gross Domestic Product.
[a] http://www.who.int/countries/uga/en/ Accessed on 13 July 2018,
[b] http://www.who.int/countries/zaf/en/ Accessed on 13 July 2018,
[c] http://www.who.int/countries/usa/en/ Accessed on 13 July 2018.

associated levels of access to health resources. By comparing and contrasting public health-related parameters (from Table 1) for each country we can better understand practices that may benefit from local and international public health support, as well as highlight effective practices.

Table 2 provides a snapshot summary of relevant health indicators.

South Africa and Uganda

Eastern and Southern Africa have the highest prevalence of HIV among adults (7%) in the world and South Africa has the highest number of people living with HIV (7.1 million) (Kaiser Family Foundation, 2018). Uganda has experienced numerous fluctuations in HIV prevalence. In the late 1980s and early 1990s, prevalence peaked at almost 30%. Vigorous campaigns of education, testing and health promotion activities were adopted and implemented at every level of Ugandan society – schools, churches, labor unions and health centers. HIV prevalence correspondingly decreased to approximately 5–6% by 2003 (U.S. Centers for Disease Control and Prevention, 2017). Such efforts afforded Uganda the distinction of being the first country in the world to decrease HIV prevalence. Economic and social conditions changed again, however, resulting in a rise in HIV prevalence to approximately 7% in 2016 (World Bank, 2016). In the most recent assessment available, the World Bank describes

Uganda's economic status as 'volatile and unstable' with growth proceeding at a slow pace. Individual poverty and inequality persist and perpetuate inequities on every level. Uganda has been identified as one of the poorest countries in the world with 75.6% of the population living on less than the equivalent of $2 per day (World Bank, 2016). A consistently high unemployment rate accompanied by overall slow economic growth characterize South Africa's economic situation (Organization for Economic Cooperation and Development, 2017). Despite these challenges, however, the prognosis for favorable trends such as increased business and international trade provide a modicum of optimism for the 2018–2019 economic forecast.

Rates of TCIM use in these countries among the general population have been reported as between 36 and 68% (Peltzer *et al.*, 2008; Langlois-Klassen *et al.*, 2007). Individuals living with HIV use traditional healing methods related to their spiritual and cultural beliefs (Taylor *et al.*, 2008). Both Uganda and South Africa have a tradition of local healers who provide herbal medicine to mitigate symptoms of HIV/AIDS as well as many other illnesses and conditions (Littlewood and Vanable, 2011). These local healers can often provide useful health education to patients as well as collaborate with conventional medical providers. Although herbs can be somewhat easy to access and are often affordable for many patients, the potential for adverse effects or interaction with antiretroviral treatment is high (Mills *et al.*, 2005). Studies estimate that only about 10% of those patients who use herbs disclose such use to their medical providers (Langlois-Klassen *et al.*, 2008). Most patients surveyed in one study reported that they would discontinue herb use if requested to do so by their medical provider (Langlois-Klassen *et al.*, 2008).

Individuals living on disability grants were more likely to use herbal medicine according to two large surveys conducted in South Africa (Peltzer *et al.*, 2008; Peltzer *et al.*, 2009). This work also shows the cost of antiretroviral treatment and medication-related side effects to be the major drivers for herbal medicine use. Accessibility may play a more significant role in herbal use than issues related to regulatory environment, scientific evidence and training and monitoring of local traditional healers.

United States

The prevalence of TCIM use among people living with HIV/AIDS in the US has been estimated to be 55% (Lorenc and Robinson, 2013). Most commonly used are vitamins, herbal medicines and supplements, followed by prayer, meditation, spiritual practices, massage and acupuncture. Factors affecting the choice of approaches used include race and ethnicity as well as geographic location. The use of TCIM varies considerably according to race and ethnicity in terms of types of TCIM utilized by Hispanics, African-Americans and Asian Americans (Hall *et al.*, 2013). Longer duration of time since initial HIV-positive diagnosis and use of a higher number of medications have also been associated with TCIM use (Mikhail *et al.*, 2004). TCIM approaches are used to address symptoms and side effects of medication, reduce stress and to boost immunity (Bornmann *et al.*, 2009). Decisions regarding use of TCIM treatment are influenced by an individuals' social networks including family and friends. TCIM use is associated with individuals' greater levels of self-management and behaviour related to health promotion (Bornmann *et al.*, 2009; London *et al.*, 2003). Barriers to accessing TCIM care include cost, location and proximity of services, time and perceived lack of evidence (Foote-Ardah, 2004). Each state within the US has separate licensure and regulation processes for a number of TCIM providers, including acupuncturists, massage therapists, naturopathic physicians and chiropractors. Herbal medicine is largely unregulated except for Chinese herbal medicine which is generally overseen by State Boards of Acupuncture and Oriental Medicine. Cautionary evidence about the use of herbs has been investigated and continues to be a priority (Ladenheim *et al.*, 2008). Strengths of the US public health system include increased capacity to conduct research studies, regulatory overview, maintaining practitioner training and monitoring practitioner networks.

Key Differences, Challenges and a Success Story

Access to TCIM related to cost and availability are over-arching determinants of usage in the three countries examined. Social and cultural factors can predispose or limit individuals in seeking TCIM care. Although these countries differ greatly with regard to the standard of living, HIV prevalence and health-related expenditures (by their respective governments), the prevalence of antiretroviral use is approximately the same across all three jurisdictions (*viz.* 58% South Africa; 54% Uganda; 53% US) (Hall *et al.*, 2013; UNAIDS, 2015). The reasons for this are unclear. In all three countries, women bear a disproportionate burden in terms of limited access to prevention information, decreased ability to access treatment including TCIM, and greater overall morbidity (Johnson *et al.*, 2015).

Within the context of this case study, the Pan African Acupuncture Project (PAAP) is an example of successful ongoing cooperation between Uganda and the US that has been in existence for over a decade (Global Acupuncture, 2018). A physician from Uganda, Margaret Muganwa, invited acupuncturist Richard Mandell from the US to Kampala, to meet with representatives from the Ministry of Health, the national medical school, and numerous AIDS service organizations. Plans were developed to train Ugandan health workers to use acupuncture for their patients with HIV. Issues of safety, training, and ongoing monitoring were addressed and continue to be part of the ongoing training protocols. Hundreds of Ugandan health workers — physical therapists, nurses, midwives — have been trained to safely and effectively incorporate acupuncture into their clinical practice (Global Acupuncture, 2018).

Recommendations

Addressing health inequities from the perspective of TCIM will require comprehensive, multisectoral efforts involving health organizations, clinicians, health educators, funders, policymakers, community advocates and nonprofit organizations or non-governmental organizations (NGOs). As a first step, involving all these stake-holders is crucial and a number of fundamental principles require consideration. First, we must remain mindful that health inequities are not acceptable from a social justice perspective and there is a need to link social justice and inequities with policies to address health and wellbeing (de Souza and Luz, 2009). In addition there needs to be a focus on health promotion and disease prevention perspectives plus efforts to improve health must be sustained, systematic, comprehensive and engage the political will of citizens as well as governments.

Another fundamental principle is to first do no harm. Depending on a country or region's capacity, efforts to identify harmful practices are critical. Clinical evidence as well as anecdotal information can be reviewed by multidisciplinary groups (representing the stakeholders as described above) according to economic and infrastructure constraints. Areas with higher levels of resource availability can utilize literature regarding adverse effects of particular TCIM approaches. If resources allow, epidemiological studies such as case-control or retrospective cohort studies may also be conducted. These studies or assessments would focus on TCIM practices that are currently utilized in the area.

A third fundamental principle guiding future work in this area is to be clear that each country/region can develop its own matrix of relevant health priorities for addressing health care needs; there may not be one uniform standard for all nations. These priorities may be developed according to WHO guidelines and reflect current prevalent causes of morbidity and/or mortality such as: infectious disease and epidemics; maternal and child health; TB and other diseases related to poverty; and chronic conditions that are costly both in terms of national health budgets but also in terms of an individual's suffering or reduced capacity to live a fulfilling life.

Based on health needs and priorities, countries can aim to reduce prevalence by a certain percentage within a certain time-frame. Such efforts are planned to extend into the future and 5 year and 10 year plans for goals and assessments should be proposed. Likewise, countries can determine the types of TCIM available and whether these identified modalities can be applied and mobilized ('up-scaled') to address patients' health concerns. Depending on needs, development and resources, countries can identify priorities in terms of how to best incorporate TCIM into the broader health and public health fabric of society. These recommendations are meant to be broad but manageable. Each group and country can determine how to optimally operationalize its commitment to meaningfully integrate TCIM into its health infrastructure. This will require significant effort, but countries are already devoting considerable energy to improving health, promoting wellness and reducing health disparities.

Through 'thinking global, acting local', countries can develop and share best practices for utilizing TCIM in ways that are based in social justice. These practices will focus on ensuring that health care that includes wellness is a right, not a privilege. Human creativity is boundless, as is the thirst for justice - our joint efforts to achieve health equity can be global, ubiquitous and transformative in re-affirming the fundamental dignity of all human beings.

References

Abou-Rizk, J., Mohamad, A., Farah, N. (2016). Prevalence and characteristics of CAM use among people living with HIV and AIDS in Lebanon: Implications for patient care. *Evidence-Based Complementary and Alternative Medicine*, 11, 1–11.

Adams, J., Andrews, G. J., Barnes, J., Broom, A., Magin, P. (2012). *Traditional, Complementary and Integrative Medicine*. An International Reader. Palgrave Macmillan Publisher, pp. 237–244.

Amzat, J., Abdullah, A. A. (2008). Roles of traditional healers in the fight against HIV/AIDS. *Journal of Ethnobiology and Ethnomedicine*, 2(2), 153–159.

Anderson, J. M., and the World Bank (2016). *25 Years on the Path Toward Prosperity*. http://www.worldbank.org/en/news/opinion/2016/02/16/mongolia-and-the-world-bank-25-years-on-the-path-toward-prosperity, Accessed on 4 August 2018.

Arcaya, M. C., Arcaya, A. L., Subramanian, S. V. (2015). Inequalities in health: Definitions, concepts and theories. *Global Health Action*, 8, 27106.

Bornmann, J. E., Uphold, C. R., Maynard, C. (2009). Predictors of complementary/alternative medicine use and intensity of use among men with HIV infection from two geographic areas in the United State. *Journal of the Association of Nurses in AIDS Care*, 20, 468–480.

Braveman, P., Gottlieb, l. (2014). The social Determinants of Health: It's time to consider the causes of the causes. *Public Health Reports*, 129, 19–31.

Broom, A., Doron, A., Tovey, P. (2009). The inequalities of medical pluralism: Hierarchies of health, the politics of tradition and the economics of care in Indian oncology. *Social Science and Medicine*, 69, 698–706.

Burg, M. A., Uphold, C. R., Findley, K., *et al.* (2005). Complementary and alternative medicine use among HIV-infected patients attending three outpatient clinics in the Southeastern U.S. *International Journal of STDs and AIDS*, 16, 112–116.

Chan, M. (2015). Director-General of the WHO. Opening Remarks at the International Forum on Traditional Medicine in China. http://www.who.int/dg/speeches/2015/traditional-medicine/en/. Accessed on 4 August 2018.

Crombie, I. K., Irvine, L., Elliot, L., Wallace, H. (2005). Closing the health inequalities gap: An international perspective. *World Health Organization Regional Office for Europe. Publication.* 7, 1–76.

de Souza, E. F. A. A., Luz, M. T. (2009). Bases socioculturas das práticas terapêuticas alternativas. *Historia, Ciências, Saúde-Manguinhos, Rio de Janeiro, 16*(2), 393–405.

Druss, B. G., Rosenbeck, R. A. (1999). Association between the use of unconventional therapies and conventional medical services. *Journal of the American Medical Association. 282*(7), 651–656.

Elgar, F. J., Pförtner, T. K., Moor, I., De Clercq, B., Stevens, G. W., Currie, C. (2015). Socioeconomic inequalities in adolescent health 2002–2010: A time-series analysis of 34 countries participating in the health behaviour in school-aged children study. *Lancet. 385*(9982), 2088–2095.

Foote-Ardah, C. E. (2004). Sociocultural barriers to the use of complementary and alternative medicine for HIV. *Qualitative Health Research. 14*, 593–611.

Gearing, R. E., Schwalbe, G. S., MacKenzie, M. J., Brwer, K. B., Ibrahim, R. W., Olimat, H. S., *et al.* (2012). Adaptation and translation of mental health interventions in middle eastern arab countries: A systematic review of barriers to and strategies for effective treatment implementation. *International Journal of Sociology and Psychiatry, 59*(7), 671–681.

Global Acupuncture. (2018). http://www.globalacupuncture.org/about.html Accessed 17 July 2018.

Hall, H. I., Frazier, E. L., Rhodes, P., Holtgrave, D. R., Furlow-Parmley, C., *et al.* (2013). Differences in human immunodeficiency virus care and treatment among subpopulations in the US. *JAMA Internal Medicine, 173*(14), 1337–1344.

Hollenberg, D., Zakus, D., Cook, T. (2009). Re-positioning the role of traditional, complementary and alternative medicine as essential health knowledge in global health: Do they still have a role to play? *World Health Population, 10*(4), 977–991.

Hosseinpoor, A. R. (coordinator). (2013). Handbook on health inequality monitoring: With a special focus on low- and middle-income countries. *World Health Organization*, p. 6. http://apps.who.int/iris/bitstream/handle/10665/85345/9789241548632_eng.pdf;jsessionid=A1A59EBD10EB2803643D94190D2A59C0?sequence=1 Accessed on 4 August 2018.

Johnson, M., Samarina, A., Xi, H., Ramalho, M. J. V., Hocqueloux, L, Loutfy, M., *et al.* (2015). Barriers to access to care reported by women living with HIV across 27 countries. *AIDS Care, 27*(10), 1220–1230.

Kaiser Family Foundation (2018). *The Global HIV/AIDS Epidemic*. https://www.kff.org/global-health-policy/fact-sheet/the-global-hivaids-epidemic/ Accessed on 11 July 2018.

Kawachi, I., Subramanian, S. V., Almeido-Filho, N. (2002). A glossary for health inequalities. *Journal of Epidemiology and Community Health, 56*, 647–652.

Ladenheim, D., Horn, O., Werneke, U., *et al.* (2008). Potential health risks of complementary alternative medicines in HIV patients. *HIV Medicine, 9*, 653–659.

Lambert, J., Leonard, K., Mungai, G., Omindi-Ogaja, E., Gatheru, G., Mirangi, T., *et al.* (2011). The contribution of traditional herbal medicine practitioners to Kenyan health care delivery: Results from community health-seeking behavior vignettes and traditional herbal medicine practitioner survey. *World Bank Health, Nutrition and Population Discussion Paper*. http://siteresources.worldbank.org/HEALTHNUTRITIONANDPOPULATION/Resources/281627-1154048816360/HNPStrategyFINALApril302007.pdf. Accessed on 18 August 2016.

Langlois-Klassen, D., Kipp, W., Jhangri, G. S., Rubale, T. (2007). Use of traditional herbal medicine by AIDS patients in Kabarole District, western Uganda. *African Journal of Tropical Medicine and Hygiene, 77*(4), 757–763.

Langlois-Klassen, D., Kipp, W., Rubale, T. (2008). Who's talking? Communication between health providers and HIV-infected adults related to herbal medicine for AIDS treatment in western Uganda. *Society of Scientific Medicine, 67*(1), 165–176.

Lewando, H. G., Stuttaford, M., Ngoma, B. (2004). The social diagnostics of stroke-like symptoms: Healers, doctors and prophets in the Agincourt Limpopo Province, South Africa. *Journal of Biosocial Science, 36*, 433–443.

Littlewood, R. A., Vanable, P. A. (2011). A global perspective on complementary and alternative medicine use among people living with HIV/AIDS in the era of antiretroviral treatment. *Current HIV/AIDS Reports, 8*, 257–268.

London, A. S., Foote-Ardah, C. E., Fleischman, J. A., *et al.* (2003). Use of alternative therapists among people in care for HIV in the United States. *American Journal of Public Health, 93*, 980–987.

Lorenc, A., Robinson, R. (2013). A review of the use of complementary and alternative Medicine and HIV: Issues for patient care. *AIDS Patient Care and STDs*, *27*(9), 503–510.

Ludwig, A., Chittenden, E. (2008). Palliative care of patients with HIV. *HIV InSite*. http://hivinsite.ucsf.edu/InSite?page=kb-03-03-05 Accessed on 4 August 2018.

Marmot, M. (2011). Highlights From An Australian Interview With Sir Michael Marmot And His Recent Canadian Presentation To Health Economists. http://epimonitor.net/Michael_Marmot_Interview.htm Accessed on 3 August 2018.

Mikhail, I. S., DeClemente, R., Person, S., *et al.* (2004). Association of complementary and alternative medicine with HIV clinical disease among a cohort of women living with HIV/AIDS. *Journal of Acquired Immune Deficiency Syndromes*, *37*, 1415–1422.

Mills, E., Foster, B. C., vanHeeswijk, R., *et al.* (2005). Impact of African herbal medicines on antiretroviral metabolism. *AIDS*, *19*(1), 95–97.

Nissen, N., Weidenhammer, W., Schunder-Tatzber, S., Johannessen, H. (2013). Public health ethics for complementary and alternative medicine. *European Journal of Integrative Medicine*, *5*, 62–67.

Nlooto, M., Naidoo, P. (2016). Traditional, complementary and alternative medicine use by HIV patients a decade after public sector antiretroviral therapy roll out in South Africa: A cross sectional study. *BMC Complementary and Alternative Medicine*, *16*, 128.

Olshansky, S. J., Antonucci, T., Berkman, L., Binstock, R. H., Boersch-Supan, A., Cacioppo, J. T., Carnes, B. A., Carstensen, L. L., Fried, L. P., Goldman, D. P., Jackson, J., Kohli, M., Rother, J., Zheng, Y., Rowe, J. (2012). Differences in life expectancy due to race and educational differences are widening, and many may not catch up. *Health Affairs*, *31*(8), 1803–1813.

Organization for Economic Cooperation and Development (2017). *Economic Survey of South Africa*. http://www.oecd.org/eco/surveys/economic-survey-south-africa.htm Accessed on13 July 2018.

Pan American Health Organization. Announcement from General Staff. (2018). https://www.paho.org/hq/index.php?option=com_content&view=article&id=14382%3A-paho-reaffirms-the-importance-of-traditional-medicine-to-advance-towards-universal-health&catid=4669%3Aannouncements-hss&Itemid=39594&lang=en. Accessed on 19 July 2018.

Pederson, C. G., Soren, C., Bonde, A. (2009). Prevalence, socio-demographic and clinical predictors of post-diagnostic utilization of different types of complementary and alternative medicine (CAM) in a nationwide cohort of Danish women treated for primary breast cancer. *European Journal of Cancer*, *45*, 3172–3181.

Peltzer, K., Preez, N. F., Ramlagan, S., *et al.* (2009). Traditional complementary and alternative medicine and antiretroviral treatment adherence among HIV patients in Kwazulu-Natal, South Africa. *African Journal of Traditional, Complementary and Alternative Medicine*, *7*(2), 125–137.

Peltzer, K., Preez, N. F., Ramlagan, S., Fomundam, H. (2008). Use of traditional complementary and alternative medicine for HIV patients in Kwa-Zulu-Natal, South Africa. *BMC Public Health*, *8*, 255.

Pinheiro Edos, S., Antunes, O. A., Forunak, J. M. (2008). A survey of the synthesis of active pharmaceutical ingredients for antiretroviral drug combinations critical to access in emerging nations. *Antiviral Research*, *79*(3), 143–165.

Sengupta, S., Lo, B., Strauss, R. P., Eron, J., Gifford, A. L. (2010). How researchers define vulnerable populations in HIV/AIDS clinical trials. *AIDS Behavior*, 14(6), 1313–1319.

Sommers, E. (2014). *Acupuncture as an Adjuvant in the Treatment of HIV/AIDS: Examining Disparities in Access, Cost-effectiveness and Public Health Considerations.* Lambert Academic Publishing, Oxford, UK, p. 87.

Struthers, R., Nichols, L. A. (2008). Chapter 11 Utilization of complementary and alternative medicine among racial and ethnic minority populations: Implications for reducing health disparities. In Fitzpatrick, J. J., Villaruel, A. M., Comelia, P. *Annual Review of Nursing Research*, Vol. 22 Springer Publishing Co., New York.

Stuttaford, M., Al Makjamreh, S., Coomans, F., Harrington, J., Himongo, C., Hundt, G. L. (2014). The right to traditional, complementary and alternative health care. *Global Health Action*, *7*, 724121.

Taylor, T. N., Dolezal, C., Tross, S., Holmes, W. C. (2008). Comparison of HIV/AIDS-specific quality of life change in Zimbabwean patients in western medicine versus traditional African medicine care sites. *Journal of Acquired Immune Deficiency Syndrome*, 49(5), 52–56.

U.S. Centers for Disease Control and Prevention (CDC). (2017). *Global HIV and tuberculosis.* https://www.cdc.gov/globalhivtb/where-we-work/uganda/uganda.html. Accessed on 13 July 2018.

UNAIDS. (2015). Access to antiretroviral therapy in Africa. *Statistical Report 2015*, p. 10.

United Nations. (1966). International covenant on social, economic and cultural rights. Article 12. United Nations, New York. https://www.un.org/ruleoflaw/files/International%20Covenant%20on%20Economic,%20Social%20and%20Cultural%20Rights.pdf. Accessed on 4 August 2018.

United Nations (2000). The right to the highest attainable standard of health. General Comments Section 2. *General legal obligations*, p. 11. http://www.refworld.org/pdfid/4538838d0.pdf. Accessed on 4 August 2018.

World Bank (2016). http://www.worldbank.org/en/country/uganda/brief/uganda-economic-update-fact-sheet-june-2016. Accessed on 13 July 2018.

World Health Organization and Mongolian Ministry of Health. (2012). *Health Service Delivery Profile*, pp. 4–5. http://www.wpro.who.int/health_services/service_delivery_profile_mongolia.pdf. Accessed on 4 August 2018.

World Health Organization. Health and human rights (2015). *Fact sheet N°323*, p. 1 http://www.who.int/news-room/fact-sheets/detail/human-rights-and-health. Accessed on 4 August 2018.

World Health Organization (1978). *International Conference on Primary Health Care*, Alma-Ata, USSR, 6–12 September, p. 1. http://www.who.int/publications/almaata_declaration_en.pdf. Accessed on 21 July 2016.

Xu, K. T., Farrell, T. W. (2007). The complementarity and substitution between unconventional and mainstream medicine among racial and ethnic groups in the United States. *Health Research and Educational Trust*, 42(2), 811–826.

Yamin, A. E. (2016). *Power, Suffering and the Struggle for Dignity*, Chapter 3, Penn Press, Oxford, UK.

Yarney, J., Donkor, A., Opoku, S. Y., Yarney, L., Agyeman-Duah, I., Abakah, A. C., Asampong, E. (2013). Characteristics of users and implications for the use of complementary and alternative medicine in Ghanaian cancer patients undergoing radiotherapy and chemotherapy: A cross-sectional study. *BMC Complementary and Alternative Medicine*, 13, 16.

Index